OXFORD MEDICAL PUBLICATIONS

Migraine: A Spectrum of Ideas

Migraine: A Spectrum of Ideas

Edited by
Merton Sandler
and
Geralyn M. Collins

Oxford   New York   Tokyo
OXFORD UNIVERSITY PRESS
1990

Oxford University Press, Walton Street, Oxford OX2 6DP

Oxford New York Toronto
Delhi Bombay Calcutta Madras Karachi
Petaling Jaya Singapore Hong Kong Tokyo
Nairobi Dar es Salaam Cape Town
Melbourne Auckland

and associated companies in
Berlin Ibadan

Oxford is a trade mark of Oxford University Press

Published in the United States
by Oxford University Press, New York

© The various contributors
listed on pp. ix–xiii, 1990

British Library Cataloguing in Publication Data
Migraine.
1. Man. Migraine
I. Sandler, Merton II. Collins, Geralyn M.
616.8'57
ISBN 0-19-261810-5

Library of Congress Cataloging-in-Publication Data
Migraine: a spectrum of ideas / edited by Merton Sandler and Geralyn M.
Collins.
(Oxford medical publications)
Includes bibliographical references.
1. Migraine. I. Sandler, Merton. II. Collins, Geralyn M.
III. Series.
RC392.M56   1989   616.8'57—dc20   89-16265
ISBN 0-19-261810-5

Set by Graphicraft Typesetting Ltd, Hong Kong
Printed in Great Britain at
Bookcraft Ltd, Midsomer Norton, Avon.

Contents

Contents

Contributors

Angst, J.
Psychiatrische Universitatsklinik, University of Zurich, Zurich, Switzerland.

Arrang, J.M.
National Institute of Health and Medical Research, Neurobiology Unit, Centre Paul Broca de l'INSERM, 2 ter rue de'Alésia, 75014 Paris, France.

Belleroche, de J.*
Department of Biochemistry and Academic Unit of Neuroscience, Charing Cross and Westminster Medical School, Fulham Palace Road, London W6 8RF, UK.

Blau, J.N.*
The National Hospital for Nervous Diseases, Queen Square, London WC1N 3BG, UK.

Buzzi, M.G.
Stroke Research Laboratory, Department of Neurology and Neurosurgery, Massachusetts General Hospital, Harvard Medical School, Boston, MA 02114, USA.

Coppen, A.J.*
MRC Neuropsychiatry Research Unit, Clinical Investigation Ward, Greenbank, West Park Hospital, Epsom, Surrey KT19 8PB, UK.

Clifford Rose, F.*
Academic Unit of Neuroscience, Charing Cross and Westminster Medical School, Fulham Palace Road, London W6 8RF, UK.

Curzon, G.*
Department of Neurochemistry, Institute of Neurology, 1 Wakefield Street, London WC1N 1PJ, UK.

Edvinsson, L.*
Department of Internal Medicine, University Hospital of Lund, S-221 85 Lund, Sweden.

Feniuk, W.

Pharmacology Division, Glaxo Group Research Limited, Ware, Hertfordshire, SG12 0DP, UK.

Ferreira, S.H.*

Department of Pharmacology, Faculty of Medicine of Ribeirâo Preto, Ribeirâo Preto, Sâo Paulo, 14049, Brazil.

Fozard, J.R.*

Preclinical Research Department, Sandoz Ltd, CH-4002 Basel, Switzerland.

Friberg, L.

Department of Clinical Physiology, Bispebjerg Hospital, University of Copenhagen, DK-2900 Hellerup, Denmark.

Garbarg, M.

National Institute of Health and Medical Research, Neurobiology Unit, Centre Paul Broca de l'INSERM, 2 ter rue d'Alésia, 75014 Paris, France.

Gardner-Medwin, A.R.*

Department of Physiology, University College, Gower Street, London WC1E 6BT, UK.

Giros, B.

National Institute of Health and Medical Research, Neurobiology Unit, Centre Paul Broca de l'INSERM, 2 ter rue d'Alésia, 75014 Paris, France.

Glover, V.*

Bernhard Baron Memorial Research Laboratories, Queen Charlotte's and Chelsea Hospital, Goldhawk Road, London W6 0XG, UK.

Goadsby, P.J.

Department of Neurology, The Prince Henry Hospital, University of New South Wales, Little Bay, NSW 2036, Australia.

Gros, C.

National Institute of Health and Medical Research, Neurobiology Unit, Centre Paul Broca de l'INSERM, 2 ter rue d'Alésia, 75014 Paris, France.

Gross, M.*

Department of Neurology, Atkinson Morley's Hospital, Copse Hill, Wimbledon, London SW20 0NE, UK.

Gryglewski, R.J.*

Department of Pharmacology, Copernicus Academy of Medicine in Cracow, Cracow, Poland.

Humphrey, P.P.A.*

Pharmacology Division, Glaxo Group Research Limited, Ware,
Hertfordshire, SG12 0DP, UK.

Jansen, I.

Department of Experimental Research, University of Malmö, Sweden.

Kano, M.

Departments of Neurology and Neurosurgery, Massachusetts General
Hospital, Harvard Medical School, 32 Fruit Street, Boston, MA 02114,
USA.

Kennett, G.A.

Department of Neurochemistry, Institute of Neurology, 1 Wakefield Street,
London WC1N 1PJ, UK.

Kontos, H.A.

Department of Medicine, Medical College of Virginia, Richmond,
VA 23298, USA.

Lambert, G.A.

Department of Neurology, The Prince Henry Hospital, University of
New South Wales, Little Bay, NSW 2036, Australia.

Lance, J.W.*

Department of Neurology, The Prince Henry Hospital, University of
New South Wales, Little Bay, NSW 2036, Australia.

Llorens-Cortes, C.

National Institute of Health and Medical Research, Neurobiology Unit,
Centre Paul Broca de l'INSERM, 2 ter rue de'Alésia, 75014 Paris, France.

Merikangas, K.R.*

Yale University School of Medicine, Genetic Epidemiology Research Unit,
40 Temple Street, Lower Level, New Haven, CT 06510, USA.

Moskowitz, M.A.*

Departments of Neurology and Neurosurgery, Massachusetts General
Hospital, Harvard Medical School, 32 Fruit Street, Boston, MA 02114,
USA.

Olesen, J.*

Department of Neurology, Gentofte Hospital, University of Copenhagen,
DK-2900 Hellerup, Denmark.

Peatfield, R.C.*

Department of Neurology, The General Infirmary, Great George Street,
Leeds LS1 3EX, UK.

Perren, M.J.

Pharmacology Division, Glaxo Group Research Limited, Ware, Hertfordshire, SG12 0DP, UK.

Pollard, H.

National Institute of Health and Medical Research, Neurobiology Unit, Centre Paul Broca de l'INSERM, 2 ter rue d'Alésia, 75014 Paris, France.

Sakas, D.E.

Departments of Neurology and Neurosurgery, Massachusetts General Hospital, Harvard Medical School, 32 Fruit Street, Boston, MA 02114, USA.

Sandler, M.* (Chairman)

Bernhard Baron Memorial Research Laboratories, Queen Charlotte's and Chelsea Hospital, Goldhawk Road, London W6 0XG, UK.

Saxena, P.R.*

Institute of Pharmacology, Faculteit der Geneeskunde, Erasmus University, Postbus 1738 3000, DR Rotterdam, The Netherlands.

Schwartz, J.C.*

National Institute of Health and Medical Research, Neurobiology Unit, Centre Paul Broca de l'INSERM, 2 ter rue d'Alésia, 75014, Paris, France.

Shah, K.

Department of Neurochemistry, Institute of Neurology, 1 Wakefield Street, London WC1N 1PJ, UK.

Skyhøj Olsen, T.

Department of Clinical Physiology, Bispebjerg Hospital, University of Copenhagen, DK-2900 Hellerup, Denmark.

Stokes, J.F.*

Ossicles, Newnham Hill, Nr. Henley-on-Thames, Oxon RG9 5LT, UK.

Uddman, R.

Department of Oto-rhino-laryngology, University of Malmö, Sweden.

Vane, J.R.*

The William Harvey Research Institute, St Bartholomew's Hospital Medical College, Charterhouse Square, London EC1M 6BQ, UK.

Wei, E.P.

Department of Medicine, Medical College of Virginia, Richmond, VA 23298, USA.

Welch, K.M.A.*

Department of Neurology, Henry Ford Hospital, 2799 West Grand
Boulevard, Detroit, MI 48202, USA.

Whitton, P.

Department of Neurochemistry, Institute of Neurology, 1 Wakefield Street,
London WC1N 1PJ, UK.

Zagami, A.S.

Department of Neurology, The Prince Henry Hospital, University of
New South Wales, Little Bay, NSW 2036, Australia.

Ziegler, A.*

Department of Pharmacology, University of Kiel, Hospitalstrasse 4–6,
D2300 Kiel, West Germany.

* Participant in the Migraine Workshop (Leeds Castle, Maidstone, UK,
18–21 October 1988).

1. Introduction

Merton Sandler (Chairman)

Our knowledge of migraine is clouded by a vast anecdotal literature, top-heavy with speculation and dominated by the cult of personality (for example, Wolff 1948). The disease is difficult to get to grips with because its main manifestation, headache, is subjective and there are no animal models of it, which makes available research approaches less than straightforward.

Migraine in a crippling illness: it does not kill, but its high morbidity poses a massive economic problem and gives rise to considerable individual suffering. Despite the 'background noise', there has also been considerable and valuable research effort — if one combs the literature hard enough to find it. Even so, the international migraine scene tends to be dominated by large set-piece meetings, weak on innovative science but strong on drug-trial reports. This approach may be good for the market analysts but does little for our understanding of migraine. The Migraine Trust therefore decided that a 'brain-storming' type of meeting, as recorded in this present volume, might be timely, to try to decide what precisely we are up to, and where we are going.

Despite an appearance of furious activity, the migraine research scene is curiously static. People still tend to measure the things they measured 20 years ago when I first came on the scene. Rao and Rao (1988), for example, recently published data on urinary 5-hydroxyindoleacetic acid output in migraine and we were turning our hand to that in the mid-1960s (see Curzon 1968). It refuses to go away. This tenacity probably reflects the widespread feeling that some disturbance in 5-hydroxytryptamine (5-HT) economy lies at the heart of migraine. The first migraine meeting I myself attended was in 1969, the Third Migraine Symposium (Cochrane 1970) of the Migraine Trust. I have been looking again at the proceedings and they are very interesting, not least because many of the participants are contributors to this present volume and still dominate the field. Many of the questions were the same as those we are tackling here. Lance *et al.* (1970) spoke about migraine and 5-HT and, at that time, Saxena (1970) remarked rather prophetically, 'I am not quite sure whether 5-HT release or its depletion is responsible for triggering migraine attacks'. We may still be uncertain on this point; things have not changed. There have been massive recent advances, of course, in our knowledge of 5-HT receptors and, with luck, this research will lead to the most effective treatments of the disorder that have yet appeared. Nevertheless, many parts of the canvas are blank, and we need all our ingenuity to paint them in. At that time, 20 years ago, Blau (1970) was very properly questioning revealed truth *à la* Wolff (1948). The concept of extracranial vasodilatation then held sway as a cause of migraine headache, and the question is still debated today. Diamond (1970) also spoke, somewhat anecdotally, on the relationship between migraine and depression. The connection is surfacing once again but in a more investigative manner, and new data on this line of research are recorded in this volume. And, most tantalizing of all, Heyck (1970) spoke about arteriovenous shunts. He had first propounded his theory about their role in migraine more than a decade earlier (Heyck 1956) and the theory is just as relevant and controversial today (see within)!

What we could not have anticipated 20 years ago was the advent of powerful, non-invasive machines to provide information about what goes on in what can only be viewed as an archetypal 'black box'. As a result of positron emission tomography and magnetic resonance scan techniques, to mention two of the most powerful instrumental assemblies available to us, we are for the first time in a position to monitor intracerebral chemical events and receptor localization with some precision.

We debated, 20 years ago, the *aura* of classical migraine. At that time, nobody had invoked Leão's (1944) spreading depression as an explanation for it. The matter is still controversial but the evidence grows stronger that the two phenomena can be equated, and the topic is well aired in this volume.

Another puzzling problem is the question of vulnerability to the disorder — what factors decide who gets migraine and who doesn't? And there are many more questions: how do migraine-triggering agents work? What is the nature of the associated peripheral chemical changes? And, of course, why is migraine headache largely unilateral? We are still unable to answer this last question, and it remains a key one.

The 25 participants at the Leeds Castle Migraine Workshop were handpicked, from all over the world. From their track records, as you might expect, they generated much fertile discussion, which is recorded in this volume. They have not, of course, provided all the answers but have tried to formulate a set of further questions and to devise further experiments that may well take us through to the year 2000!

References

Blau, J.N. (1970). Discussion remark. In *Background to migraine*, (ed. A.L. Cochrane), p. 27. Heinemann, London.

Cochrane, A.L. (ed.) (1970) *Background to migraine*, Heinemann, London.

Curzon, G. (1968). 5-Hydroxyindoles and migraine. In *Advances in Pharmacology*, Vol. 6B, (eds E. Costa and M. Sandler), Academic Press, New York. pp. 191–200.

Diamond, S. (1970). The psychiatric aspects of headache. In *Background to migraine*, (ed. A.L. Cochrane), pp. 60–4. Heinemann, London.

Heyck, H. (1956). Neue Beitrage zur Klinik und Pathogenese der Migräne. Thieme, Stuttgart.

Heyck, H. (1970). The importance of arterio-venous shunts in the pathogenesis of migraine. In *Background to migraine*, (ed. A.L. Cochrane), pp. 19–25. Heinemann, London.

Lance, J.W., Anthony, M., and Hinterberger, H. (1970). Migraine and 5-hydroxytryptamine. In *Background to migraine*, (ed. A.L. Cochrane), pp. 155–61. Heinemann, London.

Leão, A.A.P. (1944). Spreading depression of activity in the cerebral cortex. *Journal of Neurophysiology*, **7**, 359–90.

Rao, A. and Rao, S.N. (1988). Urinary excretion of biogenic amine metabolites in migraine. *Biochemical Archives*, **4**, 141–4.

Saxena, P. (1970). Discussion remark. In *Background to migraine*, (ed. A.L. Cochrane), p. 164. Heinemann, London.

Wolff, H.G. (1948). *Headache and other head pain*. Oxford University Press, New York.

2. The nature of migraine: do we need to invoke slow neurochemical processes?

J.N. Blau

Introduction

'What is migraine?' That was the question posed by our organizer to open this workshop designed to contribute and provoke new ideas in migraine research. So that we are discussing the same topic, the word 'migraine' needs clarifying because it can be used in two senses: (1) clinical attacks; and (2) the underlying migraine processes. In considering which to put first it is worth recalling Newton's dictum (Harré 1969)

> 'We must learn from the Phaenomena of Nature what bodies attract one another and what are the Laws and Properties of Attraction, before we enquire the Cause by which the Attractions is perform'd'.

I shall therefore describe the clinical phenomena of migraine (first in outline and then in detail), followed by the life-cycle of migraine in individuals, and end with some implications of clinical migraine on possible mechanisms.

Migraine in outline and defined

Because we do not know, and are trying to find out, the mechanism of migraine, I believe we can describe the condition only by its clinical features. A widely accepted delineation has been Vahlquist's criteria (1955). These were: (1) paroxysmal headaches separated by free intervals; and (2) at least two of the four following points: unilateral headache, nausea, visual aura, and family history. I have tried to define migraine more strictly (Blau 1984), the novel feature of this definition being that it included timing, which has been incorporated in the International Headache Society's (IHS) Classification (Headache Classification Committee 1988). The definition I proposed was (Blau 1984):

> 'Episodic headaches lasting 2–72 hours with total freedom between attacks. The headache must be associated with visual or gastro-intestinal disturbances, or both. The visual symptoms occur as an aura before, and/or photophobia during, the

headache phase. If there are no visual but only alimentary disturbances, then vomiting must feature in some attacks.

Migraine attacks in detail

Migraine attacks can be divided into five phases.

1. Premonitory symptoms
2. Aura
3. Headache phase
4. Recovery phase
5. Postdromes

Premonitory phase

When patients have had migraine headaches for a number of years they, and particularly their close relatives, if observant, can recognize warning symptoms several hours, or often the day or evening before, the headache begins. Premonitory symptoms manifest in about 50 per cent of migraineurs, and consist of excitatory or inhibitory symptoms and signs (Table 2.1) in the mental or neurological state, the intestines, muscles, or fluid balance of the individual; their appearance averages at about three hours before the aura or onset of headache.

Aura

A neurological aura constituting classical migraine (migraine with aura, in the IHS classification; (Headache Classification Committee 1988) must last 5–60 minutes: flashing lights for a few seconds is inadequate for a diagnosis. The slow rate of migration of the visual aura (Fig. 2.1a) across the visual field, or the paraesthesiae ascending from the hand up the arm to the face, are important features in distinguishing migraine from cerebrovascular disease or epilepsy. This slow migration demands a special neuropharmacological process for which Leão's spreading depression may be a model (Lauritzen and Olesen 1987), but there is no evidence so far that Leão's spreading depression occurs in the human cortex.

   The unique feature of the visual aura is the simultaneity of a scotoma (an inhibitory phenomenon) adjacent in the visual field to scintillations (excitation); inhibition and excitation of the nervous system are characteristic of other phases of migraine attacks.

Headache phase

Headache is the essence of migraine attacks and the most troublesome aspect for the patient. The headache may be unilateral or bilateral; it can move from one part of the head to the other in the same attack; it is throbbing in only 47 per cent of patients — in a series of 750 (Olesen 1978) — but even then the pulsatile quality is present only in part of the attack.

TABLE 2.1. *Premonitory symptoms and signs in 40 migraineurs*

Symptoms and signs	Excitatory		Inhibitory	
Mental state	Irritable	18	Withdrawn	18
	High	12		
	High then low	4		
Altered behaviour	Irritable	2	Sluggish	3
(often observed	Hyperactive	2	Clumsy	2
first or only by	Obsessional	1		
relatives)	Witty	1		
	Singing	1		
Altered appearance			Eyes dark, heavy or sunken	3
			Pale face	1
Neurological				
symptoms and signs	Yawning	8	Tired	17
	Light-sensitive	17	Focusing difficulty	13
	Noise-sensitive	11	Speech slurred	5
	Irritable skin	5	Dysphasia (word selection)	10
	Hyperosmia	1	Talking less	1
			Concentration impaired	5
			Slower thinking	3
Muscular symptoms	Stiff neck	16	General muscle weakness or	
and signs			sluggishness	6
			Feeling cold	2
Alimentary symptoms	Craving for foods	9	Anorexia	3
	Increased bowel frequency	3	Constipation	7
			Abdomen bloated	3
Altered fluid balance	Increased urinary frequency	4	Fluid retention	1
	Thirst	5		

Total symptoms in 40 patients were 223: average 5–6 per patient.

Patients say the headache develops slowly, often taking several hours before reaching its maximum intensity. At the beginning, patients are frequently unsure whether it is going to be and 'ordinary headache' or the beginning of a migraine.

The site of origin of the pain is disputed: Wolff (1963) argued that it arose from extracranial vasodilatation, but patients most often say the pain is deeply seated. Furthermore, they lie still because movement accentuates the headache, a characteristic of pain that arises from inside the skull. Blau and Dexter (1981) observing patients during their migraine attacks found that in 49 out of 50 there was evidence of an intracranial component, because

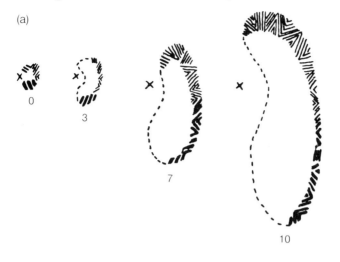

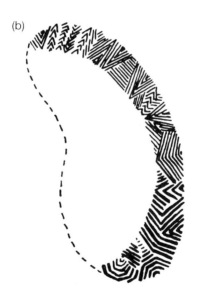

FIG. 2.1. (a) Successive maps of a scintillating scotoma to show characteristic distribution of the fortification figures. The × in each case indicates the fixation point. (b) Sketch to show apparent differences in fortification figures. The coarser and more complicated figures are generally in the lower part of the field.

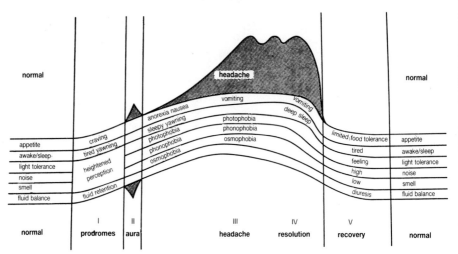

FIG. 2.2. Diagram to illustrate major symptoms and signs during various phases of migraine attacks and their relationship to normality. (Reproduced, with permission, from Blau 1986.)

coughing, breath holding, or sudden head movement from side to side increased the pain. They concluded that the pain arose from inside the skull.

Symptoms and signs accompanying the headache

Symptoms and signs concomitant with the headache are illustrated in Fig. 2.2. In addition, patients are commonly pale in the face, which may also be sunken; they have haptophobia, not liking to be touched; their extracranial and cervical muscles may be tender; and although constipation is frequently reported a few patients experience increased bowel movements. All these symptoms and signs indicate excitatory and inhibitory features of the central nervous system which may be primarily affected by, but could be secondary to, vascular changes.

Resolution of migraine attacks

Attacks of migraine end in different ways (Blau 1982), sleeping being the most common. Of 28 out of 50 whose attacks resolved in sleep, 14 went to bed by day, with 1–2 hours of sleep often ending their attacks. It may be significant that a cycle of deep/rapid-eye-movement (REM) sleep is 90–120 minutes. Five out of 50 patients in this series found that a meal could end an attack. In the remainder the migraine headaches 'just fade away slowly', a frequently heard remark. Some patients end their attack by vomiting, sometimes encouraged by putting their fingers to the back of the tongue.

Sleep and vomiting are neurological events. But eating dilates blood vessels, and hunger and nausea are associated with pallor and feeling cold.

Postdromes

'Hangover symptoms' the day after a migraine attack are common, and they were found to affect 47 out of 50 patients (Blau 1982). Symptoms include: (1) limited food tolerance; (2) mood variation — feeling low or occasionally 'high'; (3) tiredness — lack of physical and mental energy; (4) aching muscles; and (5) occasionally diuresis.

These symptoms after the headache has finished are the counterpart of prodromes and may be the diminution of symptoms that accompanied the headache, although some of these postdromal symptoms could arise from not eating, vomiting, or taking tablets during the headache phase.

Migraine precipitants also provoke other headaches

Harold Wolff's researches (Wolff 1963) showed that a broad study of headaches could illuminate those of migraine. Thus:

hunger → hunger headache;
alcohol → 'hangover headaches';
premenstrual tension → premenstrual headache;
physical stimuli (heat, light, and noise) → cinema headache, for example;
local pain in eyes, teeth, sinuses, or neck → headache, local or generalized;
travel and exercise → coital headache, for example;
stress → tension headache;
sleep excess → a 'lie-in headache'.

Other currently accepted migraine precipitants do not induce headache. Thus, allergy does not cause headaches unless allergic rhinitis produces a blocked nose. Cheese does not give rise to headache, although in folklore is said to cause nightmares. Chocolate does not induce headaches but patients eating chocolate when they experience cravings have already begun a migraine attack and therefore the eating of chocolate is not the cause but a manifestation of the beginning of an episode (see prodromes in Table 2.1).

Migraine in the life cycle of individuals

Inheritance

The inheritance of migraine has been estimated to range from 60–80 per cent (Bille 1962; Heyck 1981). In a subgroup of severely affected children with migraine, Bille (1962) found that migraine occurred in the mother in 72.6 per cent and in the father in 20.5 percent, a highly significant difference. But if a family history is a diagnostic criterion (Vahlquist 1955, see earlier) then these figures are based on a circular argument. Nevertheless a positive family history of migraine amongst immediate relatives (parents,

TABLE 2.2.(a)   *Physical initiation*

Case no.	Age now	Age at initiation	Sex	Migraine type	Initiating mechanism
1	39	29	F	Cl	Started on contraceptive pill.
2	29	25	F	Cm	After birth of baby.
3	26	16	F	Cl	After birth of baby and starting on contraceptive pill.
4	45	37	F	Cm	Vaginal haemorrhage, cause unknown.
5	8	6	M	Cm	Knocked down by van, not unconscious but dazed and shaken.
6	39	20	M	Cl	Head injury, not unconscious but dazed and large swelling on head.
7	13	6	F	Cm	Meningitis three months and head injury three weeks earlier.
8	39	28	F	Cp	Lack of sleep for 18 months with difficult child. Head injury one year earlier.
9	23	14	F	Cl	Six weeks after onset of Scheuermann's disease with spinal and neck pain.
10	15	14	M	Cl	'Shooting up', grew 3 inches in 6 months

TABLE 2.2.(b)   *Emotional initiation*

Case no.	Age now	Age at initiation	Sex	Migraine type	Initiating mechanism
11	25	23	F	Cl	Within minutes of hearing that both parents sentenced to prison.
12	50	24	M	Cm	Patient with brother who drowned on holiday abroad. Had to find and bring body back to England.
13	47	32	M	Cp	Promoted in his company.
14	53	36	F	Cl	Married, moved house to troubled N. Ireland, father died.
15	40	32	F	Cm	Fighting by own noisy children.
16	24	16	F	Cp	First time away from home, and examinations.
17	42	20	F	Cl	Difficult final year at college.

TABLE 2.2.(c)   *Emotional and physical initiation*

Case no.	Age now	Age at initiation	Sex	Migraine type	Initiating mechanism
18	50	14	M	Cl	Head injury aged 8 provoked aura. Schoolmaster attempted to touch genitalia aged 14 produced first attack within minutes.
19	34	24	F	Cm	Weight loss. Failure in acting profession. Had to change to teaching. Death of mother.
20	33	12	F	Cm	Started menstruation for which unprepared: felt 'dirty and deeply embarrassed' at boarding school.
21	58	11	F	Cm	First period a great shock, thought 'something terrible was happening'.
22	22	12	F	Cl	Onset of periods and difficulty with step-father.
23	27	12	M	Cm	Difficult puberty.
24	55	30	F	Cp	Emotionally and physically low after third miscarriage.
25	37	21	F	Cm	Four months after marriage, moved home, started on the pill.
26	62	16	M	Cm	Started work; long hours without food or drink.
27	34	22	F	Cp	Excess alcohol intake. Learning to live on her own in London.
28	44	26	F	Cm	Two to three months after birth of baby, depressed, started the contraceptive pill.
29	36	17	F	Cp	Studying Russian very hard on her own. Painful swollen neck.

Reproduced, with permission, from Blau (1985). Cl, classical; Cm, Common; Cp, complete migraine.

siblings, or children) is so common clinically that no-one doubts a genetic basis, and currently a recessive gene of approximately 70 per cent penetrance is reasonably assumed.

Initiation of migraine

Migraine frequently begins without a reason. However, in 29 of 60 patients studied (Blau 1985), a physical, emotional, or a combined physical and emotional stimulus were found (see Table 2.2, a, b, and c). These stimuli were closely associated with the first migraine attack. It was believed that the initial triggering mechanism would be related to subsequent precipitants: this was not the case. Hence the suggestion was made that a person's genetic inheritance enabled a subsequent neural pathway to be established in them.

This is comparable with a learning capacity: a coordinated muscle movement needs to be learnt, for example, in learning to ride a bicycle, or a series of notes in learning a tune. Once learnt, these processes are never to be forgotten.

Sex and hormonal variations

Although migraine typically begins in the teenage years, attacks can start in childhood. The incidence of migraine in boys and girls is the same at age 7–9 years (Bille 1962), but from then onwards girls have an increased incidence (1.5:1) that persists throughout female reproductive life.

The evidence that female hormones play a role includes the following.

1. The menarche can initiate migraine.
2. Some women have attacks only during the premenstrual phase of their cycle.
3. Migraine can increase in frequency and severity in those taking he contraceptive pill.
4. 60–80 per cent of pregnant woman lose their migraine totally in the second and third trimester.
5. The menopause can coincide with cessation of migraine (see 'Loss of migraine', below).

The influence of the menopause is, however, variable and migraine can increase at that time. Migraine after the menopause needs further study.

Loss of migraine

An advertisement in an issue of the British Migraine Association newsletter produced 52 patients who had 'lost' their migraine; that is, they had not had migraine for at least three years (Blau 1987). The causes attributed to this loss are listed in Table 2.3; whether these are all correct is doubtful, but the loss of migraine after the menopause is part of folklore. The mean age of 55 years in the above series corresponds to the time of lessening of headache in general (Espir *et al.* 1988) and is associated with a radiologically demonstrable reduction of neuronal substance, a further argument in favour of a neurological basis for migraine pathogenesis.

Those favouring a vascular basis for migraine have used this point as an argument that the vessels of the brain become less contractile: but angina or transient ischaemic attacks become more frequent at this age.

Implications of clinical migraine on possible mechanisms

The clinical picture needs a unifying theory. However, a simple or single chemical derangement for a process so complex as migraine attacks seems unlikely. How then can we tackle the problem?

TABLE 2.3.   *Patients' attribution to migraine disappearing*

Psychological		
Retirement (2 male, 2 female)		4
Relaxation or less responsibility		4
Change of occupation		2
Moving home		1
		11
Physical		
Avoiding specific foods		9
Cheese	(2)	
Gluten	(1)	
Coffee	(1)	
'Very restricted diet'	(1)	
Not stated	(4)	
Menopause (10) Hormonal therapy (1)		11
Postoperative		3
Hysterectomy	(2)	
Peritonitis	(1)	
Hypotensive therapy		4
Propranolol	(2)	
Spironolactone	(1)	
Bendrofluazide	(1)	
Other measures		
Tolazamide for diabetes		1
Chiropraxis		1
Acupuncture		1
Half pint water in the morning		1
		31
Unknown or not stated		10
		Total 52

Comparison with other complex biological processes

Fig. 2.3, showing other slow, biological processes, albeit highly selected ones, suggests a comparison with appetite developing into hunger, or with tiredness ending in sleep; that is, a comparison with other circadian rhythms. Arguing by analogy is fraught with danger, but gastrointestinal disturbances, as well as tiredness and sleep, feature in — and provoke — migraine attacks. Even if the comparison is not valid, the timing of these biological processes indicates the tempo of migraine attacks — all are slow, taking minutes or hours rather than milliseconds or seconds.

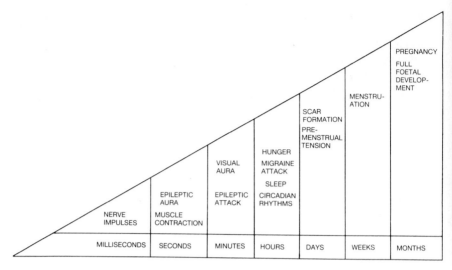

FIG. 2.3. Timing of selected biological processes.

Biological cycles

Another approach is to think of other biochemical cycles, such as the Krebs cycle (where a chain of reactions is required to metabolize glucose), or cutaneous reactions, such as the immediate hypersensitivity to histamine, as a model for migraine.

The site of the lesion

A standard question in neurology is: 'what is the site of the disturbance?' So we may say: 'where does the headache arise?' because the brain is insensitive to painful stimuli; or 'where does the aura arise?' and 'how does it give rise to simultaneous blank areas adjacent to scintillations?' I propose that this simultaneous excitation and inhibition are characteristic of disturbances in the *nervous system* and are not a feature of *blood vessel* changes.

With these difficulties in mind I have raised some questions and their possible answers in Table 2.4.

Tentative conclusions for migraine pathogenesis

The only migraine symptom to develop suddenly is the onset of the aura, although even that can be slow, the patient being unsure of the visual disturbance in the peripheral field of vision. All other symptoms wax and wane slowly, taking minutes or even hours. Hence, slow biochemical processes, whether these involve the accumulation or the exhaustion of chemicals, seem to be essential.

TABLE 2.4. *Some possible answers to questions about migraine*

Questions	Possible answers
The site of premonitory symptoms?	?Frontal lobe ?Hypothalamus ?Whole brain with selected portions being affected
Site of aura?	Occipital cortex Lateral geniculate body Retina
Mechanism of spread? Lashley's questions (1941) about the visual aura Maintenance of characteristic shape of scotoma as it drifts across visual field and away from the fixation point Yet it becomes magnified Scintillating edge remains the same width Rate of scintillations about 10 per second	?Leão's spreading depression
Pattern of scintillations fine and less complicated in upper than in lower quadrants (see Fig. 2.1b)	Lashley (1941) suggests the pattern is a function of the anatomical substratum rather than the nature of the propagated disturbance
Mechanism of positive scintillations and negative blindspot	Characteristic of neural disturbances
Site of origin of headache	?Extracranial ?Meningeal
Mechanism of slow build-up of headache Movement of pain site Change of quality	Increasing transmitters Decrease of inhibitors Brain swelling Increased vessel dilatation or constriction
Site of origin of accompanying symptoms of headache namely nausea, vomiting, photo and phonophobia	Hypothalamus Brainstem Meninges Peripheral — hence relief by vomiting
Why is there variability in individuals of photophobia, phonophobia and osmophobia	Different individual threshold

TABLE 2.4. (*cont.*)

Questions	Possible answers
Resolution How does sleep resolve attacks? How does vomiting resolve attacks?	
Hangover symptoms — what is their cause?	Attacks *per se* Effect of attack by not eating, by impairing sleep or taking tablets.
Why so many triggers?	Anything that can produce a headache may cause a migraine in those predisposed
Hormonal changes in female, do they affect the central nervous system or blood vessels?	?Act on hypothalamus ?Act on veins

Is migraine pathogenesis primarily vascular or primarily neural? (Here a circulating agent is considered to be vascular but if it acts directly on the central nervous system, rather than blood vessels, it would be a neurological stimulus.) This is a major problem. But if stress is the most common trigger of migraine, then a neurological cause would seem to be primary. Furthermore, if prodromes affect 50 per cent of patients, these also provide a further argument for a neurological basis for migraine.

If the above points are correct, then I believe a slow, primary neurochemical process or processes is what we should be seeking, to account for the complexity of migraine episodes.

References

Bille, B. (1962). Migraine in school children. *Acta Paediatrica*, **51**, Suppl. 156, 71.

Blau, J.N. (1982). Resolution of migraine attacks: sleep and the recovery phase. *Journal of Neurology, Neurosurgery and Psychiatry*, **45**, 223–6.

Blau, J.N. (1984). Towards a definition of migraine. *Lancet*, **i**, 444–5.

Blau, J.N. (1985). Pathogenesis of migraine: initiation. *Journal of the Royal College of Physicians of London*, **19**, 166–8.

Blau, J.N. (1986). Clinical characteristics of premonitory symptoms in migraine. In *The prelude to the migraine attack*, (ed. W.K. Amery and A. Wauquier), pp. 39–45. Ballière Tindall, London.

Blau, J.N. (1987). Loss of migraine: when, why and how. *Journal of the Royal College of Physicians of London*, **21**, 140–2.

Blau, J.N. and Dexter, S.L. (1981). The site of pain origin during migraine attacks. *Cephalalgia*, **1**, 143–7.

Espir, M.L.E., Thomason, J., Blau, J.N., and Kurtz, Z. (1988). Headaches in civil servants: effect on work and leisure. *British Journal of Industrial Medicine*, **45**, 336–40.

Harré, R. (1969). *Scientific thought 1900–60. A selective survey.* (see p. 127), Clarendon Press, Oxford.

Headache Classification Committee of the International Headache Society (Jes Olesen, chairman). (1988). Classification and diagnostic criteria for headache disorders, cranial neuralgias and facial pain. *Cephalalgia*, **8**, Suppl. 7, 1–96.

Heyck, H. (1981). *Headache and facial pain* (4th edn). (see p. 43). George Thieme, Stuttgart.

Lashley, K.S. (1941). Patterns of cerebral integration indicated by the scotomas of migraine. *Archives of Neurology and Psychiatry*, **46**, 331–9.

Lauritzen, M. and Olesen, J. (1987). Leão's spreading depression. In Migraine: clinical therapeutic, conceptual and research aspects (ed. J.N. Blau), pp. 387–402. Chapman and Hall, London.

Olesen, J. (1978). Some clinical features of the acute migraine attack. An analysis of 750 patients. *Headache*, **18**, 268–71.

Vahlquist, B. (1955). Migraine in children. *International Archives of Allergy and Applied Immunology*, **7**, 348–55.

Wolff, H.G. (1963). *Headache and other head pain* (2nd edn). (see p. 269). Oxford University Press, New York.

Discussion

FOZARD: I have to question Dr Blau's difficulty in accepting that molecules such as 5-hydroxytryptamine or similar neurohormones cannot induce a sustained response. Blood pressure, for example, is maintained by such molecules reacting with the vasculature. If the neurohormone is there for long enough and does not induce tachyphylaxis, it can surely sustain a response over hours rather than seconds. Furthermore, in the context of migraine, one has to think in terms of these simple molecules initiating responses that set in train a sequence of positive feedback activity over a period of hours. So, the relatively short action of some neurohormones in the gut bath is misleading, may be irrelevant, and should not be a source of concern in implicating these molecules in the pathological symptoms.

LANCE: I have a comment about the site of origin of the visual hallucinations in migraine. Hubel and Wiesel (1968) demonstrated that columns of cells in the primary visual cortex respond to the orientation of bars of light. If one looks at their illustrations one could easily imagine a phase of excitation followed by inhibition passing over the visual cortex, and exciting one after another of these columns of cells, each of which responds to angled moving edges. This would cause the shimmering zig-zags that migraine patients describe, followed by a phase of inhibition associated with scotomas. Nothing of this sort could be produced from the lateral geniculate ganglion, which has six layers, three of which are connected with each retina.

BLAU: But we need real experimental evidence that the visual cortex can produce these shapes. We now have plenty of acutely observed information about visual disturbances from patient's own drawings. As I showed in Lashley's drawings (Fig.

2.1) the visual field is sometimes the shape of a kidney; at other times, it is rounded. So we need to ask how this can be explained anatomically, and how different patterns can occur.

LANCE: Brindley and Lewin (1968) have shown that stimulation of the visual cortex in humans will give rise to scintillations. These are not fortification spectra, but scintillations across the entire visual field. There is no ethical, experimental way that one could induce scotomas in humans. Cerebral blood flow studies in rats (Lauritzen *et al.* 1982) show a wave of depression, sometimes preceded by excitation, moving across the visual cortex. This wave travels across columns of cells that respond to orientation at different angles. It is not difficult to see how this could be responsible for the classical fortification spectra.

BLAU: But the visual disturbances are often more complex than that. Part of the field is more excited than the other; for example, the upper is brighter than the lower part. One has to explain the mode of spread of this phenomenon, too. If the visual field disturbances fit with the concept of cortical stimulation we need to ask which areas of, or layers within, the cortex need to be excited.

LANCE: Cortical stimulation by Penfield and Perot (1963) did not replicate fortification spectra, but it did evoke the sensation of unformed hallucinations or flashes of light.

OLESEN: Kölmel (1984), in Germany, has studied the photopsias, as they are called, or visual hallucinations seen by persons with an occipital lobe lesion. His book contains many drawings of hallucinations which are very similar to the fortification spectra seen by migraine patients, but these were fixed hallucinations that did not spread. Another point, as Professor Lance mentioned, is that our blood flow studies in humans, confirmed by some electroencephalographic studies, have made it quite clear that the migraine aura are generated in the cortex. I was very interested, Dr Blau, in your implications that the hypothalamus and other areas are involved. Do you have any proposals about how one could analyse these phenomena further?

BLAU: A colleague in the laboratory has suggested that patients could measure the specific gravity of their urine, until they get an attack, to see whether there is evidence of a change. A lot of information is available now about antidiuretic hormone, for example.

SANDLER: Another candidate might be atrial natriuretic peptide. Perhaps people could attempt to measure that in migraine.

BLAU: In the first instance one has to select patients who have this postulated specific gravity change as a demonstrable phenomenon. Having found the phenomenon, one can then chase it. But one might well find migraineurs who do not have fluid retention or a diuresis.

VANE: You listed a tremendous number of side-effects of migraine, ranging from excitatory to inhibitory; for example, either increased motions or constipation. Can you say that a particular patient will only get constipation or will only get an increased frequency of motions, or do all people demonstrate many varying side-effects at different times? If both sorts of effects are observed in all patients, it sounds as though they could be experiencing a normal kind of life.

BLAU: No; individual people tend to be typically constipated or typically to have diarrhoea before an attack. This is analogous to the different responses to anxiety experienced, for example, by people standing outside an examination hall: some will become talkative, others silent; some will want to pass urine, others to open their bowels; some will get sweaty hands, and so on. All these are responses to anxiety. What you say about inhibition and excitation is simply a feature of the way the nervous system works. For example, a dental anaesthetic first produces numbness, which wears off and leaves the area feeling 'tingly' and excited before it returns to normal. Perhaps the patients who are more sensitive to sound, or more musical, are the very ones who may be phonophobic during an attack. Some individuals who are more visually artistic may be the ones who are more sensitive to light. Others may be more sensitive to smell, and so on. Perhaps a patient's natural propensities will simply be excited or inhibited, depending on their state. Whether they show an excitatory or inhibitory response may, however, depend on the severity of the attack.

VANE: But in a particular individual is there a propensity for them to have the same *kind* of effect?

BLAU: Yes. Some patients will never notice a disturbance of the sense of smell, for example. They are simply not aware of any change.

VANE: You mentioned the infrequency of migraine during pregnancy. Does anyone know what happens at the end of pregnancy, when the baby is born, and there are violent hormonal changes?

PEATFIELD: There has been a study of women in the first week or so after they have given birth, which found that a lot of them experienced migraine attacks in that first week (Stein *et al.* 1984).

VANE: What about during the birth process?

PEATFIELD: No. The higher incidence of attacks was about four to six days afterwards.

MOSKOWITZ: I want to extend a point that Dr Blau made about pain. There are lots of parallels between the pain of migraine headache and other, visceral pains. Perhaps we can learn a great deal about migraine by studying visceral pain in general, that is, pain from the heart, the gall bladder, or urinary tract (Cervero and Morrison 1986). Both types of pain can be referred to superficial structures, including the skin. For example a headache arising from intracranial blood vessels causes a pain that is projected to the forehead. When the diaphragm is injured, the pain is referred to the shoulder. In both instances, this referral of pain is mediated by a neurophysiological phenomenon called viscerosomatic convergence. That is, a pain fibre from the skin and a visceral afferent can converge onto a postsynaptic neurone. (Convergence may also occur at thalamic and cortical levels.) When the postsynaptic neurone fires, the central nervous system does not distinguish the site of origin of the pain as visceral or somatic. This is one of the bases of referred pain. Furthermore, visceral pain — like migraine headache — tends to be rather diffuse and dull; it is not sharp like the epicritic type of pain in response to a pin-prick (Cervero and Morrison 1986). Visceral pain can be accompanied by muscle contractions in the overlying structures. For example, with abdominal pain, there is often a rigidity of the abdominal muscles. Some of the muscular complaints that we observe in migraine patients might arise from a similar neurophysiological phenomenon. Lastly, the site of termination in the brain of pain fibres from blood vessels is in the trigeminal nucleus caudalis, in the brainstem. Interestingly, the termination sites of visceral afferents are similar, but distinguishable, from cutaneous afferent fibres (de Groat 1986). Cutaneous pain fibres more commonly terminate in the superficial laminae, in Rexed's laminae II–V of the dorsal horn of the spinal cord. Visceral afferents, on the other hand, terminate in laminae I, V, VII, VIII, and so too do afferents from the blood vessels, which are therefore very similar to the visceral afferents from organs in the rest of the body.

ROSE: When you divided your symptoms into excitatory and inhibitory you were not referring, neurophysiologically, to electrical activity, so I wonder whether positive and negative phenomena might be better than excitatory and inhibitory?

BLAU: I accept that.

ROSE: My other question concerns the initiation of migraine. You extracted a selected series of patients whose initiation of migraine attacks was linked with highly significant life events. Any of those events could have been a provocative or trigger factor for any migraine attack. If a study is to have any value epidemiologically one needs a case-controlled approach. All you could say about these patients is that those events were trigger factors at a certain time. Surely you are not suggesting that without that life event these patients would not have developed migraine later on?

BLAU: One has to speculate in this sphere and be aware that migraine is a very complicated process. I had expected that if there was a psychological initiation to migraine attacks, then ever afterwards only a psychological trigger would operate, but that was not the case. I am really looking for new avenues of approach, here. How can the birth of a child initiate migraine? One tends to believe that the hormonal changes are involved — this is supported by the observation that the contraceptive pill can initiate, or aggravate, migraine. We may assume that a person is born with the genetic capacity to develop migraine and yet does not develop an attack until they are 25, or even older. One cannot have a case-controlled study for this sort of thing.

ROSE: Understanding this may be relevant to Dr Ferreira's concept (Ferreira, this volume) of learned pain impulses. Migraine is a cyclical disease: there are times when it is frequent, and there are times of remission. Often, we are treating the patient over that high frequency of episodes, which somehow break the 'learned' pattern. Remission may then continue when medication has been stopped.

BLAU: That is behind my notion of an 'internal level'. If this internal level in some way goes down — and the best example is in pregnancy — then no stimulus can provoke an attack. The suggestion, therefore, is that if the internal level is quantity A, and the trigger is quantity B, then A plus B reaches a threshold level that will give rise to an attack. But if A, for some reason, is very low, then the addition of the trigger will have no effect.

References

Brindley, G.S. and Lewin, W.S. (1968). The sensations produced by electrical stimulation of the visual cortex. *Journal of Physiology (London)*, **196**, 479–93.

Cervero, F. and Morrison, J.F.B. (ed.) (1986). *Visceral sensation*, Progress in Brain Research, Vol. 67. Elsevier, Amsterdam.

de Groat, W.C. (1986). Spinal cord projections and neuropeptides in visceral afferent neurons. In *Visceral sensation*, Progress in Brain Research, Vol. 67., (eds F. Cervero and J.F.B. Morrison), pp. 165–88. Elsevier, Amsterdam.

Hubel, D.H. and Wiesel, T.N. (1968). Receptive fields and functional architecture of monkey striate cortex. *Journal of Physiology (London)*, **195**, 215–43.

Kölmel, H.W. (1984). *Vizuelle Halluzinationen im hemianopen Feld bei homonymer hemianopsie*. Springer, Berlin.

Lauritzen, M. *et al*. (1982). Persistent oligaemia of rat cerebral cortex in the wake of spreading depression. *Annals of Neurology*, **12**, 469–74.

Penfield, W. and Perot, P. (1963). The brain's record of auditory and visual experience. *Brain*, **86**, 595–696.

Stein, G., *et al*. (1984). Headaches after childbirth. *Acta Neurologica Scandinavica*, **69**, 74–9.

3. Contribution of experimental studies to understanding the pathophysiology of migraine

J.W. Lance, G.A. Lambert, P.J. Goadsby, and A.S. Zagami

Introduction

For any hypothesis to be truly satisfying, it must be compatible with all known facts. The manifestations of migraine are so diverse that one must resist the temptation to seize on some and reject others in an attempt to justify a tenuous theory. Certain symptoms that can be recognized within the conceptual framework of migraine may be present in some episodes and not others, and may recur in certain phases of each attack but not in others. Each of these symptoms or groups of symptoms may have a different neurovascular basis.

What do we have to explain?

Any attempt to explain the pathophysiology of migraine has to account for the following components.

Premonitory symptoms   Changes in mood, increased appetite and excessive yawning may precede migraine by some 24 hours on at least some occasions in about one-third of migraineurs (Blau 1980; Drummond and Lance 1984). A feeling of elation, of being 'on top of the world' and 'flying through the day's work', is the most common mood change, while increased appetite may embrace a craving for sweet foods (including chocolates and other putative precipitants of migraine headache). This constellation of symptoms suggests a hypothalamic origin (Herberg 1975).

Focal neurological symptoms and signs (aura)   The migrainous aura may develop as a 'slow march' of symptoms, for example the spread of fortification spectra across one visual field, or may be diffuse from the outset, suggesting the simultaneous but patchy involvement of large areas of the cerebral cortex.

Headache   Headache is unilateral in two-thirds of patients and commonly starts as a dull ache at the occipito-nuchal junction, or in one temple, which then spreads over that side of the head or the whole head, or which may remain localized as a 'bar of pain' extending from eye to occiput. The pain is usually constant and unremitting but assumes a pulsatile or 'throbbing' quality when severe. It may consistently affect the same side of the head or may move from side to side, even in the one migrainous episode, and it bears no constant relationship to the hemisphere giving rise to the aura (Peatfield *et al.* 1981). Pain may radiate down the neck to the shoulder or, in some cases, to the arm and even the leg on the same side of the body, suggesting that the spinothalamic tract has collaborated with trigeminal pathways in the production of pain.

Prominent scalp vessels   The frontal branches of the superficial temporal artery become distended in about one third of patients: venous engorgement may be seen and heat loss increases from the affected area, while pressure over the prominent vessels eases the headache to some extent (Drummond and Lance 1983). Most patients appear pale and 'dark under the eyes' as the headache worsens, although exceptional patients flush before or during the attack.

Sensory hyperacuity   Light may be perceived as dazzling by both eyes or may provoke pain in the eye on the side of headache (Drummond 1986). Sounds may appear unnaturally loud and smells more intense during (or even before) the headache phase. Sensitivity of the scalp to touch and muscular hyperalgesia may develop during, and outlast, the headache phase.

Gastrointestinal symptoms   Nausea sometimes precedes the onset of headache but commonly evolves as the attack progresses, and may culminate in vomiting. Diarrhoea is associated in about 20 per cent of patients (Lance and Anthony 1966).

Fluid retention   Fluid retention and oliguria is common early in the attack with polyuria developing as the attack eases.

Precipitating factors   The injection of a contrast medium into the cerebral blood vessels during arteriography, or the administration of vasodilator drugs, may trigger a migraine attack through a presumably vascular mechanism. Excessive afferent stimuli such as flickering light, noise, or strong smells may induce migraine by their impact on the central nervous system. Excitement, stress, and relaxation after stress are most likely to act through a central mechanism. Other precipitants like a sharp blow to the head, alcohol intake, or hypoglycaemia could exert their effect peripherally or centrally. Many patients have their migraine attacks at regular intervals as though the attacks are governed by an internal clock, irrespective of emotional or environmental change.

Relieving factors   Simple methods of alleviating pain, such as the application of pressure or cold packs to the head and warming the hands, abdomen and feet might act by constricting some vessels and dilating others. The induction of vomiting and the onset of sleep are natural remedies in many cases.

Ergotamine tartrate and dihydroergotamine were thought to shorten or abort migraine headache by constriction of arteries and capacitance vessels, respectively, but recent work in our laboratory has shown that both these agents suppress the discharge of cells in the central connections of pain afferents from cerebral vessels (G.A. Lambert, A.S. Zagami, N. Bogduk, R.W. Adams, and J.W. Lance, unpublished results). Most of the medications that have proved beneficial in the management of migraine have an action on receptors for 5-hydroxytryptamine (5-HT, serotonin), noradrenaline (norepinephrine) or dopamine although the non-steroidal anti-inflammatory and calcium-channel blocking agents are apparent exceptions. Intravenous lignocaine and the new 5-HT agonist GR43175C (Doenicke *et al.* 1988) probably act peripherally on the vascular system in alleviating migraine headache.

What facts do we have to explain these phenomena?

Clinical studies

Cerebral cortex   Some differences have been demonstrated between the reactions of the migrainous brain and those of control subjects. The migrainous patient reacts more to stress (Henryk-Gutt and Rees 1973). The *contingent negative variation*, a slow event-related potential which is thought to be mediated by noradrenergic pathways, is enhanced in migrainous patients and is reduced by the administration of β-blockers (Maertens de Noordhout *et al.* 1985). The amplitude difference between the primary positive and negative waves of the visual evoked response is increased in migrainous subjects (Gawel *et al.* 1983). Variations in the visual evoked responses are not related to the duration or severity of migraine attacks and probably reflect a predisposition to migraine (Winter and Cooper 1985). Patients with 'essential headache' (including migraine) are more responsive to hallucinogenic agents than control subjects (Fanciullacci *et al.* 1974) and are more susceptible to hypotension when given bromocriptine (Fanciullacci *et al.* 1980).

Neuroendocrine changes   Premenstrual migraine is related to the fall in blood levels of oestradiol that takes place at this time (Somerville 1972). Suppression of prolactin secretion by dopaminergic agents was found to be diminished in migrainous women, a result possibly indicating reduced dopamine activity and hyperactivity of dopamine receptors (Nappi and Savoldi 1985). The thyrotropin response to thyrotropin releasing hormone is diminished in some migrainous patients (Daras *et al.* 1987).

Innervation of the pupil   Pupillary changes noted by Fanciullacci (1979) and Gotoh *et al.* (1984) suggested a sympathetic deficit in the iris of migrainous patients with peripheral adrenoceptor supersensitivity. Drummond (1987) demonstrated that the pupil was smaller on the symptomatic side in patients during unilateral headache.

Cerebral blood flow   Since the introduction of radioactive xenon techniques of measurement 15 years ago, cerebral blood flow has been known to diminish by about 20 per cent during the aura phase of migraine. Meticulous studies by the Copenhagen group have shown that the diminution in flow ('cerebral oligaemia') spreads forwards from the occipital region over the cortex at 2.2 mm per minute, irrespective of arterial territories, and it stops short at the central and lateral sulci, although patches of oligaemia may also develop in the frontal lobes (Olesen *et al.* 1981*a*; Lauritzen *et al.* 1983). The spreading oligaemia in these studies typically began before the patient noticed focal neurological symptoms, reached the sensorimotor area only after the appropriate symptoms had started, and outlasted these symptoms. The headache usually started while cerebral blood flow was still diminished. The authors concluded that cortical oligaemia was a reflection of the 'spreading depression of Leão' responsible for the 'slow march' of fortification spectra and other neurological symptoms previously calculated to traverse the cortex at about 3 mm per minute. Lauritzen *et al.* (1982) showed that induced spreading depression in the rat was accompanied by a transient hyperaemia for some three minutes, followed by a 20–25 per cent depression of cerebral blood flow for 60 minutes or more.

Re-evaluation of cerebral blood flow studies to allow for the influence of scattered radiation on the recording from areas of low flow has shown that flow dropped to 16–23 ml 100 g^{-1}min^{-1}, (below the critical level for cortical function) in the most under-perfused areas in the majority of patients (Skyhøj Olsen *et al.* 1984). This degree of ischaemia is sufficient to explain transient and possibly persistent neurological deficits. No change in regional cerebral blood flow was found in cases of migraine without aura — 'common migraine' (Olesen *et al.* 1981*b*; Lauritzen and Olesen 1984). Patchy involvement of cortical function during the aura phase of migraine may result from diffuse cortical ischaemia following vasoconstriction in the cortical microcirculation, while the 'slow march' of symptoms in other cases is correlated with spreading depression of cortical function.

It is clear that the presence or absence of headache does not depend upon changes in cerebral blood flow.

The extracranial circulation The concept that migraine headache arises from distension of branches of the external carotid artery (middle meningeal and scalp arteries) derives from the classical studies of Wolff and his colleagues. On re-reading the work of Tunis and Wolff (1953) we noted that 10 of 75 migrainous patients were selected for special analysis, and that the correlation in their paper between the headache intensity and the pulsation amplitude of the frontal branch of the superficial temporal artery was based on this limited sample. To reinvestigate this question, Drummond and Lance (1983) examined 66 patients during unilateral migrainous headache, finding that the pulsation of the main trunk of the temporal artery was not altered but the pulsation of its frontal branch increased in amplitude on the affected side. This increase was significant for a subgroup comprising about one-third of patients. In this subgroup, thermographic studies showed increased heat loss from the frontotemporal area on the headache side, and compression of the superficial temporal artery relieved the pain. In another third of patients, headache was eased by pressure on the common carotid artery, while the final third was not helped by any form of vascular compression. This is consistent with the observation of Blau and Dexter (1981) that the extracranial circulation did not contribute to headache in 21 of 50 patients examined. It is thus evident that distension of extracranial arteries is not essential for migraine headache although it appears to add a throbbing component of pain when the headache is well advanced. Extracranial blood flow is increased during migraine attacks (Sakai and Meyer 1978), possibly as a secondary phenomenon.

Monoamines Estimation of catecholamine levels in migrainous patients have given conflicting results. Schoenen *et al.* (1985) found that noradrenaline levels were significantly higher in headache-free migrainous patients than in patients with tension headache, while Gotoh *et al.* (1984) reported that the noradrenaline levels were lower in migraine patients than in a control group. Anthony (1981) demonstrated a significant increase during the headache phase, in contrast to the earlier finding of Fog-Moller *et al.* (1978).

Reports of changes in 5-HT levels have been more consistent. The main metabolite of 5-HT, 5-hydroxyindoleacetic acid, is excreted in excess in the urine of some patients during migraine attacks (Sicuteri *et al.* 1961; Curran *et al.* 1965). Furthermore, 5-HT levels drop at the onset of headache in blood taken from the cubital vein (Anthony *et al.* 1967) and from the external jugular vein (Somerville 1976). This apparently applies to patients with common migraine rather than classical migraine (Ferrari *et al.* 1987). The release of 5-HT from platelets appears to depend upon a substance of low relative molecular mass that is present during the migraine attack but not at other times (Anthony *et al.* 1969; Dvilansky *et al.* 1976; Mück-Seler *et al.* 1979). Such changes are probably relevant to the cause of migraine

headache because a characteristic headache may be precipitated in susceptible subjects by the intramuscular injection of reserpine, which lowers
platelet 5-HT levels, and is relieved by the intravenous injection of 5-HT
(Kimball *et al.* 1960; Lance *et al.* 1967*b*).

Experimental studies

Research in our laboratories, on anaesthetized cats and monkeys, has been
designed to answer the following questions.

1. What effect do vasoactive agents have on the internal and external
carotid circulations, and could such changes replicate those of migraine?
2. What effect do the monoaminergic nuclei of the brainstem exert on the
cerebral and extracranial circulations? Do the effects of noradrenergic projections from locus coeruleus differ from the serotoninergic projections of
the raphé nuclei?
3. Does activity in trigeminal pain pathways induce vascular changes?
4. What are the pathways mediating vascular pain from the head? Are
they subject to modulation by the endogenous pain control system?
5. What are the neurotransmitters involved in the pathway for perception
of vascular pain and what transmitter agents mediate constriction and dilatation of cephalic blood vessels?

The cranial circulation of the monkey (*Macaca nemstrina*), which closely
resembles the human cranial circulation, has been used for studies of differential effects on the internal and external carotid arterial tree. The
regional cerebral blood flow and the pain pathway studies have been done in
cats. The results of our investigations may be summarized as follows.

Vasoactive agents   All humoral agents had a greater effect on the external than on the internal carotid circulation of the monkey. The external
vasculature was constricted by adrenaline, noradrenaline, 5-HT and prostaglandins F1 and F2 and was dilated by prostaglandin E, bradykinin, histamine, and acetylcholine (Spira *et al.* 1976). The results suggested that the
amount of 5-HT liberated from platelets during migraine would be unlikely
to exert any significant effect on the circulation (Spira *et al.* 1978).

*Effects of stimulation of the trigeminal nerve and brainstem nuc-
lei on the external carotid circulation*   Extracranial blood flow increases by about 20 per cent during stimulation of the locus coeruleus
(Goadsby *et al.* 1982, 1983), the dorsal raphé nucleus (Goadsby *et al.* 1985*a*,
b, *c*) or the trigeminal nerve (Lambert *et al.* 1984). This vasodilator pathway
leaves the brainstem in the facial nerve and traverses the greater superficial
petrosal branch of that nerve to the pterygopalatine (sphenopalatine) and
otic ganglia, from which vasodilator fibres are distributed to branches of the
external carotid artery (Goadsby *et al.* 1983, 1984). The resulting vasodilata-

tion depends upon the release of vasoactive intestinal polypeptide (Goadsby and Macdonald 1985). It has thus been shown that dilatation of extracranial arteries can be caused by stimulation of the trigeminal nerve. Such dilatation may therefore develop as a phenomenon secondary to the activation of pain pathways in migraine headache. We have termed this the 'trigeminovascular reflex'.

Effects of the trigeminal nerve and brainstem nuclei on the internal carotid circulation   Low-frequency stimulation (less than 20 per second) of locus coeruleus reduces total cerebral blood flow ipsilaterally by about 20 per cent (Goadsby *et al.* 1982). This is a direct effect of the projection from locus coeruleus to the cerebral cortex and is mediated by α_2-adrenoceptors since it is blocked selectively by yohimbine in the monkey (Goadsby *et al.* 1985*a*). Regional cerebral blood flow is also diminished, particularly in the occipital cortex of the cat (Goadsby and Duckworth 1989). This effect of locus coeruleus stimulation is presumably exerted on the microcirculation since stimulation does not produce any consistent change in the resting discharge frequency of cells in the cat occipital cortex (Adams *et al.* 1989).

Stimulation of the dorsal raphé nucleus does not exert a direct effect on cerebral blood flow but does increase flow by about 20 per cent indirectly, by means of the greater superficial petrosal nerve pathway described above. Trigeminal nerve stimulation does not alter bulk cerebral blood flow in the monkey (Goadsby *et al.* 1986) but regional cerebral blood flow studies in the cat have shown an increase in perfusion of the frontal and parietal cortex (Goadsby and Duckworth 1987). The effect is even greater when the superior sagittal sinus is stimulated (Lambert *et al.* 1988).

Catecholamine release   Stimulation in the region of the locus coeruleus causes a pressor effect that is associated with a 260 per cent increase in blood levels of noradrenaline and a 196 per cent increase in adrenaline; the increases are reversibly blocked by clamping the adrenal hilum bilaterally (Goadsby 1985). This indicates that brainstem activity may liberate catecholamines from the adrenal glands and may thus provide a '5-HT-releasing factor' of relevance to migraine.

The central pathway for vascular pain from the head   We have recently found that cells in the region of the lateral cervical nucleus of the cat, in the second cervical cord segment, receive a convergent input from the superior sagittal sinus, the middle meningeal artery and the superficial temporal artery (G.A. Lambert *et al.* unpublished results). The cell discharge evoked by such stimulation of vascular pain fibres is inhibited by concurrent stimulation of the periaqueductal grey matter and is also suppressed by the intravenous injection of ergotamine tartrate and dihydroergotamine. This area may act as a visceral afferent centre, for the mediation of vascular pain, that complements the trigeminal nucleus caudalis which receives both vascular and somatic afferents (Davis and Dostrovsky 1986; Strassman *et al.* 1986). The dorsolateral area of the upper cervical cord therefore warrants further study as an alternative pathway for the mediation of headache.

Can we fit these facts together as a neurovascular hypothesis?

What are the arguments for and against a vascular and a neural theory of migraine?

The vascular/humoral hypothesis

Factors in favour   Migraine headache throbs when severe and is relieved temporarily by carotid compression in two-thirds of patients. Branches of the superficial temporal artery become dilated in one-third of patients and pressure on these branches often eases the headache. Ligation of one temporal artery may relieve pain in the temporal area for weeks or months.

Migraine is precipitated by vascular irritation (angiography) and by the administration of vasodilator substances.

Noradrenaline promotes platelet aggregation and release of 5-HT, which is a feature of the migraine attack. Bradykinin and 5-IIT potentiate one another in inducing vascular pain (Sicuteri 1967). Peptides released from trigeminal nerve terminals may also contribute to the genesis of vascular pain. These include substance P in the rat (Moskowitz 1984), and calcitonin gene-related peptide and substance P in both cats and humans (Goadsby *et al.* 1988). Migraine headache is relieved by the intravenous administration of lignocaine, 5-HT, and the new 5-HT agonist, GR43175C.

Factors against   Compression of the common carotid artery does not ease headache in one third of patients and produces only temporary benefit in the remaining two-thirds. Headache is not associated with increased cerebral blood flow and may develop in classical migraine while the flow is still diminished.

Cortical ischaemia or spreading depression does not cause headache since a classical aura may not be followed by headache.

Platelet aggregation and 5-HT release would have to take place consistently on each occasion in a particular region of the carotid or vertebrobasilar circulation to produce an habitual aura. If such a reaction (or the release of peptides from trigeminal nerve terminals) were responsible both for the aura and the ensuing headache, the latter should develop on the side of the cerebral hemisphere that produces the aura, whereas some 50 per cent of headaches are on the inappropriate side (Peatfield *et al.* 1981).

Infusion of 5-HT into the carotid circulation of the monkey has shown that the changes in 5-HT level observed in migrainous patients would not have significant effects on the circulation.

The neural hypothesis

Factors in favour Hypothalamic symptoms (elation, hunger) may precede headache by 24 hours or more. Specific afferent input to the nervous system may lead to an aura involving the appropriate part of the cortex. For example, flickering sunlight may induce fortification spectra within minutes. An emotional stimulus such as an unpleasant letter from a lawyer may have the same effect.

'Ice-pick' pains and 'ice-cream headache' are more common in migrainous patients (Raskin and Knittle 1976; Raskin and Schwartz 1980) and pain is localized to the habitual site of migrainous headache in about 40 per cent of patients (Drummond and Lance 1984), suggesting a segmental defect in a pain-inhibitory system. Headache may be provoked by the implantation of electrodes in the human periaqueductal grey matter (Raskin *et al.* 1987).

A dull ache may precede migraine by hours or days. Some patients state that the pain of migraine radiates to the ipsilateral neck, shoulder, arm or even the whole side of the body, suggesting a spinothalamic distribution. Hyperalgesia and hyperaesthesia are often unilateral and may be segmental in distribution. Headache may change from one side to the other, even in the one attack, suggesting a neural switching mechanism at brainstem level.

Our laboratory studies in cat and monkey have shown that brainstem structures can induce ipsilateral cerebral and extracranial vascular changes of the same order as those in migraine. The same brainstem structures play a part in the endogenous pain control system, so that one could propose a phase of excitation of brainstem nuclei that initiates headache together with the associated vascular changes, followed by a phase of monoamine depletion that opens the pain gates (Lance *et al.* 1983).

Factors against The neural concept is theoretical and based on animal experimentation although there are compatible observations in human patients. Perhaps the advent of positron emission tomography (PET) scanning with 5-HT binding ligands may clarify the central role of monoaminergic transmitters in migraine headache. Distension and sensitivity of extracranial arteries can be demonstrated in about one-third of migrainous patients, so that vascular factors cannot be ignored, whether they be primary or secondary to neural discharge. Moreover, many of the triggers for migraine appear to act primarily on blood vessels.

A compromise hypothesis: complementary neural and vascular mechanisms

The genetic susceptibility to migraine must depend upon an hereditary instability of pain control mechanisms and neurovascular reflexes.

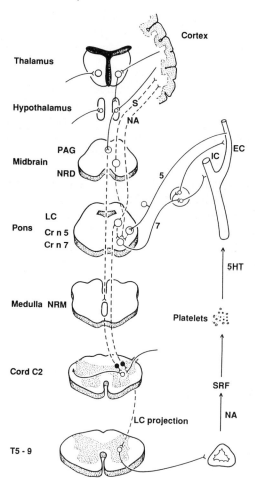

FIG. 3.1. The neurovascular hypothesis for migraine. Brainstem mechanisms are triggered by descending pathways from the cerebral cortex (in response to emotion or stress), from the thalamus (in response to excessive afferent stimulation, light, noise, or smells), or from the hypothalamus (in response to changes in the internal environment or 'internal clocks'). Nucleus raphé dorsalis (NRD) and locus coeruleus (LC) project diffusely to the cerebral cortex, employing 5-HT, that is, serotonin (S), and noradrenaline (NA), respectively, as transmitter agents. LC causes constriction of the ipsilateral cortical microcirculation through this direct pathway. Stimulation of NRD , LC, or the trigeminal nerve (5) induces dilatation of the extracranial circulation (EC), by connections with the parasympathetic component of the facial nerve (7), the greater superficial petrosal nerve and the sphenopalatine and otic ganglia, and releases vasoactive intestinal peptide as a peripheral transmitter agent ('the trigeminovascular reflex'). NRD causes dilatation in the internal carotid circulation (IC) through the same indirect pathway. Stimulation of the LC

The increasing prevalence of migraine with increasing age during child-hood and the doubling of prevalence in females during the reproductive years of life implicate hypothalamopituitary factors in reducing the safety factor of normal control mechanisms.

The episodic recurrence of migraine and the nature of the symptoms (such as hunger, drowsiness, or elation) that may precede headache suggest that 'internal clocks' of the hypothalamic region play an important role. Some patients undergo cycles of susceptible and refractory periods, with patients responding to trigger factors in the former but not the latter. In a susceptible period, migraine may be triggered by neural mechanisms as the result of excitement or stress, or when the brain is subjected to an intense afferent stimulus (visual, auditory, or olfactory). The cranial circulation itself becomes an important source of afferent stimuli when vessels: (1) are dilated by exercise, alcohol, or medications; (2) are sensitized by humoral agents; or (3) are subjected to a direct insult by head injury or by the internally applied trauma caused by contrast medium during arteriography.

The cerebral response to such stimuli is to alert the organism by activation of brainstem mechanisms and the autonomic nervous system, with the secretion of noradrenaline from the adrenal gland which, in turn, may promote platelet aggregation, 5-HT release, and vascular sensitization.

Brainstem activation can reduce or increase cerebral blood flow ipsilaterally by about 20 per cent through projections of locus coeruleus or dorsal raphé nucleus, respectively. Extracranial blood flow is increased by stimulation of these structures or the trigeminal nerve, by means of a reflex connection with the parasympathetic outflow, which traverses the facial nerve, the greater superficial petrosal nerve and the sphenopalatine and otic ganglia, and which releases vasoactive intestinal peptide at its vascular terminals (Fig. 3.1). In this way neural activity can produce the extracranial vascular changes associated with migraine.

---

area causes release of NA from the adrenal gland by its connection with the inter-mediolateral cell column of the thoracic cord (LC projection). NA, or a serotonin (5-HT) releasing factor (SRF) liberated by NA, causes a platelet release reaction. Free serotonin released from platelets increases the sensitivity of vascular receptors, thus augmenting the afferent inflow through the trigeminal nerve (5). The spinal tract of the trigeminal nerve (not illustrated) descends to the second cervical segment of the spinal cord (C2) where it converges with fibres from the second cervical root onto second order neurones in the pain pathway. Transmission at this synapse is regulated by inhibitory neurones (black circles) which, in turn, are modulated by the endogenous pain-control pathway descending from the periaqueductal grey matter (PAG) through nucleus raphé magnus (NRM), and from LC. Activity in brainstem monoaminergic pathways is thus able to replicate the vascular changes of migraine as well as to regulate the perception of pain arising from cranial vessels.

J.W. Lance et al.

Whether or not such vascular changes take place in any particular attack, the painful component of migraine must be accounted for by *either* segmental disinhibition of the trigeminal complex *or* increased afferent inflow into that segment, or both factors. The commonest sites for pain to be felt initially in migraine are the temple and the upper neck in the distribution of the second and third cervical segments. The temple is innervated by the zygomaticotemporal nerve (arising from the second trigeminal division) and the auriculotemporal nerve (from the third division). The only intracranial structures innervated by the second and third divisions of the trigeminal nerves are the dura of the anterior and middle fossa and the middle meningeal artery. While it is possible that afferent inflow from these structures, and from the upper neck, might increase in the early stages of migraine, it would seem more likely that a portion of the spinal nucleus of the trigeminal nerve (probably the nucleus caudalis), and cells of the lateral cervical nucleus that receive cranial afferents, start to discharge spontaneously and to respond excessively to a normal afferent inflow. Extracranial vasodilatation would then follow as a secondary phenomenon, induced by activity in the 'trigeminovascular reflex' pathway that we have described. If the adsorption of 5-HT or other substances to vessel walls enhanced vascular sensitivity, afferent inflow from vessels would increase and would impart a pulsatile quality to the headache.

The most likely neurotransmitters to be involved in this neurovascular reaction are noradrenaline (contained in locus coeruleus neurones) and 5-HT (in raphé nuclei) with the probable implication of dopamine (area postrema) in the mechanism of vomiting. This concept is supported by the changes reported in the levels of these monoamines in venous blood and by the beneficial effect of medications that act on adrenergic or serotoninergic receptors. This neurovascular hypothesis is illustrated in Figure 3.1.

Acknowledgements

The research work on which this review is based was generously supported by the National Health and Medical Research Council of Australia, the J.A. Perini Family Trust, the Basser Trust, and Mr and Mrs Warren Anderson. The figure was drawn by Marcus Cremonese and prepared by the Department of Medical Illustration, University of New South Wales.

References

Adams, R.W., Lambert, G.A., and Lance, J.W. (1989). Effects of brainstem nuclei on neuronal activity in the primary visual cortex of the cat. Relevance to cerebral blood flow and migraine. *Cephalalgia*, **9**, 107–18.

Anthony, M. (1981). Biochemical indices of sympathetic activity in migraine. *Cephalalgia*, **1**, 83–9.

Anthony, M., Hinterberger, H., and Lance, J.W. (1967). Plasma serotonin in migraine and stress. *Archives of Neurology*, **16**, 544–52.

Anthony, M., Hinterberger, H., and Lance, J.W. (1969). The possible relationship of serotonin to the migraine syndrome. *Research and Clinical Studies in Headache*, **2**, 29–59.

Blau, J.N. (1980). Migraine prodromes separated from the aura: complete migraine. *British Medical Journal*, **281**, 658–60.

Blau, J.N. and Dexter, S.L. (1981). The site of pain origin during migraine attacks. *Cephalalgia*, **1**, 143–7.

Curran, D.A., Hinterberger, H., and Lance, J.W. (1965). Total plasma serotonin, 5-hydroxyindoleacetic acid and *p*-hydroxy-*m*-methoxymandelic acid excretion in normal and migrainous subjects. *Brain*, **88**, 997–1010.

Davis, K.P. and Dostrovsky, J.P. (1986). Activation of trigeminal brainstem nociceptive neurons by dural artery stimulation. *Pain*, **25**, 395–401.

Daras, M., Papakostas, Y., Markianos, M., and Stefanis, C. (1987). Neuroendocrine approach to migraine: the TRH test. In *Current problems in neurology*, vol. 4, *Advances in headache research*, (ed. F. Clifford Rose), pp. 59–64, John Libbey, London.

Doenicke, A., Brand, J., and Perrin, V.L. (1988). Possible benefit of GR43175, a novel 5-HT-like receptor agonist, for the acute treatment of severe migraine. *Lancet*, **i**, 1309–11.

Drummond, P.D. (1986). A quantitative assessment of photophobia in migraine and tension headache. *Headache*, **26**, 465–9.

Drummond, P.D. (1987). Pupil diameter in migraine and tension headache. *Journal of Neurology Neurosurgery and Psychiatry*, **50**, 228–30.

Drummond, P.D. and Lance, J.W. (1983). Extracranial vascular changes and the source of pain in migraine headache. *Annals of Neurology*, **13**, 32–7.

Drummond, P.D. and Lance, J.W. (1984). Neurovascular disturbances in headache patients. *Clinical and Experimental Neurology*, **20**, 93–9.

Dvilansky, A., Rishpon, S., Nathan, I., Zolotow, Z., and Korcyn, A.D. (1976). Release of platelet 5-hydroxytryptamine by plasma taken from patients during and between migraine attacks. *Pain*, **2**, 315–8.

Fanciullacci, M. (1979). Iris adrenergic impairment in idiopathic headache. *Headache*, **19**, 8–13.

Fanciullacci, M., Franchi, G., and Sicuteri, F. (1974). Hypersensitivity to lysergic acid diethylamide (LSD-25) and psilocybin in essential headache. *Experientia*, **30**, 1441–2.

Fanciullacci, M., Michelacci, S., Curradi, C., and Sicuteri, F. (1980). Hyper-responsiveness of migraine patients to the hypotensive action of bromocriptine. *Headache*, **20**, 99–102.

Ferrari, M.D., Frolich, M., Odink, J., Tapparelli, C., Portielje, J.E.A., and Bruyn, G.W. (1987). Methionine-enkephalin and serotonin in migraine and tension headache. In *Current problems in neurology, vol. 4, Advances in headache research*, (ed. F. Clifford Rose), pp. 227–34. John Libbey, London.

Fog-Møller, F., Genefke, I.K., and Bryndum, B. (1978). Changes in concentration of catecholamines in blood during spontaneous migraine attacks and reserpine-induced attacks. In *Current concepts in migraine research*, (ed. R. Greene), pp. 115–9. Raven Press, New York.

Gawel, M., Connolly, J.F., and Clifford Rose, F. (1983). Migraine patients exhibit abnormalities in the visual evoked potential. *Headache*, **23**, 40–52.

Goadsby, P.J. (1985). Brainstem activation of the adrenal medulla in the cat. *Brain Research*, **327**, 241–8.

Goadsby, P.J. and Macdonald, G.J. (1985). Extracranial vasodilatation mediated by vasoactive intestinal polypeptide (VIP). *Brain Research*, **329**, 285–8.

Goadsby, P.J. and Duckworth, J.W. (1987). The effect of stimulation of the trigeminal ganglion on regional cerebral blood flow in the cat. *American Journal of Physiology*, **253**, R270–R274.

Goadsby, P.J. and Duckworth, J.W. (1989). Low frequency stimulation of locus coeruleus reduces regional cerebral blood flow in the spinalized cat. *Brain Research*, **476**, 71–7.

Goadsby, P.J., Lambert, G.A., and Lance, J.W. (1982). Differential effects on the internal and external carotid circulation of the monkey evoked by locus coeruleus stimulation. *Brain Research*, **249**, 247–54.

Goadsby, P.J., Lambert, G.A., and Lance, J.W. (1983). Effects of locus coeruleus stimulation on carotid vascular resistance in the cat. *Brain Research*, **278**, 175–83.

Goadsby, P.J., Lambert, G.A., and Lance, J.W. (1984). The peripheral pathway for extracranial vasodilatation in the cat. *Journal of the Autonomic Nervous System*, **10**, 145–55.

Goadsby, P.J., Lambert, G.A., and Lance, J.W. (1985a). The mechanism of cerebrovascular constriction in response to locus coeruleus stimulation. *Brain Research*, **326**, 213–7.

Goadsby, P.J., Piper, R.D., Lambert, G.A., and Lance, J.W. (1985b). Effect of stimulation of nucleus raphé dorsalis on carotid blood flow. I. The monkey. *American Journal of Physiology*, **28**, R257–R262.

Goadsby, P.J., Piper, R.D., Lambert, G.A., and Lance, J.W. (1985c). Effect of stimulation of nucleus raphé dorsalis on carotid blood flow. II. The cat. *American Journal of Physiology*, **248**, R263–R269.

Goadsby, P.J., Lambert, G.A., and Lance, J.W. (1986). Stimulation of the trigeminal ganglion increases flow in the extracranial but not the cerebral circulation of the monkey. *Brain Research*, **381**, 63–7.

Goadsby, P.J., Edvinsson, L., and Ekman, R. (1988). Release of vasoactive peptides in the extracerebral circulation of humans and the cat during activation of the trigeminovascular system. *Annals of Neurology*, **23**, 193–6.

Gotoh, F., Komatsumoto, S., Araki, N., and Gomi, S. (1984). Noradrenergic nervous activity in migraine. *Archives of Neurology*, **4**, 951–5.

Henryk-Gutt, R. and Rees, W.L. (1973). Psychological aspects of migraine. *Journal of Psychosomatic Research*, **17**, 141–53.

Herberg, L.J. (1975). The hypothalamus and aminergic pathways in migraine. In *Modern Topics in migraine*, (ed. J. Pearce), pp. 85–95. Heinemann, London.

Kimball, R.W., Friedman, A.P., and Vallejo, E. (1960). Effect of serotonin in migraine patients. *Neurology*, **10**, 107–11.

Lambert, G.A., Bogduk, N., Goadsby, P.J., Duckworth, J.W., and Lance, J.W. (1984). Decreased carotid arterial resistance in cats in response to trigeminal stimulation. *Journal of Neurosurgery*, **61**, 307–15.

Lambert, G.A., Goadsby, P.J., Zagami, A.S., and Duckworth, J.W. (1988). Comparative effects of stimulation of the trigeminal ganglion and the superior sagittal sinus on cerebral blood flow and evoked potentials in the cat. *Brain Research*, **453**, 143–9.

Lance, J.W. and Anthony, M. (1966). Some clinical aspects of migraine. *Archives of Neurology*, **15**, 356–61.

Lance, J.W., Anthony, M., and Gonski, A.G. (1967a). Serotonin, the carotid body and cranial vessels in migraine. *Archives of Neurology*, **16**, 553–8.

Lance, J.W., Anthony, M., and Hinterberger, H. (1967b). The control of cranial arteries by humoral mechanisms and its relation to the migraine syndrome. *Headache*, **7**, 93–102.

Lance, J.W., Lambert, G.A., Goadsby, P.J., and Duckworth, J.W. (1983). Brainstem influences on the cephalic circulation: experimental data from cat and monkey of relevance to the mechanism of migraine. *Headache*, **23**, 258–65.

Lauritzen, M. and Olesen, J. (1984). Regional cerebral blood flow during migraine attacks by xenon-133 inhalation and emission tomography. *Brain*, **107**, 447–61.

Lauritzen, M., Jorgensen, M.B., Diemer, N.H., Gjedde, A., and Hansen, A.J. (1982). Persistent oligemia of rat cerebral cortex in the wake of spreading depression. *Annals of Neurology*, **12**, 469–74.

Lauritzen, M., Skyhoj Olsen, T., Lassen, N.A., and Paulson, O.B. (1983). Changes in regional cerebral blood flow during the course of classical migraine attacks. *Annals of Neurology*, **13**, 633–41.

Maertens de Noordhout, A., Timsit-Berthier, M., and Schoenen, J. (1985). Contingent negative variation (CNV) in migraineurs before and during prophylactic treatment with beta-blockers. *Cephalagia*, **5**, Suppl. 3, 34–5.

Moskowitz, M.A. (1984). The neurobiology of vascular head pain. *Annals of Neurology*, **16**, 157–68.

Mück-Šeler, D., Deanović, Ž., and Dupelj, M. (1979). Platelet serotonin (5-HT) and 5-HT releasing factor in plasma of migrainous patients. *Headache*, **19**, 14–7.

Nappi, G. and Savoldi, F. (1985). *Headache: diagnostic system and taxonomic criteria*. pp. 53–9. John Libbey, London.

Olesen, J., Larsen, B., and Lauritzen, M. (1981a). Focal hyperemia followed by spreading oligemia and impaired activation of rCBF in classical migraine. *Annals of Neurology*, **9**, 344–52.

Olesen, J., Tfelt-Hansen, P., Henricksen, L., and Larsen, B. (1981b). The common migraine attack may not be initiated by cerebral ischaemia. *Lancet*, **ii**, 438–40.

Peatfield, R.C., Gawel, M.J., and Clifford Rose, F. (1981). Asymmetry of the aura and pain in migraine. *Journal of Neurology Neurosurgery and Psychiatry*, **44**, 846–8.

Raskin, N.H. and Knittle, S.C. (1976). Ice-cream headache and orthostatic symptoms in patients with migraine headache. *Headache*, **16**, 222–5.

Raskin, N.H. and Schwartz, R.K. (1980). Ice pick-like pain. *Neurology*, **30**, 203–5.

Raskin, N.H., Hosobuchi, Y., and Lamb, S. (1987). Headache may arise from perturbation of the brain. *Headache*, **27**, 416–20.

Sakai, F. and Meyer, J.S. (1978). Regional cerebral hemodynamics during migraine and cluster headaches measured by the 133 Xe inhalation method. *Headache*, **18**, 122–32.

Schoenen, J., Maertens de Noordhout, A., and Delwaide, P.J. (1985). Plasma catecholamines in headache patients: clinical correlations. *Cephalalgia*, **5** (Suppl. 3), 28–9.

Sicuteri, F. (1967). Vasoneuroactive substances and their implication in vascular pain. *Research and Clinical Studies in Headache*, **1**, 6–45.

Sicuteri, F., Testi, A., and Anselmi, B. (1961). Biochemical investigations in headache: increase in hydroxyindoleacetic acid excretion during migraine attacks. *International Archives of Allergy and Applied Immunology*, **19**, 55–8.

Skyhøj Olsen, T., Lauritzen, M., and Lassen, N.A. (1984). Focal ischaemia during migraine attacks in patients with classical and complicated migraine. *Acta Neurolo-gica Scandinavica*, **69**, (Suppl. 98), 258–9.

Somerville, B.W. (1972). The role of estradiol withdrawal in the etiology of men-strual migraine. *Neurology*, **22**, 355–65.

Somerville, B.W. (1976). Platelet-bound and free serotonin levels in jugular and forearm venous blood during migraine. *Neurology*, **26**, 41–5.

Spira, P.J., Mylecharane, E.J., and Lance, J.W. (1976). The effects of humoral agents and antimigraine drugs on the cranial circulation of the monkey. *Research and Clinical Studies in Headache*, **4**, 37–75.

Spira, P.J., Mylecharane, E.J., Misbach, J., Duckworth, J.W., and Lance, J.W. (1978). Internal and external carotid vascular responses to vasoactive agents in the monkey. *Neurology*, **28**, 162–73.

Strassman, A., Mason, P., Moskowitz, M., and Maciewicz, R. (1986). Response of brain stem trigeminal neurons to electrical stimulation of the dura. *Brain Research*, **379**, 242–50.

Tunis, M.M. and Wolff, H.G. (1953). Studies on headache; long-term observations of the reactivity of the cranial arteries in subjects with vascular headache of the migraine type. *Archives of Neurology Neurosurgery and Psychiatry*, **70**, 551–7.

Winter, A.L. and Cooper, R. (1985). Neurophysiological measures of the visual system in classic migraine. In *Migraine: clinical and research advances*, (ed. F. Clifford Rose), pp. 11–16. Karger, Basel.

Discussion

VANE: When you showed the vasoactive intestinal peptide (VIP) effect of the antibody, were you suggesting that the VIP is released into the circulation? That is the only place where the antibody will be found. Or is the VIP underneath the endothelial cells, directly affecting the smooth muscle below them?

LANCE: Perhaps you could suggest an answer to this. We simply know that the injection of the anti-VIP serum will prevent this vasodilator reaction, but we have not studied the site of the interaction.

VANE: My interpretation of that would be that the VIP has to be within the circulation; the antibody is such a large molecule that it will not get through the endothelial cells to the underlying smooth muscle.

MOSKOWITZ: In your studies of substance P levels in the plasma, it was interesting to see the increased levels in response to thermocoagulation of the trigeminal ganglia, or to electrical stimulation of the trigeminal nerve in the cat. Yet I know that the measurement of substance P levels in the blood is fraught with technical difficulties. I was particularly concerned that the calcitonin gene related peptide (CGRP) and substance P data changes reported by your group with Dr Edvinsson (Goadsby *et al.* 1988) were not reproduced by Bloom and his group (Schon *et al.* 1987). Could this be because of a methodological difference?

LANCE: Didn't the Bloom group study venous blood taken from the cubital fossa?

EDVINSSON: That was the difference, and we have discussed this with them (Schon *et al.* 1987). The difference is that we took our blood samples from the jugular vein, which is close to the site of the release of cranial peptides (Goadsby *et al.* 1988). When you dilute the concentration of these peptides in the whole circula-tion (seven litres of blood) by sampling elsewhere, you will not detect any change from the cubital fossa measurement.

SCHWARTZ: I am interested in your comment that the unilateral symptoms in migraine can be explained by the mostly ipsilateral projection of the mono-aminergic systems. It is not only the noradrenergic and the 5-HT (5-hydroxy-tryptamine; serotonin) systems that are organized in this way but also the histaminergic system. The cholinergic system could have a similar role. Is there any evidence of a left/right dissociation in the pattern of activity of, say, the locus coeruleus or the raphé nucleus, in specific circumstances, in animals or in humans?

LANCE: We have not studied the interaction between sides. We have shown that all the vascular changes I have spoken of are predominantly unilateral. Buda *et al.* (1975) showed that a lesion of one locus increases tyrosine hydroxylase activity in the contralateral locus and therefore, by implication, normally inhibits activity of the opposite locus. We could envisage a sort of 'flip-flop' arrangement in the brainstem so that, if one side is active, the other is inhibited. By analogy, in Parkinson's disease, impulses come down the pyramidal tract at four to five per second. It is only at the spinal cord level that these are transmuted into an alternating tremor. Hypothalamic or frontal lobe projections may activate brain-stem mechanisms, which could then transform them into an alternating system, with cortical phenomena produced on one side and headache on the other side. We do not yet have good evidence about this, but we plan to investigate it. Such study is difficult because the two locus coeruleus areas are so very close to one another. It would be difficult, physiologically, to stimulate one and to study what is happening on the other without problems of artefact. At least by chemical inves-tigation it has been shown that one does seem to inhibit the other (Buda *et al.* 1975).

SCHWARTZ: One could also attempt to record simultaneously the activity at each locus, to see if there are any circumstances in which there is a dissociated activa-tion.

LANCE: That would be interesting. I am not aware that anyone has attempted it.

GLOVER: Have you looked at the interactions between the locus coeruleus and the raphé nucleus? I believe there are projections from the locus to the raphé. You said that when you stimulated the locus coeruleus, an α_2-adrenergic blocking agent prevented the vasoconstrictor effect of the stimulation. Have you tried to see if any antiserotoninergic drugs block the effect?

LANCE: Antiserotonin agents such as methysergide do not block the effect of locus coeruleus or raphé stimulation.

GLOVER: If an antiserotonin drug can be shown to block the raphé, one could see if that also works for locus coeruleus. Why do you think that methysergide does not block the effect of raphé stimulation? Surely some antiserotonin drug should block it?

LANCE: One would think so, but we have not yet tested all the available drugs. It would be interesting to study the new preparations now available, such as the 5-HT$_1$ agonist GR43175, and the 5-HT$_3$ antagonists.

GARDNER-MEDWIN: It is known that the 5-HT and noradrenaline (norepinephrine) systems are much involved in the control of neural function during sleep and arousal. Could some component of the changes in vascular resistance that you observed be secondary to changes in metabolic activity?

LANCE: We have stimulated the dorsal raphé nuclei, locus coeruleus, and reticular formation, and have studied the effect on both evoked and spontaneous elec-trophysiological activity in the visual cortex of the cat (Lance *et al.* 1986). The evoked responses were potentiated from all those stimulation sites but we found no consistent change in the spontaneous discharge of cells in the visual cortex — even from the area of visual cortex where we have demonstrated an increase in blood flow in response to stimulation of the trigeminal nucleus. We observed phases of both inhibition and excitation of resting discharge, but no clear trend. We concluded that the changes we have observed after stimulating locus coeruleus or raphé nucleus almost certainly act on the microcirculation, but we have not demonstrated any primary effect on cellular discharge in the visual cortex. One deduces that vascular changes are not simply following a metabolic demand but are probably the result of a direct vasoconstrictor action.

GARDNER-MEDWIN: Do you yet have any direct metabolic measurements?

LANCE: No, but we are currently doing metabolic measurements as part of our study of regional cerebral blood flow.

WELCH: You say that when you stimulated the locus coeruleus and the dorsal raphé nucleus you saw an increase in the evoked responses but no change in spontaneous activity. One could infer from this that you have probably changed the threshold for the evoked responses in some way, which may have happened because of a shift in DC (direct current) potential. This may relate to an influence of these brainstem centres over the threshold for spontaneous depolarization or spreading depression. It would be interesting to check that in your experiments.

LANCE: I agree. There are many things we would like to do.

SAXENA: It is intriguing that ergotamine administered intravenously, but not when applied locally on blood vessels, could block the neuronal responses evoked from blood vessels. You use this as an argument to suggest that ergotamine acts within the central nervous system. However, ergotamine is a polar substance with a large molecule and therefore does not seem to cross the blood–brain barrier readily (Perrin 1985). It is therefore important to know the *exact* doses of ergotamine that you used in your experiments. You may also know that small doses $(1-5~\mu\mathrm{g~kg^{-1}}$, intravenously) of ergotamine have a profound vasoconstrictor action (Saxena and de Vlaam Schluter 1974). Furthermore, I have some doubts that ergotamine applied from outside the blood vessels would reach the place from where you are evoking neuronal responses. Finally, have you tried other vasoconstrictor agents, for example noradrenaline? The very fact that the blood vessel tone changes after ergotamine administration may influence the neuronal responses that you elicit.

LANCE: We have not studied the effect of noradrenaline. The ergotamine and dihydroergotamine dosage (Lambert *et al.* 1988) that we have used in the cat $(4-40~\mu\mathrm{g~kg^{-1}}$, intravenously) is comparable to that given in humans for migraine. Humans readily experience nausea and other central phenomena very quickly after ergotamine. This indicates to me that the drug does enter the human central nervous system. Admittedly, nausea could be mediated by the area postrema, which is outside the blood–brain barrier, but I suspect that ergotamine has a central action.

FOZARD: If ergotamine is an effective treatment for migraine because it suppresses the firing of neurones that are *perceiving* the pain, then one might expect ergotamine to be analgesic in conditions other than migraine. Is there any evidence for this?

LANCE: I have only anecdotal experience to draw on here. An Italian patient, who had been investigated thoroughly and diagnosed as having migraine, came to Sydney, where I saw him. He had typical episodic pain, which radiated from the right eye, over the head, and was associated with nausea and dilatation of blood vessels in the right temple. He responded well to ergotamine. We treated him for some time as a migraineur. I was suspicious because he subsequently developed an area of numbness over the right forehead. He had frequent computer assisted tomography (CAT) scans and X-rays, which were negative. He eventually developed a typical Gradenigo's syndrome, with a loss of sensation in the distribution of the first division of the fifth cranial nerve and a sixth nerve palsy. A nasopharyngeal carcinoma was then demonstrated by CAT scan. Even at that stage his pain was eased by the injection of ergotamine.

MOSKOWITZ: In contrast to the neural firing in the lateral cervical nucleus, we have recently observed that the firing rate of the neurones in the trigeminal nucleus caudalis does not show the same dramatic decrease following the peripheral administration of ergotamine (A. Strassman, R. Maciewicz, and M.A. Moskowitz, unpublished results). (We have sometimes wrongly identified a suppression in discharge, until we have established that our microelectrode has moved in reference to the cell we are recording from.) So our results indicate that these two nuclei are apparently processing their information very differently.

LANCE: In our studies on the suppression of cellular discharge in the laterocervical nucleus by ergotamine, we consider only those cells in which the discharge returns, and in which the inhibition is therefore reversible. If one loses the recording from a cell, one obviously cannot assume that the loss of firing is due to any administered medication. It is, nevertheless, difficult to hold a microelectrode close to a cell for a long period of time.

References

Buda, M., Roussel, B., Renaud, B., and Pujol, J.-F. (1975). Increase in tyrosine hydroxylase activity in the locus coeruleus of the rat brain after contralateral lesioning. *Brain Research*, **93**, 564–9.

Goadsby, P.J., Edvinsson, L., and Ekman, R. (1988). Release of vasoactive peptides in the extracerebral circulation of humans and the cat during activation of the trigeminovascular system. *Annals of Neurology*, **23**, 193–6.

Lambert, G.A., Zagami, A.S., and Lance, J.W. (1988). Effect of ergotamine on the spinal cord processing of sensory information from the cranial vasculature. *Society for Neuroscience Abstracts*, **14**, 695.

Lance, J.W., Adams, R.W., and Lambert, G.A. (1986). Bulbocortical pathways and their possible relevance to migraine and epilepsy. *Functional Neurology*, **1**, 357–61.

Perrin, V.L. (1985). Clinical pharmacokinetics of ergotamine in migraine and cluster headache. *Clinical Pharmacokinetics*, **10**, 334–52.

Saxena, P.R. and de Vlaam-Schluter, G.M. (1974). Role of some biogenic substances in migraine and relevant mechanism in antimigraine action of ergotamine. Studies in an animal experimental model for migraine. *Headache*, **13**, 142–63.

Schon, F., Thomas, D.T., Jewkes, D.A., Ghatei, M.A., Muldery, P.K., and Bloom, S.R. (1987). Failure to detect plasma neuropeptide release during trigeminal thermocoagulation. *Journal of Neurology, Neurosurgery and Psychiatry*, **50**, 642–3.

4. Genetic epidemiology of migraine

Kathleen R. Merikangas

Introduction

The hereditary nature of migraine has been reported consistently since it was first noted by S.A. Tissot in the 18th century. Indeed, the association between migraine and family history was believed to be so strong that it was included as a criterion for diagnosing migraine in the definition adopted by the Ad Hoc Committee on the classification of headache, in 1962. The most recent catalogue of Mendelian diseases in humans lists migraine as an autosomal dominant condition. Nevertheless, both the role of genetic factors in the pathogenesis of migraine and its mode of inheritance continue to be elusive.

Family history of migraine

More than 30 studies have described a positive family history among patients with migraine, with a range of 10–92 per cent of patients reporting such a family history. However, there are only seven controlled studies from which the relative magnitude of the increase in the proportion of probands with a positive history may be assessed (Ely 1930; Lennox 1941; Ask-Upmark 1953; Childs and Sweetnam 1961; Bille 1962; Waters 1971; Couch *et al.* 1986). The results of these studies are presented in Table 4.1. The relative risk, when one compares the proportion of probands with a positive family history of migraine to that among the controls, ranged from 1.4 to 13.1, with an average of 6.2. This indicates that migraine subjects have, on average, a six-fold greater family history of migraine compared with controls.

With the exception of the study by Waters (1971), the probands in all these studies were ascertained from treatment settings and the information about a history of migraine in the relatives was collected via non-blind reports from the probands. These methods have been shown to alter dramatically the estimates of familial aggregation of human diseases. Whereas non-blind assessment or ascertainment solely from clinical samples may falsely elevate the degree of familial aggregation, the 'family history method' — as opposed to direct interviews — generally leads to a two-to-three fold underestimation of disease prevalence in relatives. Waters (1971) collected

TABLE 4.1. *Controlled family studies of migraine*

Author (year)	Number		Percentage of positive family history		Relative risk[‡]
	Probands	Controls	Probands	Controls	
Ely (1930)	104	100	71.1	17.0	4.2
Lennox (1941)	425	1000	61.0	11.0	5.5
Childs and Sweetnam (1961)	104	103	36.5	5.8	6.3
Bille (1962)	73	73	58.0	13.0	4.5
Waters (1971)	75	40	10.0	7.0	1.4
Couch et al. (1986)	730	300	34.0*	2.6	13.1
			13.9[†]	1.6	8.6

*Mothers; [†]Fathers; [‡]Average relative risk is 6.2.

TABLE 4.2. *Twin studies of migraine*

Author (year)	Monozygotic		Dizygotic		Heritability*
	No. of pairs	%Concordance	No. of pairs	%Concordance	
Spaich and Ostertag (1936)	10	60	5	40	0.40
Harvald and Hauge (1956)	24	33	60	5	0.56
Ziegler (1975)	9	22	14	7	0.30
Lucas (1977)	86	26	75	13	0.26

*Average heritability is 0.38.

information about a family history of migraine from subjects in an epidemiological survey of Wales. Relatives were interviewed directly, with the interviewer remaining blind to the presence of migraine in the proband. However, the use of one-year prevalence rates of migraine, both in the probands and in the relatives, limits the utility of the data for investigating familial transmission of a condition whose expression varies greatly with age.

Twin studies of migraine

There are only four twin studies of migraine, all of which reveal an increase in the concordance rates among monozygotic as compared to dizygotic twins (Table 4.2). The monozygotic concordance rates range from 22 to 60 per cent, and the dizygotic twin concordance rates range from 5 to 40 per cent. The heritability, the degree of variance that can be attributed to genetic factors, computed from these figures ranges from 0.26 to 0.56. These results indicate that genetic factors play a major role in the transmission of migraine.

Lucas's (1977) study found lower concordance for classical than for common migraine, and little evidence for shared symptom patterns among concordant monozygotic twins. The four symptoms that tended to have a high heritability were the presence of a neurologic prodrome, the 'throbbing' and 'steady' nature of the headaches, and gastrointestinal symptoms. No difference was found in the concordance rates between male and female pairs. Moreover, there was a direct relationship between the degree of concordance within twin pairs and the family history of migraine.

Differential family history of migraine has been found according to both the age at onset and the sex of the proband. A strong inverse relationship has been found between the age at onset of migraine and a positive family history (Barolin and Sperlich 1969; Steiner et al. 1980; Baier 1985; DeVoto et al. 1986). The childhood onset of migraine is related to a substantial increase in the familial aggregation of migraine, with a two-to-three-fold increase in the proportion of families with a history of migraine compared to people with adult onset of migraine.

There is a three-fold increase in the proportion of probands who report a positive family history among maternal relatives as compared to paternal relatives (Mobius 1894; Bille 1962; Dalsgaard-Nielsen 1965; Barolin and Sperlich 1969; Couch et al. 1986). However, Couch et al. (1986) did not find an increase in the proportion of probands with maternal transmission among male probands; nearly equal proportions of positive family history in the maternal and paternal ascendants of male probands were found. Dalsgaard-Nielsen (1965) also found an interesting sex difference in family history. Whereas the mother was always the affected relative on the maternal side, only 16 per cent of the fathers were the affected relative when migraine was present on the paternal side. Furthermore, all these studies had nearly three times as many female migraine subjects as male subjects. These findings suggest that there may be ascertainment bias with respect to under-reporting of migraine in male relatives by female probands, or that males may either transmit migraine without expressing it themselves (that is, non-penetrance) or that males express it, but with variations in symptoms.

Bilineal inheritance has also been associated with an increased risk of migraine in offspring (Buchanan 1920; Allan 1928; Bassoe 1933; Devoto et al. 1986; Baier 1986). When both parents had migraine, the average rate of migraine in their offspring was 78 per cent. In contrast, if only one or neither parent had migraine, the rates in offspring were 44 and 14 per cent, respectively. However, the presence of assortative mating for migraine cannot be determined because the proportion of spouses concordant and discordant for migraine was not presented in any of the above-cited family studies. Current epidemiological data suggest that approximately two per cent of couples should exhibit concordance for migraine by chance alone.

Factors that impede genetic studies of migraine

There are numerous factors that have hampered genetic studies of migraine.

Definition

The lack of a valid definition of migraine and of reliable, standardized methods for eliciting the necessary criteria for the diagnosis have been a major impediment to the conduct of family and genetic studies of migraine. The studies already cited exhibit extreme variation in the definitions used to diagnose migraine, and some provide no definition of migraine at all in the published report. The issue of the definition is less problematical in studies that use a control group that is diagnosed in the same way as the proband group. Many of the family studies have included a positive family history as a diagnostic criterion for migraine in their patient samples, and have then investigated family history as an outcome as well.

Lack of a diagnostic test

The lack of an objective diagnostic test with which a presumptive diagnosis of migraine can be made has complicated not only the genetic studies of migraine but also studies of most other aspects of migraine. The lack of a one-to-one correspondence between the genotype and phenotype — as reflected in such phenomena as variable expressivity, penetrance, genetic heterogeneity, pleiotropy, and gene–environment interactions — tends to be the rule rather than the exception for most disorders for which the role of genetic factors has been well-established. It is not unexpected, then, that these factors will also characterize the expression of genetic factors in the pathogenesis of migraine.

Ascertainment bias

The vast majority of studies that have investigated the role of familial transmission of migraine have included patients who were selected from treatment settings. This has resulted in an over-representation of females, and of people who may not be representative of the 50 per cent of migraineurs in the general population who do not seek treatment for migraine *per se*. There is only one family study in which probands were selected from the general population (Waters 1971). Unfortunately, as noted above, the use by Waters of one-year prevalence rates of migraine in probands and relatives precluded the determination of accurate familial recurrence risks.

High population prevalence

Estimates of the lifetime prevalence of migraine from epidemiological studies range from four to 29 per cent of the population. Even the lower rates within this range are quite high when compared to the rates of diseases traditionally in the domain of classical genetics. As the prevalence of a disease within the population increases, detection of patterns of genetic transmission becomes more difficult owing to the increased probability that the disease will be present within pedigrees by chance. Moreover, the probability of bilineal transmission, which obscures patterns of disease transmission, is directly related to gene frequency in the population.

Sex- and age-dependent expression

There are important differences in the patterns of expression of migraine across the life span, particularly among females. Because cross-sectional assessment of families is used, relatives of different ages may express differently the underlying factors involved in the pathogenesis of migraine. This difference may complicate the specification of affectional status in family studies. Prospective studies of symptom expression by sex and age are therefore indicated, to help clarify who should be characterized as affected, in family and genetic studies. Several genetic models have been proposed as the mode of transmission of migraine. The mode of transmission most compatible with an increased risk in female relatives, X-linked transmission, has been excluded because of the high frequency of male-to-male transmission of migraine. Other postulated modes of transmission of migraine include: autosomal dominant transmission (Allan 1928; Dalsgaard-Nielsen 1965; Barolin 1970; Raskin and Appenzeller 1982); autosomal recessive transmission (Goodell *et al.* 1954); polygenic transmission (Dalsgaard-Nielsen 1965; Barolin and Sperlich 1969; Baier 1985); and lack of fit to any classical model (Pratt 1968; Devoto *et al.* 1986). This variability in the findings indicates that migraine is truly a complex human disorder because it is highly prevalent in the population and exhibits no clear-cut mode of transmission.

Maternal transmission of migraine

One of the most important clues about the role of genetic factors in the transmission of migraine is the consistently observed increase in a positive family history deriving from the maternal rather than paternal side (Table 4.3). The following predictions derive from conventional genetic models if the sex difference in a trait (that is, the increased prevalence in women) is involved in transmission of the trait:

1. the population prevalence should be lower in males;
2. the prevalence should be greater in female than in male relatives;
3. the prevalence of migraine should be equal in maternal as compared to paternal relatives;
4. the risk in first- and second-degree relatives of male probands should be greater than that in female probands.

TABLE 4.3. *Comparison of maternal and paternal transmission of migraine*

Author (year)	Percentage with positive family history	
	Maternal	Paternal
Mobius (1894)	62	18
Bille (1962)	73	21
Dalsgaard-Nielsen (1965)	70	19
Barolin and Sperlich (1969)	52	10
Couch *et al.* (1986)	40*	15
	24[†]	21

*Females; [†]Males.

An alternative explanation to the conventional genetic models for the transmission of migraine is provided by maternal inheritance. This form of inheritance may result from transmissible agents, such as viruses, pre- or perinatal complications, or mitochondrial inheritance. Alternatively, patterns consistent with maternal inheritance may result from artefacts such as sex bias in ascertainment, reporting bias by sex, non-paternity, or selective fertility. Whereas selective fertility and non-paternity do not appear to explain the vast majority of family studies of migraine, there is substantial evidence for sex biases related to ascertainment, or reporting, or both.

The expectations that derive from the maternal transmission model are as follows.

1. Offspring of female probands should have increased rates over those of male probands.
2. Siblings and parents of both male and female probands should exhibit equal prevalence rates.
3. The prevalence of migraine should be equal among brothers and sisters or between sons and daughters.
4. Fathers should have lower rates than mothers.
5. Maternal relatives should have higher rates than paternal relatives.
6. The population prevalence of migraine should be equal in males and females (Ottman *et al.* 1985).

Data from Baier's family study of migraine (1985), the only study that presented recurrence risks in relatives separately by sex of the proband and according to generation of the relative (that is, parent, sibling, or offspring), do not suggest that the sex of the proband is involved in the transmission of migraine according to conventional polygenic or single major locus genetic models. This model is excluded for two reasons: the prevalence of migraine is *not* greater among the relatives of males, the less frequently affected sex, and maternal and paternal relatives do not have equal rates of migraine. These findings do not suggest that the transmission of migraine is X-linked or that the sex of the affected person is related to transmission of the disorder. Therefore, some other factor unique to women, such as endocrine factors, may lead to sex differences in the expression of the same underlying genetic factors in males and females.

Similarly, the data are inconsistent with the maternal transmission model, because brothers and sisters of migraineurs do not have equal rates of migraine, and the population incidence is not equal in males and females. Thus, the currently available data do not suggest that sex differences are involved in the transmission of migraine.

Although the above results suggest a strong degree of heritability, the specific mechanism involved in the transmission of migraine is unknown. Instability of the autonomic vasculature, of an enzyme system, or of psychic constitution have all been suggested as the underlying heritable factors in migraine (Dalsgaard-Nielsen 1965). The application of family studies to the investigation of migraine may help to discriminate between underlying transmissible factors and environmental precipitants of migraine.

Recommendations for further studies

Although some of the parameters associated with familial transmission have been defined, the role of genetic factors in migraine is still an enigma. Future studies should proceed at three levels: the phenotype, the genotype, and the pathway between the two. Using the conceptual framework of genetic epidemiological study, which systematically controls for the genotype while varying the phenotype or the converse, provides a powerful tool with which to study the validity of diagnostic definitions and the patterns of transmission of migraine. To date, no published family study has used a control group, blind, direct interviews of relatives, and specification of the recurrence risks in relatives of each class.

At the level of the genotype, the techniques of molecular genetics should be applied cautiously in the study of families with migraine. Although linkage studies may provide the key to identification of the phenotype of migraine, they are also the most difficult method to apply because of the problems of high population prevalence, bilineal transmission, and lack of knowledge about the mode of inheritance and the penetrance for statistical linkage analysis. There is not a single example of the successful application of linkage studies to a complex human disorder to date.

Genetic methods may also be applied to studying the complex pathway between the genotype and the phenotype. These might include animal breeding experiments on traits, including photosensitivity and motion sickness, which may be associated with migraine; studies of the activity of the central nervous system within families rather than within heterogeneous groups of patients; and challenge studies to detect subthreshold cases of migraine within families.

These three levels of study could ultimately lead to more accurate specification of both the disease and the variation in its expression, to markers with which to identify vulnerability and, ultimately, to the underlying pathogenesis of the disease.

Summary

Migraine is a complex human disorder that is familial, common, and exhibits no clear-cut mode of inheritance. About 30 to 50 per cent of the variance in migraine can be attributed to genetic factors, which suggests that non-transmissible factors explain at least half of the variance as well. Familial aggregation of migraine is greater among probands with an early age of onset and a bilineal family history of migraine. Although migraine is more common in females, and more frequently transmitted on the maternal side of the family, this difference cannot be explained by transmissible genetic factors, nor by maternal transmission. However, the specific factors that may be inherited in migraine are not known.

Knowledge about the role of genetic factors in migraine has been impeded by the lack of a valid definition of the syndrome, the lack of standardized methods for ascertaining symptomatic criteria, the high prevalence of migraine within the population, and the sex- and age-specific expression of the syndrome. Not a single published family study of migraine has incorporated the usual methodological standards for the conduct of family studies. These standards include blind diagnosis of spouses and relatives via a direct interview, consideration of ascertainment bias in the selection of probands, inclusion of a control group of probands without migraine, and the use of analytical methods that yield age-corrected recurrence risks amongst the relatives.

Using the conceptual framework of genetic epidemiology can provide a powerful method for validating the diagnostic criteria for migraine, and allows both transmissible and non-transmissible causes to be specified.

Acknowledgements

This work was supported in part by the United States Public Health Service, Alcohol, Drug Abuse, and Mental Health Administration grants AA07080, DA50348, and Research Scientist Development Award MH00499.

References

'Ad Hoc' committee of the National Institute of Neurological Disease and Blindness: classification of headache. (1962). *Archives of Neurology*, **6**, 173–6.

Allan, W. (1928). The inheritance of migraine. *Archives of Internal Medicine*, **13**, 590–9.

Ask-Upmark, E. (1953). Inverted nipples and migraine. *Acta Medica Scandinavica*, **167**, 191–7.

Baier, W.K. (1985). Genetics of migraine and migraine accompagnee: a study of eighty-one children and their families. *Neuropediatrics*, **16**, 84–91.

Barolin, G.S. (1970). In *Background to migraine*, (ed. A.L. Cochrane), pp. 28–37. Heinemann, London.

Barolin, G.S. and Sperlich, D. (1969). Migranefamilien. *Fortschritte der Neurologie-Psychiatrie und ihrer Grenzgebiete*, **37**, 521–44.

Bassoe, P. (1933). Migraine. *Journal of the American Medical Association*, **101**, 599–605.

Bille, B. (1962). Migraine in schoolchildren. *Acta Paediatrica*, **51**, Suppl. 136, 1–151.

Buchanan, J.A. (1920). The mendelianism of migraine. *Medical Research*, **98**, 45–7.

Childs, A.J. and Sweetnam, M.T. (1961). A study of 104 cases of migraine. *British Journal of Industrial Medicine*, **18**, 234–6.

Couch, J.R., Bearss, C., and Verhulst, S. (1986). Importance of maternal heredity in the etiology of migraine. *Neurology*, **36**, Suppl., 99.

Dalsgaard-Nielsen, T. (1965). Migraine and heredity. *Acta Neurologica Scandinavica*, **41**, 287–300.

Devoto, M., Lozito, A., Staffa, G., D'Allessandro, R., Sacquengna, T., and Romeo, G. (1986). Segregation analysis of migraine in 128 families. *Cephalalgia*, **6**, 101–5.

Ely, F.A. (1930). The migraine–epilepsy syndrome. *Archives of Neurology and Psychiatry*, **24**, 943.

Goodell, H., Lewontin, R., and Wolff, H. (1954). The familial occurrence of migraine headache: a study of heredity. *Archives of Neurology and Psychiatry*, **72**, 325–34.

Harvald, B. and Hauge, M. (1956). A catamnestic investigation of Danish twins: a preliminary report. *Danish Medical Bulletin*, **3**, 150–8.

Lennox, W.G. (1941). *Science and seizures: new light on epilepsy and migraine*. Harper, New York.

Lucas, R.N. (1977). Migraine in twins. *Journal of Psychosomatic Research*, **20**, 147–56.

Mobius, P.J. (1894). *Die Migraine*, pp. 14–7. Holder, Vienna.

Ottman, R., Hauser, W.A., and Susser, M. (1985). Genetic and maternal influences on susceptibility to seizures: an analytic review. *American Journal of Epidemiology*, **122**, 923–9.

Pratt, R.T.C. (1968). *The genetics of neurological disorders*, p. 122. London University Press, London.

Raskin, N. and Appenzeller, O. (1982). *Headache*, p. 36. Fischer, Stuttgart.

Spaich, D. and Ostertag, M. (1936). Untersuchungen uber allergische erkranitungen beizwillingen. *Zeitschrift fuer Menschliche Vererbungs- und Konstitutionslehre*, **19**, 730 (cited in Lucas 1977).

Steiner, T.J., Guha, P., Capildeo, R., and Rose, F.C. (1980). Migraine in patients attending a migraine clinic: an analysis by computer of age, sex, and family history. *Headache*, **20**, 190–5.

Waters, W.E. (1971). Migraine: intelligence, social class, and familial prevalence. *British Medical Journal*, **2**, 77–81.

Ziegler, D.K. (1975). The epidemiology and genetics of migraine. *Research and Clinical Studies in Headache*, **5**, 21–33.

Discussion

BLAU: Patients often say they do not have migraine. Yet, if a further history is taken, some of these patients will give a typical description: headaches occurring once or twice a year; having to retire to bed and draw the curtains; and vomiting. But because they 'do not get the flashing lights', they fail to recognize that they suffer from migraine. Here then is one cause of *under*estimating migraine. However, in population surveys, migraine is easily *over*estimated: Waters (1971) gave a prevalence figure of 23 per cent, which seems unduly high, and the basic validation of his data (Waters and O'Connor 1970) may have been faulty; a figure of 10 per cent seems much more likely (for review see Linet and Stewart 1987). Regarding the genetics of migraine, each person has enough relatives for a positive family history to be very easily obtained, as you say. Indeed, one of Vahlquist's (1955) criteria for delineating migraine includes a positive family history, so one is immediately confronted with a circuitous argument.

MERIKANGAS: Yes, and such ascertainment bias would automatically yield biased segregation ratios compatible with autosomal dominant inheritance because at least two or more family members would be affected.

COPPEN: How should one ascertain a case of migraine, by current standards? Are there any generally accepted ways of doing this? We are aware of the sort of self-rating approach that W.E. Waters developed. Sometimes 'raters', without a medical background, may be carrying out the investigation. In psychiatry, we have had to face this question and have now developed research diagnostic criteria, which are generally accepted. We use ratings of severity, the Hamilton rating scale, and so on. Yet for migraine we seem to have had no universally accepted means of ascertaining cases.

OLESEN: The results of our international committee were recently published, after about three years' work (Headache Classification Committee of the International Headache Society 1988). Our new classification is hierarchical, and uses up to four digits. It also provides operational diagnostic criteria for all headache disorders.

COPPEN: This classification should certainly prove to be a key factor in the development of genetic studies of migraine.

References

Headache Classification Committee of the International Headache Society. (Jes Olesen, chairman). (1988). Classification and diagnostic criteria for headache disorders, cranial neuralgias and facial pain. *Cephalalgia*, **8**, Suppl. 7, 1–96.

Linet, S.L. and Stewart, W.F. (1987). The epidemiology of migraine headache. In *Migraine: clinical, therapeutic, conceptual and research aspects*, (ed. J.N. Blau), pp. 451–77. Chapman and Hall, London.

Waters, W.E. (1971). Migraine: intelligence, social class, and familial prevalence. *British Medical Journal*, **2**, 77–81.

Waters, W.E. and O'Connor, P.J. (1970). Clinical validation of a headache question-naire. In *Background to migraine*, (ed. A.L. Cochrane), pp. 1–8. Heinemann Medical, London.

Vahlquist, B. (1955). Migraine in children. *International Archives of Allergy and Applied Immunology*, **7**, 348–55.

5. A possible role of endothelial vasorelaxants in the pathogenesis of migraine

Ryszard J. Gryglewski and John R. Vane

There have been many attempts to explain the pathophysiological mechanism of migraine — for example, the platelet theory (Hanington *et al.* 1981), the biogenic amine theory (Sandler *et al.* 1974; Anthony and Hinterberger 1975), the vascular (Meyer *et al.* 1985), the vaso-neurogenic (Moskowitz 1984; Fozard 1985), or the neural (Pearce 1984) theories. There is still general agreement that the migraine aura is associated with a regional vasoconstriction, whilst the headache phase is accompanied by a localized vasodilatation of the cranial arteries. It is also a generally held concept that 5-hydroxytryptamine (5-HT, serotonin) is somehow involved in the pathogenesis of the disease.

We hypothesize that the vasodilator phase of migraine is mediated by two powerful vasorelaxants, which are generated by the endothelium, namely prostacyclin (PGI_2; Moncada *et al.* 1976) and the 'endothelium-derived relaxing factor' (EDRF; Furchgott and Zawadzki 1980) which has been identified as nitric oxide (NO) (Palmer *et al.* 1987; Ignarro *et al.* 1987). PGI_2 and EDRF are chemically and biologically unstable and, therefore, they are good candidates for local vasorelaxants in migraine and cluster headache. PGI_2 and EDRF through cAMP and cGMP, respectively, exert not only vasodilatation but also a platelet-suppressive action (Vane *et al.* 1987). Therefore, their release in cranial arteries that are affected with migrainous 'sterile' inflammation (Fozard 1985) may be considered as an excessive defense against localized thrombogenesis in these blood vessels.

Indeed, vasodilatation that is produced by the systemic administration of PGI_2 (Szczeklik *et al.* 1978), or of its stable analogue — Iloprost (Gryglewski and Stock 1987), or of nitroglycerine (GTN, a prodrug for NO) appears mainly in the cranial region. Moreover, high doses of PGE_1 (Carlson *et al.* 1968), PGI_2 (Szczeklik *et al.* 1978), or GTN (Drummond and Anthony 1985) cause headache.

The overproduction of PGI_2 by the endothelium of cranial arteries has already been suggested as one of the fundamental abnormalities in migraine (Meyer *et al.* 1985). The significance of arterial prostaglandins in migraine has been recognized (Parantainen *et al.* 1985), and migraine is treated with a number of cyclo-oxygenase inhibitors which suppress vascular biosynthesis of PGI_2 and other prostaglandins (Peatfield *et al.* 1986). There are good reasons to propose that the endothelial release of EDRF might be equally relevant for the development of migraine. Firstly, as already noted, the vasodilatation of cranial blood vessels and the migraine-like symptoms are produced both by PGI_2 and by organic nitrates which mimic the effects of EDRF on vascular smooth muscle. Secondly, the stimulation of the endothelial purinergic and peptidergic receptors is followed by a coupled release of PGI_2 and EDRF (de Nucci *et al.* 1988*a*). Finally, in certain types of blood vessels, 5-HT which seems to be intimately involved in the pathogenesis of migraine (Fozard 1985) triggers the endothelial production of both PGI_2 (Kokkas and Boeynaems 1988) and EDRF (Cocks and Angus 1983; Stewart *et al.* 1987; Yamamoto *et al.* 1987), thus bringing about vasorelaxation.

The influence of 5-HT on blood vessels is complex; it depends on the species, the vascular region in question, the initial arterial tone, the pathophysiological state of the blood vessel, and on interactions with other vascular mediators. In most animal species, an intravenous injection of 5-HT results in a triphasic response. The initial, transient hypotension reflects the Bezold–Jarisch reflex which is mediated by $5-HT_3$ receptors on afferent vagal fibres in the right heart. The subsequent pressor response is mediated by $5-HT_2$ receptors on vascular smooth muscle. The long-lasting hypotension is due to excitation of endothelial $5-HT_1$ receptors (van Zwieten 1987) most probably resulting in a coupled release of PGI_2 and EDRF (Furchgott *et al.* 1984; Vane *et al.* 1987).

During the migraine or cluster headache, 5-HT may derive from excited vascular serotonergic nerves that originate in the nuclei raphé (MacKenzie and Scatton 1987), or from activated platelets (Hanington *et al.* 1981) with a deficient monoamine oxidase (Sandler *et al.* 1974), or from impaired mechanisms for uptake, storage, and release of 5-HT (Lingjaerde and Monstad 1986; Pletscher 1987). The balance between the vasodilator and vasoconstrictor actions of 5-HT on isolated, perfused, resistance blood vessels depends on the ratio of potencies of 5-HT to evoke $5-HT_2$-mediated stimulation of vascular smooth muscle or $5-HT_1$-mediated release of EDRF from the endothelium (Stewart *et al.* 1987). *In vivo*, this balance is even more complex; on the vasoconstrictor side, there are both $5-HT_2$-mediated sensitization to other endogenous spasmogens and a presynaptic release of noradrenaline whereas, on the vasodilator side, there are also $5-HT_1$-mediated release of PGI_2 from intima, media, and leukocytes, a direct inhibition of vascular smooth muscle, and an inhibition of adrenergic transmission at the presynaptic level (Vanhoutte 1987).

Inhalation of 100 per cent oxygen may interrupt an attack of migraine (Drummond and Anthony 1985). A plausible explanation for the mechanism of oxygen therapy is that at high P_{O_2} the monovalent reduction of oxygen occurs; small amounts of superoxide anions are generated and they destroy EDRF (Gryglewski *et al.* 1986). If the overproduction of EDRF were responsible for the pulsating pain in the vasodilator phase of migraine then the removal of EDRF by superoxide anions might be expected to bring relief. *In vivo*, topical administration of acetylcholine generates EDRF and dilates canine cerebral arterioles. A short period of noradrenaline-induced hypertension in these animals is associated with the production of super-oxide anions within the cerebral arterial walls. Therefore, after the infusion of noradrenaline a topical application of acetylcholine does not generate EDRF, and that is why, instead of vasodilatation, a vasoconstriction occurs (Wei *et al.* 1985). These observations suggest cautious clinical trials with scavengers or inhibitors of EDRF such as dithiothreitol, BW 755C, pheni-done, or even haemoglobin (Moncada *et al.* 1986) for the treatment of migraine.

A total removal of PGI_2 and EDRF from the migraine syndrome may be dangerous. Pain relief may be replaced by intra-arterial thrombosis. The therapeutic effects in migraine of antagonists at $5\text{-}HT_2$ receptors, such as pizotifen or methysergide (Peatfield *et al.* 1986), may partially depend on the blockade by these drugs of endothelial $5\text{-}HT_1$ and histamine H_1 recep-tors, the stimulation of which is responsible for the release of EDRF (Fur-chgott *et al.* 1984), with consequent vasodilatation (Gross *et al.* 1981). Selective antagonists at $5\text{-}HT_1$ receptors are not in clinical use, but some β-adrenolytic drugs such as propranolol or pindolol may act therapeutically in migraine (Peatfield *et al.* 1986), perhaps by blocking endothelial $5\text{-}HT_1$ receptors. As early as in 1971 we reported on the anti-5-HT action of pindolol (Gryglewski and Kulig 1971).

Apart from 5-HT, other mediators are released in migraine, and they may bring about vasodilatation through a coupled endothelial release of EDRF and PGI_2. First of all, cerebral, meningeal, and extracranial arteries are innervated not only by serotonergic nerves but also by cholinergic fibres of the facial nerve, substance P-ergic fibres of the trigeminal nerve, and by adrenergic fibres from the superior cervical stellate ganglia (MacKenzie and Scatton 1987). Acetylcholine and substance P are among the most potent releasers of EDRF (Furchgott *et al.* 1984) and an excessive excitation of these nerves is claimed to be a typical feature of migraine (Pearce 1984). Noradrenaline is also an EDRF releaser from the arterial endothelium (Cocks and Angus 1983), and the release of prostaglandins (probably PGI_2) may be responsible for the acute vascular tolerance to noradrenaline *in vivo* (Gryglewski and Ocetkiewicz 1974). Secondly, in the plethora of mediators that are released at a site of 'sterile' inflammation of the arterial wall during migraine there are also found ADP and ATP (Rydzewski and Wachowicz 1978) released from platelets, as well as bradykinin generated from tissue or plasma kininogen (Fig. 5.1). Again, ADP, ATP, and bradykinin are relea-sers of EDRF and of PGI_2 (Furchgott *et al.* 1984; de Nucci *et al.* 1988).

Recently, Yanagisawa *et al.* (1988) have isolated from endothelial cells a

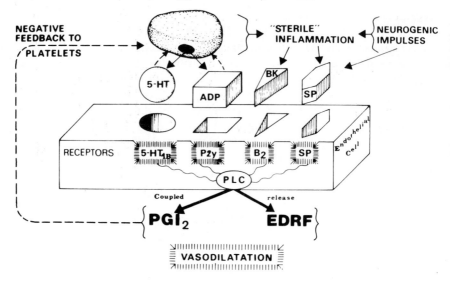

FIG. 5.1. A hypothetical mechanism for the coupled release of prostacyclin (PGI$_2$) and endothelium-derived relaxing factor (EDRF) from the arterial endothelium during the headache phase of migraine. Mediators such as serotonin (5-HT), adenosine diphosphate (ADP), bradykinin (BK) and substance P (SP) not only evoke local 'sterile' inflammation of the arterial wall but also, through stimulation of appropriate receptors (5-HT$_{1B}$, P$_{2y}$, SP), activate phospholipase C in the endothelium. Breakdown products of inositolphosphatides induce a coupled release of PGI$_2$ and EDRF — two powerful vasorelaxants which are also platelet suppressants. Pulsating pain from inflamed, vasodilated segments of the cranial artery is the cost of a synergistic antithrombotic action of PGI$_2$ and EDRF.

vasoconstrictor peptide which they named endothelin. Endothelin is also a potent releaser of PGI$_2$ and EDRF (de Nucci *et al.* 1988*b*) and, therefore, *in vivo* it may play the double role of a regional vasoconstrictor and vasodilator. Further studies on endothelin might be relevant to understanding the role of the vascular endothelium in the pathogenesis of migraine.

In conclusion, it is proposed that mediators which appear locally during the headache phase of migraine not only induce 'sterile' inflammation of the vascular wall, and not only mediate or modulate pain but also stimulate endothelial receptors which trigger a coupled release of two vasorelaxants and platelet-suppressants — EDRF and PGI$_2$. Their combined action brings about painful, pulsating vasodilatation of cranial arteries but, at the same time, prevents a thrombotic obliteration of these arteries. Therefore, a rational therapeutic approach to migraine should not aim at a total removal of PGI$_2$ and EDRF but, rather, at a selective antagonism of their vasorelaxant action.

Acknowledgement

The William Harvey Research Institute is supported by a grant from Glaxo Group Research Limited.

References

Anthony, M. and Hinterberger, H. (1975). Amine turnover in migraine. *Proceedings of the Australian Association of Neurology*, **12**, 43–7.

Carlson, L.A., Ekeland, L.G., and Oro, L. (1968). Clinical and metabolic effects of different doses of prostaglandin E_1 in man. *Acta Medica Scandinavica*, **183**, 423–30.

Cocks, T.M. and Angus, J.A. (1983). Endothelium-dependent relaxation of coronary arteries by noradrenaline and serotonin. *Nature*, **305**, 627–30.

de Nucci, G., Gryglewski, R.J., Warner, T.D., and Vane, J.R. (1988a). Receptor-mediated release of endothelium-derived relaxing factor (EDRF) and prostacyclin from bovine aortic endothelial cells is coupled. *Proceedings of the National Academy of Sciences USA* , 85, 2334–8.

de Nucci, G., Thomas, R., D'Orleans-Juste, P., Antunes, E., Walder, C., Warner, T., and Vane, J.R. (1988b). The pressor effects of circulating endothelin are limited by its removal in the pulmonary circulation and by the release of prostacyclin and EDRF. *Proceedings of the National Academy of Sciences USA* **85**, 9797–800.

Drummond, P.D. and Anthony, M. (1985). Extracranial vascular responses to sublingual nitroglycerin and oxygen inhalation in cluster headache patients. *Headache*, **25**, 70–4.

Fozard, J.R. (1985). 5-Hydroxytryptamine in the pathophysiology of migraine. In *Vascular neuroeffector mechanisms*, (ed. J.A. Bevan), pp. 321–8. Elsevier, Amsterdam.

Furchgott, R.F. and Zawadzki, J.V. (1980). The obligatory role of endothelial cells in the relaxation of arterial smooth muscle by acetylcholine. *Nature*, **288**, 373–6

Furchgott, R.F., Cherry, P.D., Zawadzki, J.V., and Jothianandan, D. (1984). Endothelial cells as mediators of vasodilation of arteries. *Journal of Cardiovascular Pharmacology*, **6**, S336–S343.

Gross, P.M., Harper, A.M., and Teasdale, G.M. (1981). Cerebral circulation and histamine: 1. Participation of vascular H_1 and H_2 receptors in vasodilatory responses to carotid artery infusions. *Journal of Cerebral Blood Flow and Metabolism*, **1**, 97–108.

Gryglewski, R.J. and Kulig, H. (1971). Beta-adrenolytic, sympathomimetic and antiserotonin properties of LB 46. *Dissertationes Pharmaceuticae et Pharmacologicae*, **23**, 481–93.

Gryglewski, R.J. and Ocetkiewicz, A. (1974). A release of prostaglandins may be responsible for acute tolerance to norepinephrine infusions. *Prostaglandins*, **8**, 31–42.

Gryglewski, R.J. and Stock, G. (1987). *Prostacyclin and its stable analogue Iloprost*. Springer, Berlin.

Gryglewski, R.J., Palmer, R.M.J., and Moncada, S. (1986). Superoxide anion is involved in the breakdown of endothelium-derived vascular relaxing factor. *Nature*, **320**, 454–6.

Hanington, E., Jones, R.J., Ameess, J.A.L., and Wachowicz, B. (1981). Migraine — a platelet disorder. *Lancet*, **ii**, 721–3.

Ignarro, L.J., Byrns, R.E., Buga, G.M., and Wood, K.S. (1987). Endothelium-derived relaxing factor from pulmonary artery and vein possesses pharmacologic and chemical properties identical of those of nitric oxide radical. *Circulation Research*, **61**, 866–79.

Kokkas, B. and Boeynaems, J.M. (1988). Release of prostacyclin from the dog saphenous vein by 5-hydroxytryptamine. *European Journal of Pharmacology*, **147**, 473–6.

Lingjaerde, O. and Monstad, P. (1986). The uptake, storage and efflux of serotonin in platelets from migraine patients. *Cephalalgia*, **6**, 135–9.

MacKenzie, E.T. and Scatton, B. (1987). Cerebral circulatory and metabolic effects of perivascular neurotransmitters. *CRC Critical Reviews in Clinical Neurobiology*, **2**, 419.

Meyer, J.S., Nance, M., Walker, M., Zetusky, W.J., and Dowell, R.E. (1985). Migraine and cluster headache treatment with calcium antagonists supports a vascular pathogenesis. *Headache*, **25**, 358–67.

Moncada, S., Gryglewski, R.J., Bunting, S., and Vane, J.R. (1976). An enzyme isolated from arteries transforms prostaglandin endoperoxides to an unstable substance that inhibits platelet aggregation. *Nature*, **263**, 663–5.

Moncada, S., Palmer, R.M.J., and Gryglewski, R.J. (1986). Mechanism of action of some inhibitors of endothelium-derived relaxing factor. *Proceedings of the National Academy of Sciences USA*, **83**, 9164–8.

Moskowitz, M.A. (1984). The neurobiology of vascular head pain. *Annals of Neurology*, **16**, 157–68.

Palmer, R.M.J., Ferridge, A.G., and Moncada, S. (1987). Nitric oxide release accounts for the biological activity of endothelium-derived relaxing factor. *Nature*, **327**, 524–6.

Parantainen, J., Vapaatalo, H., and Hokkanen, E. (1985). Relevance of prostaglandins in migraine. *Cephalalgia*, Suppl., **2**, 93–7.

Pearce, J.M.S. (1984). Migraine: a cerebral disorder. *Lancet*, **ii**, 86–9.

Peatfield, R.C., Fozard, J.R., and Rose, F.C. (1986). Drug treatment of migraine. In *Handbook of Clinical Neurology*, Vol. 4. (ed. F.C. Rose), pp. 173–216. Elsevier, Amsterdam.

Pletscher, A. (1987). The 5-hydroxytryptamine system of blood platelets: physiology and pathophysiology. *International Journal of Cardiology*, **14**, 177–88.

Rydzewski, W. and Wachowicz, B. (1978). Adenine nucleotides in platelets in and between migraine attacks. In *Current concepts of migraine research*, (ed. R. Greene), pp. 153–8. Raven, New York.

Sandler, M., Youdim, M.B.H., and Hanington, E. (1974). A phenylethylamine oxidising defect in migraine. *Nature*, **250**, 335–7.

Stewart, D.J., Holtz, J., Pohl, U., and Bassenge, E. (1987). Balance between endothelium-mediated dilating and direct constricting actions of serotonin on resistance vessels in the isolated rabbit heart. *European Journal of Pharmacology*, **143**, 131–4.

Szczeklik, A., Gryglewski, R.J., Nizankowski, R., Musia, J., Pieton, R., and Mruk, J. (1978). Circulatory and antiplatelet effects of intravenous prostacyclin in healthy men. *Pharmacological Research Communications*, **10**, 545–56.

Vane, J.R., Gryglewski, R.J., and Botting, R.M. (1987). The endothelial cell as a metabolic and endocrine organ. *Trends in Pharmacological Sciences*, **8**, 491–6.

Vanhoutte, P.M. (1987). Serotonin and the vascular wall. *International Journal of Cardiology*, **14**, 189–203.

Van Zwieten, P.A. (1987). Pathophysiological relevance of serotonin. *Journal of Cardiovascular Pharmacology*, **10**, Suppl. 3, S19–S25.

Wei, E.P., Kontos, H.A., Christman, C.W., De Witt, D.S., and Povlishock, J.T. (1985). Superoxide generation and reversal of acetylcholine-induced cerebral arteriolar dilatation after acute hypertension. *Circulation Research*, **57**, 781–7.

Yamamoto, Y., Tomoike, H., Egashira, K., and Nakamura, M. (1987). Attenuation of endothelium-related relaxation and enhanced responsiveness of vascular smooth muscle to histamine in spastic coronary arterial segments from miniature pigs. *Circulation Research*, **61**, 772–8.

Yanagisawa, M. *et al.* (1988). A novel potent vasoconstrictor peptide produced by vascular endothelial cells. *Nature*, **332**, 411–5

Discussion

PEATFIELD: I infused prostacyclin into myself some years ago (Peatfield *et al.* 1981). In addition, we used prostacyclin in patients who had migraine or who were in the active phase of cluster headache. The patients went pink, and had a throbbing headache, just as I did, but I was quite unable to trigger a cluster attack in these patients. Clearly, this type of trial is artificial. Our original experiment was a development from Professor Sandler's hypothesis (Sandler 1972) that migraine was caused by the release of prostaglandins from the lungs. Although that hypothesis could not be supported, one cannot discount the concept that prostacyclin may be released at a very local level. your evidence points towards the endothelium-derived relaxing factor (EDRF; or nitric oxide) being a much more likely mediator than prostacyclin of the vasodilatation if, indeed, headache can be attributed merely to vascular factors at all.

GRYGLEWSKI: I believe that the synergism between nitric oxide (NO) — a stimulator of guanylate cyclase — and prostacyclin, which is acting via cAMP, might be of importance. EDRF (NO) and prostacyclin are representatives of endogenous vasodilators with different biochemical mechanisms of action and both may contribute to a vascular-mediated headache.

CURZON: Why did you specifically invoke a role of 5-HT$_{1B}$ sites in releasing the vasodilators?

GRYGLEWSKI: Indeed it is questionable (Vanhoutte 1987; Van Zwieten 1987); some people are in favour of 5-HT$_{1A}$ sites for triggering the release of endothelial vasodilators. I have no experience of this.

MOSKOWITZ: As well as NO, other EDRF-like materials can be found in the endothelium, such as free radicals (Kontos *et al.* 1984). Loesch and Burnstock (1988) have now shown the presence of substance P itself within a proportion of endothelial cells. In thinking about your concept of vasodilatation and pain, it seems to me that the neuronal release must be the starting point for the pain. The vasodilatation that results is a secondary phenomenon mediated by the depolarization of the sensory nerve which, in itself, is the painful event. Many people here subscribe to the notion that vasodilatation equals pain, but can anybody give me an example of a vasodilatation of any normal blood vessel in the body that is painful?

VANE: If one infuses vasodilators, one produces headaches.

MOSKOWITZ: But are the vasodilators working on the nerves or on the smooth muscle? The vasodilator may have actions at both.

HUMPHREY: I myself have also been infused with prostacyclin and it certainly does not give rise to a migraine-like headache, but to a pulsatile, mild pain in the head. Incidentally, the pain can be rapidly abolished by administration of another vasodilator, alcohol, in the form of a pint of beer! With a hypothesis such as yours, Professor Gryglewski, one needs really good clinical observations to test it scientifically. Many hypotheses about migraine have never been properly evaluated by reliable observations from clinical studies performed to good scientific standards. Published work in human volunteers strongly suggests that prostaglandin E_1 (PGE_1) does cause migraine-like symptoms, but that prostacyclin does not. Yet the two have not, as far as I am aware, been properly compared on a scientific basis.

GRYGLEWSKI: I agree that clinical studies should be orientated to test this hypothesis. In Cracow, since 1979, we have infused prostacyclin to over 500 patients with peripheral vascular disease. The patients with a history of migraine symptoms were particularly sensitive to one side-effect of prostacyclin (5 ng kg^{-1} min^{-1}), which was the headache. Ideally, of course, a double-blind study should be attempted in order to verify this observation statistically.

HUMPHREY: Having identified those patients, one would like to know how they are affected by other vasodilators, such as PGE_1, glyceryl trinitrate, and histamine.

GRYGLEWSKI: Yes; this phenomenon certainly deserves a systematic study.

HUMPHREY: Perhaps then, on the basis of the known pharmacology of the different vasodilators, one could begin to address the issue that Dr Moskowitz has mentioned about the site of origin of vascular head pain.

References

Kontos, H.A., Wei, E.P., and Povlishock, J.T. (1984). Oxygen radicals mediate the cerebral arteriolar dilation from arachidonate and bradykinin in cats. *Circulation Research*, **55**, 295–303.

Loesch, A. and Burnstock, G. (1988). Ultrastructural localization of serotonin and substance P in vascular endothelial cells of rat femoral and mesenteric arteries. *Anatomy and Embryology*, **178**, 137–42.

Peatfield, R.C., Gawel, M.J., and Rose, F.C. (1981). The effect of infused prostacyclin in migraine and cluster headache. *Headache*, **21**, 190–5.

Sandler, M. (1972). Migraine: a pulmonary disease? *Lancet*, **i**, 618–9.

Vanhoutte, P.M. (1987). Serotonin and the vascular wall. *International Journal of Cardiology*, **14**, 189–203.

Van Zwieten, P.A. (1987). Pathophysiological relevance of serotonin. *Journal of Cardiovascular Pharmacology*, **10**, Suppl. 3, S19–S25.

6. A classification of peripheral analgesics based upon their mode of action

Sérgio H. Ferreira

Introduction

The aim of this review is to discuss current ideas about the mechanism of action of peripheral analgesics, and to provide a rational basis both for their therapeutic use and for the development of new drugs.

The classical explanation for the mechanism of inflammatory hyperalgesia is that it results from excitatory actions of endogenous mediators that are released by inflamed or damaged tissues (Lynn 1984). This concept implies that there are many mediators present, in what might be called a 'mediator soup'. If the concentration of one or several agonists in this 'mediator soup' is increased, as a result of further stimulation, activation of the nociceptor is achieved. The concept also implies that all types of nociceptive mediator are qualitatively similar — that is, that they are all equally capable of activating the nociceptors.

The nociceptor normally involved in inflammatory pain is a high-threshold polymodal nociceptor (Handwerker 1976; Perl 1976), which is normally down-regulated. A minor thermal, mechanical, or chemical nociceptive stimulus, which can activate the nociceptor if it has been previously sensitized, is unable to do so when the nociceptor is in the normal (down-regulated) state. As a result of our early studies, we propose that inflammatory pain mediators should be classified into two types: direct activators of nociceptors, and nociceptor up-regulators (those that directly sensitize the nociceptors; Moncada *et al.* 1978). Admittedly, it is possible for a stimulus of high intensity to activate the nociceptor even in its normal state. However, we believe that in most cases the concentration of the mediators responsible for direct nociceptor activation is too low to be effective, and that there exists within this 'mediator soup' up-regulatory mediators that allow 'subthreshold' concentrations of activating mediators, or normally non-effective mechanical or thermal stimuli, to produce nociceptor activation.

The technical term to describe the state of up-regulation of the nociceptor is *allodynia*. However, in this review, I shall use the term *hyperalgesia*, because it is more commonly used by clinicians and scientists.

Inflammatory mediators that directly stimulate nociceptors

Histamine has been shown to be a direct activator of nociceptors. Although the release of histamine is mainly associated with pruritus, it is considered to be a pain mediator because it causes overt pain when applied on top of a blister base (Keele and Armstrong 1964), or when given as a subdermal infusion in areas made hyperalgesic by prostaglandins (Ferreira 1972; Greaves and MacDonald-Gibson 1973). However, its role in nociception during chronic human diseases is unclear.

The most powerful endogenous mediator is bradykinin, which has been shown to activate nociceptors directly in several animal models and in humans (Keele and Armstrong 1964; Ferreira 1972; Lim *et al.* 1967). Patients suffering from headaches present high sensitivity to bradykinin injections (Sicuteri 1968). Unfortunately, the overall contribution of bradykinin to inflammatory pain is still obscure, owing to the lack of specific antagonists.

Inflammatory mediators that cause up-regulation of the nociceptors

5-Hydroxytryptamine (serotonin, 5-HT), which is released from platelets, was first suspected of being an up-regulator when it was observed that it sensitized vascular pain receptors to the action of bradykinin. From these findings, it was suggested that 5-HT was an important agonist of migraine headaches (Sicuteri *et al.* 1965; Sicuteri 1968). This hypothesis was supported by the fact that 5-HT potentiated the algogenic effect of bradykinin, when 5-HT was injected intravenously in humans. 5-HT can also potentiate other types of pain, because when it was injected intra-arterially in dogs (Moncada *et al.* 1975), it enhanced the nociceptive response due to bradykinin.

The products of arachidonic acid metabolism by cyclo-oxygenase (prostaglandins PGE_2, PGI_2, and PGD_2) are well-established hyperalgesic mediators. Their ability to sensitize pain receptors has been demonstrated in humans and animals by the use of both behavioural and electrophysiological techniques (Ferreira 1983). An injurious stimulus promotes prostaglandin release from damaged local cells. More importantly, it also stimulates phagocytes (macrophages or neutrophils) to release prostaglandins directly or to release substances such as interleukin 1 (IL-1; Dinarello 1984) and platelet activating factor (PAF, Vargaftig *et al.* 1980a) which, in turn, cause the release of prostaglandin from phagocytes. We have recently tested IL-1α and IL-1β in rats for hyperalgesic activity. Our results show that IL-β, given systemically, is an extremely potent hyperalgesic. IL-1α is 3000 times less active than 1L-1β (Ferreira 1983; Francischi *et al.* 1988; Ferreira *et al.* 1988). PAF is known to cause many biological effects, in particular platelet aggregation and bronchoconstriction (Vargaftig *et al.* 1980*b*). In hyperalgesia in rats, PAF acts indirectly by causing the release of cyclo-oxygenase and sympathomimetic amines (Vargaftig and Ferreira 1981; S.H. Ferreira and B.B. Lorenzetti, unpublished results). Carrageenan causes the release of platelet activating factor–acether, which then contributes to carrageenan-induced hyperalgesia in rats.

The arachidonic acid metabolites formed by the action of lipoxygenase, such as leukotrienes B4, have also been described as causing hyperalgesia in the rat paw (Levine *et al.* 1986), but confirmatory evidence from other experiments has not yet been presented.

Extensive physiological, pharmacological, and clinical evidence supports the existence of a sympathetic modulatory influence on somatosensory input. Recently, sympathomimetic amines (noradrenaline, dopamine, and 5-hydroxytryptamine) have been shown to up-regulate the nociceptors (Nakamura and Ferreira 1987). We have reported that depletion, by guanethidine, of peripheral sympathomimetic amines, or treatment with adrenergic antagonists (beta-blockers), or with a dopamine (DA)-1 antagonist (SCH 23390), significantly reduced carrageenan-induced hyperalgesia. These antagonists also abolished the rat paw hyperalgesia induced by several sympathomimetic amines as well as that induced by a selective DA-1 agonist, SKF 38393. Blockade of neural uptake by cocaine potentiated the hyperalgesia induced by carrageenan or by sympathomimetic amines. From these results, we conclude that there is a sympathetic component, possibly mediated by a DA-1-type receptor, in carrageenan-induced hyperalgesia. We believe that this component may predominate in certain types of pain. A contribution by the sympathetic system has also been demonstrated in other animal models (Coderre *et al.* 1984; Duarte *et al.* 1988). Thus, it is conceivable that different types of injury release different types of mediators which require different types of drugs to control the resultant pain (Moncada *et al.* 1975; Ferreira *et al.* 1978; Nakamura and Ferreira 1987).

Among the stimuli know to cause pain, it is important to mention two conditions which are also responsible for pain. The lack of oxygen (angina) or a drop in pH (as happens in the inflammatory exudate) are frequently considered to be pain stimuli. We are yet uncertain, however, whether these stimuli act directly or indirectly via the release of endogenous mediators.

The mechanism of hyperalgesia

The biochemical mechanism of up-regulation is not yet completely understood. However, there is evidence that an increase in the concentration of cAMP and Ca^{2+} many play a role in the process. Prostaglandins and dopamine (via a DA1 receptor) are the most potent stimulators of neuronal-tissue adenylate cyclase and are the most active up-regulators of nociceptors. It has been shown that inhibitors of cAMP inactivation potentiate the up-regulation of the nociceptor. An increase in the cytosolic Ca^{2+} concentration by the use of a calcium ionophore causes hyperalgesia, and calcium antagonists prevent the effect of hyperalgesic mediators (Ferreira and Nakamura 1979a). We also observed in animals that nociceptor sensitization by prostaglandins is blocked by treatment with a protein synthesis inhibitor, cycloheximide. However, intraplantar injection of dibutyryl cAMP (dibutyryl cAMP), which bypasses adenylate cyclase activation, produced hyperalgesia in cycloheximide-treated animals. From the above results, we believe that adenylate cyclase activation depends on the neosynthesis of a regulatory protein (Ferreira and Lorenzetti 1981). Thus, the mechanism by which the nociceptors are up-regulated differs substantially from that of the membrane ionic fluxes responsible for the nociceptor activation.

It appears that nociceptor up-regulation can be memorized by the nociceptors. Recently, we reported experimental findings which support the idea that a state of persistent hyperalgesia is generated by prolonged periods of pain stimulation, as experienced in the initial stage of chronic pain (S.H. Ferreira, J.N. Francischi and B.B. Lorenzetti, unpublished results; S.H. Ferreira, B.B. Lorenzetti and D.I. Campos, unpublished results). Daily injections of PGE_2, dopamine or isoprenaline for 14 days caused the development of a persistent hyperalgesic state. In contrast, rats receiving injections of dibutyryl cAMP for 14 days — at doses sufficient to cause an intense, acute, and hyperalgesic response — did not show any persistent hyperalgesia. In addition, we found that the duration of the persistent hyperalgesic state depends strongly on the length of the hyperalgesic treatment. Noxious stimulation applied for less than seven days caused a short-lived hyperalgesic state (1–3 days). However, when the treatment was given for 14 days, the hyperalgesic state was markedly extended (by up to a month). We believe that this state of persistent hyperalgesia also depends on *de novo* protein synthesis, because experimental results show that two treatments with cycloheximide reduced the intensity of the persistent hyperalgesic state by about 40 per cent. The formation of a regulatory protein, which we believe controls adenylate cyclase activation, might be important in the persistence of chronic pain.

Classification of the peripheral analgesics

If we consider the two complementary mechanisms of nociceptor activation (excitation and up-regulation) described above, it is possible to define three general classes of peripheral analgesic. These are indicated in Table 6.1.

TABLE 6.1.   *Classification of the peripheral analgesics*

TYPE 1   Drugs that are receptor antagonists of nociceptor excitation
     A   Antihistaminics
TYPE 2   Drugs that prevent nociceptor up-regulation
     A   Cyclo-oxygenase inhibitors:
          non-steroidal anti-inflammatory drugs
     B   Antagonists of prostaglandin releasers:
          Interleukin 1 antagonists;
          platelet activating factor–acether antagonists
     C   Phospholipase A2 inhibitors:
          Glucocorticoids
     D   Sympatholytics:
          β-blockers;
          dopamine-1 antagonists;
          blockers of the release of sympathomimetic amines
TYPE 3   Drugs that down-regulate the nociceptor
     A   Analgesics that directly down-regulate the nociceptor:
          dipyrone;
          peripheral opiates
     B   Analgesics that indirectly down-regulate the nociceptors:
          clonidine

Type 1: Drugs that are receptor antagonists of nociceptor excitation

In this class, the only group of antagonists that have a clinical application are the H1-antihistaminics. This group of drugs is effective in blocking the activation of a special class of nociceptor associated with pruritus (that is, those responsible for inflammatory itching; Ferreira 1972; Greaves and MacDonald-Gibson 1973). However, prevention of nociceptor stimulation can be achieved without the use of drugs. The most frequent nociceptor excitatory stimulus is mechanical stimulation such as increased tissue tension (excess exudate in a closed cavity) or body movements. The most popular clinical treatment of choice for alleviating inflammatory pain of this origin is drainage of the exudate and rest.

Type 2: Drugs that prevent nociceptor up-regulation

Cyclo-oxygenase inhibitors   This is one of the most commonly prescribed groups of analgesics, the non-steroidal anti-inflammatory drugs (Vane 1971; Ferreira *et al.* 1971; Smith and Willis 1971). At therapeutic doses, they inhibit prostaglandin synthesis, thus preventing the development of nociceptor up-regulation (hyperalgesia).

A hyperalgesia characterized by a delayed onset and a long duration has been observed in nociceptive tests on human skin (Ferreira 1972), rat paw and dog knee joint (Ferreira et al. 1978). These tests involve the soma-tosensory system. In visceral pain tests, such as the dog spleen test or the mice contortion test (Moncada et al. 1978; Smith et al. 1985), sensitization to prostaglandin is immediate and of short duration, probably lasting only while the agonist is stimulating the receptors. When one considers the somatosensory type of hyperalgesia (long-lasting), it is difficult to explain the relatively rapid analgesic effect of aspirin-like drugs in certain pains, such as some types of headache. However, we believe that the effectiveness of the drug reflects the type of prostaglandin involved in the process. It was found that prostacyclin (PGI_2), a major arachidonic acid cyclo-oxygenase metabolite generated by endothelial cells, produced a nociceptor sensitiza-tion of much shorter onset and duration than did PGE_2 (Ferreira et al. 1978). We believe that in processes in which the injury is predominantly vascular, the up-regulation of the nociceptor is caused by prostacyclin. In contrast, when more extensive tissue lesions take place, with substantial participation of phagocytes (neutrophils and macrophages), PGE_2 is re-leased. Under these circumstances, a long-lasting sensitization of the nociceptor occurs, making ineffective a single administration of a short-lived (half-life less than 12 hours), non-steroidal anti-inflammatory drug. Recent-ly, work has been done with patients undergoing surgical procedures that result in extensive tissue trauma. In order to prevent the development of a hyperalgesic state, aspirin-like drugs are administered before, during and after surgery. The rationale is that if the release of PGE_2 due to tissue trauma is prevented, sensitization will not take place and the patient will not experience the pain of surgery. However, with this treatment, the stress due to surgery could cause an intense sympathetic response, and the use of an aspirin-like drug could abolish the prostaglandin vasodilatory feedback mechanism in the vessels of the kidney. Both situations cause vasoconstric-tion and, of course, can cause serious injury to the kidney.

The mechanism of analgesic action of the non-acidic, non-steroidal drugs — acetaminophen (paracetamol) and dipyrone — is still controversial (Flower and Vane 1972; Dembinska-Kiec et al. 1976; Lanz et al. 1986a,b). It is difficult to explain how the blockade of prostaglandin synthesis can cause analgesia without a parallel anti-oedematogenic effect. It has been suggested (Flower and Vane 1972; Dembinska-Kiec et al. 1976; Campos et al. 1988) that prostaglandin synthesis by the nervous tissues is specifically sensitive to non-acidic analgesics. This suggestion would imply that hyper-algesia is caused by prostaglandins originating from the nociceptor itself or from its immediate vicinity. We now have experimental evidence that sup-ports this view. In the rat model, interleukin 1β produces a strong hyper-algesia without causing oedema, and a tripeptide interleukin-1β antagonist blocks carrageenan-induced hyperalgesia, without affecting the oedematogenic response (Ferreira *et al.* 1988). We also found that paracetamol is an effective blocker of interleukin 1β-induced hyperalgesia (S.H. Ferreira personal observation).

Antagonists of prostaglandin releasers As mentioned earlier, interleukin 1β may be an important mediator of inflammatory pain, and particularly of chronic inflammatory pain. We have delineated the region of interleukin 1β that mediates hyperalgesia and have developed an analgesic tripeptide analogue of interleukin 1β (lysine-D-proline-threonine) which antagonizes the hyperalgesia evoked by interleukin 1β and by the inflammatory agent carrageenan. This molecule may constitute a prototype for the development of a new class of analgesics.

Until recently, it was accepted that PAF induced a hyperalgesia in rats by causing the release of cyclo-oxygenase metabolites (Vargaftig and Ferreira 1981). However, we have found that PAF causes the release of endogenous amines which are also responsible for hyperalgesia. The hyperalgesic effect caused by PAF is abolished by PAF antagonists like BN25021 and RP 48740 (B.B. Lorenzetti and S.H. Ferreira, unpublished results). However, we have no indication that PAF antagonists are analgesic in humans.

Phospholipase A₂ inhibitors It is generally believed that the analgesic action of glucocorticoids is a consequence of their 'anti-inflammatory activity'. It is now well established that corticoids stimulate macrophages to secrete lipocortin, a phospholipase A_2 inhibitor (Blackwell *et al.* 1982) and that one of the mechanisms involved in the anti-inflammatory activity of corticoids is the blockade of the release of prostaglandin via lipocortin. These agents also inhibit the release of interleukin 1 (Dinarello 1984). This indicates that another mechanism is probably responsible for the analgesic activity of corticoids.

Sympatholytics There are only a few physiopathological events (erythema, oedema, phagocyte migration, and nociceptor stimulation) which characterize an inflammatory response and produce the clinical symptoms. However, the number and type of mediators responsible for a single symptom are great and depend on the type of injurious stimulus. Sympathomimetic amines mediate some peripheral pain states in humans. Interestingly enough, it has been observed that when hyperalgesia is accompanied by pain, analgesia is achieved by local sympathetic blockade with the aid of guanethidine (Hannington-Kiff 1974; Loh and Nathan 1978; Loh *et al.* 1980). The β-blocker propranolol is useful in the management of migraine, but we do not know if its beneficial effect is due to a central or a peripheral mechanism.

Type 3: Drugs that down-regulate the nociceptor

Analgesics that directly down-regulate the nociceptors   As already pointed out, when the nociceptor is up-regulated, drugs that block the release of prostaglandin or sympathomimetic amines are not effective analgesic agents. However, Lorenzetti and Ferreira (1985) and Marques and Ferreira (1987) recently found that dipyrone (also classified as a type 2 analgesic) was able to counteract established hyperalgesia that was induced by either PGE_2, isoprenaline, or calcium chloride, thus indicating a direct effect on hyperalgesia. Type 2 drugs (which act by inhibiting prostaglandin formation) block oedema and are antinociceptive, while type 3 drugs do not block oedema but are antinociceptive. Dipyrone is known to inhibit cyclo-oxygenase at concentrations greater than the plasma concentrations of dipyrone reached during analgesic therapy (Lanz *et al.* 1986*b*). We have described above that repeated administration of nociceptor up-regulatory stimuli induces a state of persistent hyperalgesia. This state is not altered by treatment with standard cyclo-oxygenase inhibitors (non-steroidal anti-inflammatory drugs) but it is down-regulated by dipyrone or peripherally acting opiates, such as quarternary morphine (see below). Once down-regulated, the nociceptor remains as such if there are no additional hyperalgesic stimuli. However, if a new hyperalgesic stimulus takes place, the persistent state of up-regulation of the nociceptor is restored. We believe that this peripheral memory of nociceptor up-regulation may be one of the missing pieces in the puzzle of chronic pain.

Morphine has been reported to antagonize prostaglandin-induced cAMP accumulation in neural tissue (Collier and Roy 1974; Kalix 1979). Following this lead, we demonstrated that the local administration of opiates blocked an established prostaglandin-induced hyperalgesia (Ferreira and Nakamura 1979*b*). In addition, quaternary agonists and antagonists, owing to steric hindrance, are unable to cross the blood–brain barrier. The use of these agents has demonstrated unequivocally that opiates can act as peripheral analgesics (Lorenzetti and Ferreira 1982; Rios and Jacob 1982; Smith *et al.* 1982). The blockade by opiates of nociceptor up-regulation has also been demonstrated by single-neurone electrophysiological recordings in the isolated rabbit ear and in inflamed rat joints (J.W. Russell, C.G. Heapy, and M. Rance, unpublished results; 1987).

Recently, a novel peripherally acting opioid peptide (BW 443C) was developed. This peptide is based upon the enkephalin structure, and its site of action has been demonstrated (Lorenzetti and Ferreira 1987; Follenfant *et al.* 1988). We believe that this class of analgesics has the same span of clinical use as dipyrone, whose therapeutic profile as an analgesic is thought to be different from that of the non-steroidal anti-inflammatory drugs. An important difference between these drugs is that BW 443C is devoid of antipyretic action. This characteristic may make agents like BW 443C the drugs of choice for postoperative pain or for other types of pain in which the possibility of fever development is important in assessing the progress of the patient. Curiously, BW 443C, as well as quaternary morphine, has antitussive effects that result from its inhibition of vagal sensory nerve activity (Adcock *et al.* 1988). Another peculiarity of this new class of agents, in contrast with other centrally acting opiates, is that they do not induce tolerance or dependency (Lorenzetti and Ferreira 1987; Follenfant *et al.* 1988).

Analgesics that indirectly down-regulate the nociceptor We have explored the' possibility that some agents could produce peripheral anti-nociception by releasing their own enkephalin. We have found that, in addition to its central analgesic action, clonidine can induce analgesia by causing the release of enkephalin-like substances via the stimulation of an α-2-peripheral adrenoceptor. ST-91, a clonidine analogue that does not cross the blood–brain barrier, also promotes significant antinociception (Nakamura and Ferreira 1988).

References

Adcock, J.J., Schneider, C., and Smith, T.W. (1988). Effects of codeine, morphine and a novel opioid pentapeptide BW443C, on cough, nociception and ventilation in the unanaesthetized guinea-pig. *British Journal of Pharmacology*, **93**, 93–100.

Blackwell, G.J. *et al.* (1982). Glucocorticoids induce the formation and release of anti-inflammatory and anti-phospholipase proteins into the peritoneal cavity of the rat. *British Journal of Pharmacology*, **76**, 185–94.

Campos, D.I., Cunha, F.Q., and Ferreira, S.H. (1988). A new mechanism of dipyrone: blockade of the release of a nociceptive factor from macrophages. *Brazilian Journal of Medical and Biological Research*, **21**, 565–8.

Coderre, T.J., Abbott, F.V., and Melzack, R. (1984). Effects of peripheral antisympathetic treatments in the tail-flick, formalin and autotomy tests. *Pain*, **18**, 13–23.

Collier, H.O.J. and Roy, A.C. (1974). Hypothesis, inhibition of prostaglandin E sensitive adenyl cyclase as the mechanism of morphine analgesia. *Prostaglandins*, **7**, 361–76.

Dembinska-Kiec, A., Zmuda, A., and Krupinska, I. (1976). Inhibition of prostaglandin synthetase by aspirin-like drugs in different microsomal preparations. In *Advances in prostaglandin and thromboxane research*, Vol. 1. (ed. B. Samuelson and R. Paoletti), pp. 99–101, Raven, New York.

Dinarello, C.A. (1984). Interleukin-1 and the pathogenesis of the acute phase response. *New England Journal of Medicine*, **311**, 1413–8.

Duarte, I.D.G., Nakamura, M., and Ferreira, S.H. (1988). Participation of the sympathetic system in acetic acid-induced writhing in mice. *Brazilian Journal of Medical and Biological Research*, **21**, 341–3.

Ferreira, S.H. (1972). Prostaglandins, aspirin-like drugs and analgesia. *Nature New Biology*, **240**, 200–3.

Ferreira, S.H. (1983). Prostaglandins, peripheral and central analgesia. In *Advances in pain research and therapy*, Vol. 5. (ed. J.J. Bonica), pp. 627–34. Raven, New York.

Ferreira, S.H. and Lorenzetti, B.B. (1981). Prostaglandin hyperalgesia, a metabolic process. *Prostaglandins*, **23**, 789–92.

Ferreira, S.H. and Nakamura, M. (1979*a*). Prostaglandin hyperalgesia, a cAMP/ Ca^{2+} dependent process. *Prostaglandins*, **18**, 179–90.

Ferreira, S.H. and Nakamura, M. (1979*b*). II: Prostaglandin hyperalgesia, the peripheral analgesic activity of morphine, enkephalin and opioid antagonists. *Prostaglandins*, **18**, 191–200.

Ferreira, S.H. Moncada, S., and Vane, J.R. (1971). Indomethacin and aspirin abolish prostaglandin release from the spleen. *Nature New Biology*, **231**, 237–9.

Ferreira, S.H., Nakamura, M., and Castro, M.S.A. (1978). The hyperalgesic effects of prostacyclin and prostaglandin E_2. *Prostaglandins*, **16**, 31–7.

Ferreira, S.H., Lorenzetti, B.B., Bristow, A.F., and Poole, S. (1988). Interleukin-1β as a potent hyperalgesic agent antagonized by a tripeptide analogue. *Nature*, **334**, 2–4.

Flower, R.J. and Vane, J.R. (1972). Inhibition of prostaglandin synthetase in brain explains the anti-pyretic activity of paracetamol (4-acetamidophenol). *Nature*, **240**, 410–1.

Follenfant, R.L., Hardy, C.W., Lowe, L.A., and Smith, T.W. (1988). Antinociceptive effects of the novel opioid peptide BW443C compared with classical opiates; peripheral versus central actions. *British Journal of Pharmacology*, **93**, 85–92.

Francischi, J.N., Lorenzetti, B.B., and Ferreira, S.H. (1988). Interleukin-1 mimics the hyperalgesia induced by a factor obtained by macrophage lysis. *Brazilian Journal of Medical and Biological Research*, **21**, 321–31.

Greaves, M.W. and MacDonald-Gibson, W. (1973). Itch, role of prostaglandin. *British Medical Journal*, **3**, 608–9.

Handwerker, H.O. (1976). Influences of algogenic substances on the discharges of unmyelinated cutaneous nerve fibres identified as nociceptors. In *Advances in Pain Research Therapy*, Vol. 1. (ed. J.J. Bonica and D. Albe-Fessard), pp. 41–5. Raven, New York.

Hannington-Kiff, J.G. (1974). Intravenous regional sympathetic block with guanethidine. *Lancet*, **i**, 119–20.

Kalix, P. (1979). Prostaglandin E_1 raises the cAMP content of peripheral nerve tissue. *Neurosciences*, **12**, 361–5.

Keele, C.A., and Armstrong, D. (1964). Substances producing pain and itch. Edward Arnold, London.

Lanz, R., Polster, P., and Brune, K. (1986*a*) Antipyretic analgesics inhibit prostaglandin release from astrocytes and macrophages similarly. *European Journal of Pharmacology*, **130**, 105–9.

Lanz, R., Peskar, B.A., and Brune, K. (1986*b*). The effects of acidic and nonacidic pyrazoles on arachidonic acid metabolism in mouse peritoneal macrophages. *Agents and Actions Supplement*, **19**, 125–35.

Levine, J.G., Lam, D., Taiwo, Y.O., Donatoni, P., and Goetzl, E.J. (1986). Hyperalgesic properties of 15-lipoxygenase products of arachidonic acid. *Proceedings of the National Academy of Sciences USA*, **83**, 5331–4.

Lim, R.K.S. *et al.* (1967). Pain and analgesia evaluated by intraperitoneal bradykinin-evoked pain method in man. *Clinical Pharmacology and Therapeutics*, **8**, 521–42.

Loh, L. and Nathan, P.W. (1978). Painful peripheral states and sympathetic blocks. *Journal of Neurology, Neurosurgery and Psychiatry*, **41**, 664–71.

Loh, L., Nathan, P.W., Schott, G.D., and Wilson, P.G. (1980). Effects of regional guanethidine infusion on certain painful states. *Journal of Neurology Neurosurgery and Psychiatry*, **43**, 446–51.

Lorenzetti, B.B. and Ferreira, S.H. (1982). The analgesic effect of quaternary analogues of morphine and nalorphine. *Brazilian Journal of Medical and Biological Research*, **15**, 285–90.

Lorenzetti, B.B. and Ferreira, S.H. (1985). Mode of analgesic action of dipyrone, direct antagonism of inflammatory hyperalgesia. *European Journal of Pharmacology*, **114**, 375–81.

Lorenzetti. B.B. and Ferreira, S.H. (1987). On the mode of analgesic action of Tyr-D-Arg-Gly-Phe [4-NO$_2$] Pro-NH (443C). *British Journal of Pharmacology*, **90**, 69.

Lynn, B. (1984). The detection of injury and tissue damage. In *Pain*, (ed. P. Wall and R. Melzack), pp. 19–33. Churchill Livingstone, Edinburgh.

Marques, J.O. and Ferreira, S.H. (1987). Regional dipyrone nociceptor blockade, a pilot study. *Brazilian Journal of Medical and Biological Research*, **20**, 441–4.

Moncada, S. Ferreira, S.H., and Vane, J.R. (1975). Inhibition of prostaglandin biosynthesis as the mechanism of aspirin-like drugs in the dog knee joint. *European Journal of Pharmacology*, **31**, 250–60.

Moncada, S., Ferreira, S.H., and Vane, J.R. (1978). Pain and inflammatory mediators. In *Inflammation; Handbook of experimental pharmacology* Vol. 50. (ed. J.R. Vane and S.H. Ferreira), pp. 588–616. Springer-Verlag, Berlin.

Nakamura, M. and Ferreira, S.H. (1987). A peripheral sympathetic component in inflammatory hyperalgesia. *European Journal of Pharmacology*, **135**, 145–53.

Nakamura, M. and Ferreira, S.H. (1988). Peripheral analgesic effect of clonidine, mediated by release of endogenous enkephalin-like substance. *European Journal of Pharmacology*, **146**, 223–8.

Perl, E.R. (1976). Sensitization of nociceptors and its relation to sensation. In *Advances in pain research and therapy*, Vol. 1. (ed. J.J. Bonica and D. Albe-Fessard), pp. 17–34. Raven, New York.

Rios, L. and Jacob, J.J.C. (1982). Inhibition of inflammatory pain by naloxone and its *N*-methyl quaternary analogue. *Life Sciences*, **31**, 1209.

Russell, N.J.W, Schaible, H.G., and Schimidt, R.F. (1987). Opiates inhibit the discharges of fine afferent units from inflamed knee joint of the cat. *Neuroscience Letters*, **76**, 107–12.

Sicuteri, F. (1968). Sensitization of nociceptors by 5-hydroxytryptamine in man. In *Pharmacology of pain*, (ed. R.K.S. Lim, D. Armstrong, and E.G. Pardo), pp. 57–86. Pergamon, Oxford.

Sicuteri, F., Franciullacci, F., Franchi, G., and Del Bianco, P.L. (1965). Serotonin–bradykinin potentiation on the pain receptors in man. *Life Sciences*, **4**, 309–16.

Smith, J.B. and Willis, A.L. (1971). Aspirin selectively inhibits prostaglandin production in human platelets. *Nature New Biology* **231**, 236–7.

Smith, T.W., Buchan, P., Parsons, N.D., and Wilkinson, S. (1982) Peripheral antinociceptive effects of *N*-methyl morphine, *Life Sciences*, **31**, 1205.

Smith, T.W., Follenfant, R.L., and Ferreira, S.H. (1985). Antinociceptive models displaying peripheral opioid activity. *International Journal of Tissue Reactions*, **7**, 61–7.

Vane, J.R. (1971). Inhibition of prostaglandin synthesis as a mechanism of action for aspirin-like drugs. *Nature New Biology*, **231**, 232–5.

Vargaftig, B.B. and Ferreira, S.H. (1981). Blockade of the inflammatory effects

70   S.H. Ferreira

of platelet-activating factor by cyclo-oxygenase inhibitors. *Brazilian Journal of Medical and Biological Research*, **14**, 178–80.

Vargaftig, B.B., Fouque, F., and Chignard, M. (1980*a*). Interference of bromophenacyl bromide with platelet phospholipase A2 activity induced by thrombin and by the ionophore A23187. *Thrombosis Research*, **17**, 91–102.

Vargaftig, B.B., Lefort, J., Chignard, M., and Benveniste, J. (1980*b*). Platelet-activating factor induces a platelet-dependent bronchoconstriction unrelated to the formation of prostaglandin derivatives. *European Journal of Pharmacology*, **65**, 185–92.

Discussion

ZIEGLER: In your work on the peripheral memory of inflammatory pain, does the sensitizing effect of prostaglandins hold true only for nociceptors or also for other generator potentials such as those in endothelial cells?

FERREIRA: In animals with persistent hyperalgesia, there is no oedema. I have not measured potentials but there are no other apparent problems in the vessels. During this phase of nociceptor sensitization, the response of the paws to inflammation is normal.

DE BELLEROCHE: The mechanism of memory you proposed is very like that of Kandel and Schwartz (1982) to explain the mechanisms behind habituation and sensitization. In that case they have now shown the effects on the synthesis of proteins involved. It is an interesting parallel.

BLAU: I would like to expand Dr Ferreira's concept of learned pain pathways. We teach a child not to touch a fire, because it is hot, so the child learns to avoid burning itself. There must be a learning process involved in avoiding pain, and there must be a memory capacity for pain. I say this despite an awareness of the folklore that one loses one's memory for pain. But I agree with Dr Ferreira — there are mechanisms of pain memory and they merit further study. It is certainly true that people looking at particular jazzy patterns will find them uncomfortable, and these patterns may provoke a migraine in those patients.

MOSKOWITZ: I am very interested in the relationship between the peripheral sympathetic system and the pain system. One theory is that prostaglandins are synthesized by the sympathetic fibres. Is this compatible with your ideas about the sensitization phenomena?

FERREIRA: I believe that prostaglandins are released by the nociceptor, in response to the pain stimuli, and they act in the nociceptor itself. But this concept need not exclude the idea that sympathetic neurones, or macrophages, can release prostaglandins. We still have to identify the mediator involved in sympathetic injury. If noradrenaline (norepinephrine) is not a plausible candidate, dopamine may well be, because it is a potent activator of the adenylate cyclase system and it could be important for sympathetic sensitization (Nakamura and Ferreira 1987). If prostaglandin does play a part in migraine it must be at the beginning of the vasodilatation phase. Patients who are aware of a future migraine attack may take a high dose of aspirin. If this treatment is successful, with no experience of pain, there is also no vasodilatation. Does prostaglandin formation occur in the vessels? Is prostaglandin formed during the vasoconstriction phase? Since migraine is a long-lasting process, before pain appears there may be a prolonged vasoconstriction in large vessels. This event might serve to occlude the *vasa vasorum* for a long period of time, thus causing an anoxic lesion of the vessel. The *vasa vasorum* is oxygenated during diastole, not during systole, when it is usually occluded. If the vessels are also constricted during diastole, the oxygenation and nutrition of the blood vessels may be rather deficient.

PEATFIELD: You have described the antagonism of hyperalgesia induced by interleukin 1β in the control of chronic pain. Is interleukin 1 part of the pathway of neurogenic inflammation or of any immune inflammatory processes?

FERREIRA: Neither. It is part of the cellular component of inflammation. It can be released in the acute process or in the chronic process, but there is no evidence that it participates in immune or neurogenic responses.

PEATFIELD: Is it part of the pathway of the axon reflex?

FERREIRA: No. It is released in the body when macrophages recognise non-self. It is a direct recognition, not necessarily mediated by an immunological stimulus.

PEATFIELD: Is it completely unrelated to neurogenic inflammation?

FERREIRA: We believe that interleukin 1 is able to release prostaglandin either from the nerves or from the structures present in the proximity of the nerves.

MOSKOWITZ: How could you prove that interleukin 1 is working on nerves directly?

FERREIRA: By an indirect proof: exogenous prostaglandin potentiates the oedematogenic response of an inflammation. Interleukin 1 causes an intense hyperalgesia but does not potentiate inflammatory oedematogenic responses.

MOSKOWITZ: How can you establish where the prostaglandins are coming from?

FERREIRA: I believe they come from the nociceptor itself.

MOSKOWITZ: When you use as the behavioural paradigm the paw-pressing technique, could you do an operation to open up the dorsal root ganglion cells? You could then treat them locally with aspirin to block the cyclo-oxygenase enzyme selectively in those individual ganglia. There are five, I believe, that go to the front paw.

FERREIRA: We can give indomethacin, normally into the hind paws. So we know that it acts locally.

MOSKOWITZ: If you do a sympathectomy, do you still see the sensitization?

FERREIRA: I can do a sort of pharmacological sympathectomy with guanethidine and, still, interleukin 1 produces hyperalgesia. With tyramine, which produces a local release of amines, the ability to induce hyperalgesia is lost.

FOZARD: With regard to interleukin 1 hyperalgesia, can you do the memory trick in the neurones with that?

FERREIRA: I did not induce memory with interleukin 1, but with prostaglandin E_2. However, if the persistent hyperalgesia is blocked, one can fully restore it with interleukin 1.

FOZARD: Why have you not used interleukin 1 *per se*?

FERREIRA: The experiment is too expensive!

HUMPHREY: You said that the interleukin antagonist did not inhibit the oedema, and yet indomethacin does. So, one could speculate that the interleukin is stimulating the release of prostaglandins from the *nerves*, which would explain the hyperalgesia. But the oedema is still prostaglandin-dependent, and presumably that prostaglandin is coming from another cell?

FERREIRA: Yes; from the endothelial cells. The release may occur at discrete sites, where the mediator acts.

GRYGLEWSKI: Does your synthetic peptide that antagonizes hyperalgesia also have an effect on capillary permeability and on cell migration at the site of inflammation?

FERREIRA: Oedema is not blocked, and neither is cell migration affected by this interleukin 1 antagonist.

BLAU: What is the minimum dosage of aspirin that will stop prostaglandin release in humans, and how long will it last? I ask because on that must depend the extent to which prostaglandin is connected with migraine.

FERREIRA: It depends on the cell. One single dose of 50 mg to a 70 kg man for three days will produce total inhibition of prostaglandin release by platelets.

BLAU: So could you say that migraine, then, is not dependent on platelets?

MOSKOWITZ: Well, prostaglandins do not control everything in platelets, and other substances such as ADP, 5-HT (serotonin), growth factors, and calcium may be influential.

FERREIRA: There is another point. The prostaglandin that I believe to be important in migraine is being released by an injury to the vessel itself. The initial vasoconstriction in migraine is important in causing a mild damage to the vessel, and a subsequent sensitization of the nociceptors. That is why if aspirin is given in an early stage, one can abort the attack. I have a general point to make here. Normally, pharmacologists state that an effect is due to the presence of a mediator near a receptor; so when one sees an effect there must be some mediator at the receptor site. If 10 ng of prostaglandin is injected subcutaneously, after five minutes the subject will develop hyperalgesia, which lasts for four hours. And yet the disappearance of prostaglandin is immediate. The prostaglandin effect lasts so long because it induces metabolic changes in the nociceptor.

SAXENA: I couldn't agree with you more. Often, all that is measured is the plasma concentration of a drug, but it is the tissue concentration near the receptor site that is important. On other occasions, the concentration of an active metabolite, instead, may be the more relevant measurement.

References

Kandel, E.R. and Schwartz, J.H. (1982). Molecular biology of learning: modulation of transmitter release. *Science*, **218**, 433–43.

Nakamura, M. and Ferreira, S.H. (1987). A peripheral sympathetic component in inflammatory hyperalgesia. *European Journal of Pharmacology*, **135**, 145–53.

7. Vasomotor functions of trigeminovascular fibres: inferences from lesion studies

Michael A. Moskowitz, Damianos E. Sakas, Michihisa Kano, Hermes A. Kontos, and Enoch P. Wei

Introduction

The trigeminovascular system plays an essential role in the transmission of pain from cephalic blood vessels and mediates the pain of vascular headaches (Moskowitz *et al.* 1979; Moskowitz 1984; Strassman *et al.* 1986; Davis and Dostrovsky 1986). This system contains vasoactive neuropeptides which are synthesized by ganglion cells and then transported both to small unmyelinated axons (Liu-Chen *et al.* 1986) that surround cranial blood vessels and to root fibres that terminate within the trigeminal nucleus caudalis (Arbab *et al.* 1988). Experiments to date have confirmed that at least four neurotransmitter candidates reside within these fibres, including substance P (Liu-Chen *et al.* 1983*a,b*), neurokinin A (Saito *et al.* 1987), calcitonin gene-related peptide (Uddman *et al.* 1986; McCulloch *et al.* 1986), and cholecystokinin-8 (Liu-Chen *et al.* 1985; O'Connor and van der Kooy 1988). (No doubt this list is incomplete.) Of these four peptides, calcitonin gene-related peptide is the most potent vasodilator. The tachykinins substance P and neurokinin A are also vasodilators and promote vascular permeability as well, an effect not mimicked by calcitonin gene-related peptide. Release of substance P from perivascular fibres has been reported after the addition of depolarizing chemicals such as potassium or capsaicin *in vitro* by calcium-dependent mechanisms (Moskowitz *et al.* 1983). Release of substance P *in vivo* has been inferred from studies showing that vasodilatation and enhanced plasma protein permeability (for example, in the dura mater) follows electrical stimulation of the trigeminal ganglion (Markowitz *et al.* 1987).

In this report, we examined patterns of cerebral blood flow that develop in animals after unilateral trigeminal ganglionectomy. Blood flow was measured during acute severe hypertension (above 180 mmHg), and seizures. The latter two conditions are often associated with headache. From the information described above, we anticipated significant asymmetries in blood flow between the two sides, which would reflect the loss of a mechanism for cerebrovascular vasodilatation.

Materials and methods

Under general anaesthesia and with a sterile microsurgical technique, we subjected adult mongrel cats (3–4 kg) either to unilateral trigeminal ganglion lesion (Norregaard and Moskowitz 1985), to sham operation, or to a trigeminal rhizotomy via a posterior fossa approach. The animals were allowed to recover and were used for experiments after 1–3 weeks.

Bilateral cranial windows measured the responses of pial precapillary vessels after trigeminal ganglionectomy. The windows were implanted caudally to the coronal suture, over the ectosylvian and suprasylvian gyri of each hemisphere. The diameters of small (< 100 μm) and large (> 100 μm) arterioles were measured with an image-splitting device (Levasseur et al. 1975).

Cerebral blood flow was measured by radiolabelled (^{113}Sn, ^{103}Ru, ^{95}Nb, or ^{46}Sc) microspheres ($3.3–8.2 \times 10^5$, 20–50 μCi), according to Marcus et al. (1976). Measurements were made in 10 symmetrical regions including cortical grey matter of anterior, middle, and posterior cerebral arteries, subcortical white matter (in the territory of the middle cerebral artery), caudate nucleus, thalamus, midbrain, pons, medulla, and cerebellum. Blood flow determinations were based on the amount of radioactivity measured in dissected brain regions and on the total average radioactivity in blood per unit time.

Pial vessel responses were examined during hypercapnia (5 per cent carbon dioxide), hypocapnia (hyperventilation), hypoxia (10 per cent oxygen and 90 per cent nitrogen), and acute severe hypertension (after angiotensin II infusion). Cerebral blood flow was measured during normocapnia–normotension, hypercapnia, acute severe hypertension, and during generalized seizures (after bicuculline 1 mg kg^{-1} bolus i.v.; arterial blood pressure was maintained below 150 mmHg by controlled haemorrhage).

A paired t-test was used to determine the statistical significance of differences between flow values from symmetrical regions and of differences in vessel calibre during severe hypertension.

Results

Trigeminal ganglionectomy

During basal conditions, no significant differences in blood flow were found in 10 symmetrical brain regions.

Hypercapnia (P_{CO_2} approximately 50 mmHg) and hypoxia (P_{O_2} approximately 43 mmHg) caused symmetrical vasodilatation. Hypercapnia (P_{CO_2} approximately 50 mmHg) increased blood flow symmetrically in all brain regions. In addition, the responses on both sides were similar during hypocapnia (P_{CO_2} approximately 16 mmHg).

Acute severe hypertension (with blood pressure around 200 mmHg) caused

TABLE 7.1. *Effects of left trigeminal ganglionectomy (n = 10) on the responses of pial arterioles to severe hypertension*

	Diameter (μm) of small arterioles		Diameter (μm) of large arterioles		MABP (mmHg ± s.e.m.)
	I	D	I	D	
Control	58	58	140	135	126 ± 4
Hypertension					
5 min	69	68	168	156	192 ± 5*
Per cent control	119	117	117	116	
15 min	73	68	174	159	181 ± 5*
Per cent control	126	119†	125	118†	

Standard error (s.e.m.) was less than 6 per cent. I, intact side; D, deafferented side; MABP, mean arterial blood pressure. *$p < 0.0001$ compared with control level (paired t test). †$p < 0.05$ compared with I by Student's t test.

TABLE 7.2. *Mean blood flow in cortical grey matter (ml 100 g^{-1} min^{-1}) following left trigeminal ganglionectomy*

Type of cerebral artery	Control		Hypercapnia		Hypertension		Seizures	
	R	L	R	L	R	L	R	L
Anterior	48	47	86	83	145	116*	182	145*
Middle	50	48	88	84	157	122*	186	150*
Posterior	48	49	85	84	142	114*	179	143*

($n = 7$). s.e.m. was less than 10 per cent for all flow measurements. *$p < 0.01$ as compared to right side (paired t-test).

dilatation of both small (<100 μm) and large (>100 μm) arterioles when observed after 15 min of hypertension. The increase in vessel diameter was much less pronounced on the denervated side ($p < 0.05$; Table 7.1). Blood flow was attenuated only in cortical grey matter on the lesioned side ($p < 0.01$). Reductions of 29 ± 5 per cent, 31 ± 5 per cent, and 28 ± 4 per cent were measured in anterior, middle, and posterior cerebral arteries, respectively (Table 7.2).

During seizures, flow increased significantly within all brain regions. The most profound increases were found in cortical grey matter. Increases were approximately 25–30 per cent lower on the denervated side than on the

TABLE 7.3. *Mean blood flow in cortical grey matter (ml 100 g^{-1} min^{-1}) following left trigeminal rhizotomy*

Type of cerebral artery	Control		Hypertension		Seizures	
	R	L	R	L	R	L
Anterior	52	52	146	150	180	176
Middle	54	57	150	156	184	186
Posterior	54	51	150	152	169	168

($n = 8$). s.e.m. was less than 13 per cent for all flow measurements.

intact side within the territory of the three major cerebral arteries, anterior, middle, and posterior (p < 0.01) (Table 7.2).

Trigeminal rhizotomy
Blood flow values did not differ significantly between symmetrical brain regions under control conditions and during hypercapnia. Increases during acute severe hypertension or seizures were similar in magnitude to those on the intact side of ganglionectomized animals (Table 7.3). Asymmetries in flow were not observed in sham-operated animals or in animals subjected to trigeminal rhizotomy.

Discussion

There are many important findings to discuss in this study, and interested readers are referred to more detailed analyses (Moskowitz *et al.* 1988; Sakas *et al.* 1989). Nevertheless, there are several major findings worthy of note here. First, trigeminovascular axons participate in the vasodilatation and flow increases that develop during acute severe hypertension or seizures. Secondly, these effects are mediated by axonal activation of local reflex pathways and do not involve central neurotransmission. To our knowledge, this is the first study to demonstrate the phenomenon of local axonal control of cerebral blood flow. The phenomenon may not be unique to the trigeminovascular system. For example, local axonal mechanisms may prove to be important in the coupling of brain blood flow to metabolism (see review by Yarowsky and Ingvar 1981), and in the responses of cerebrovascular sympathetic projections during severe hypertension (Heistad *et al.* 1978).

How do hypertension or seizures activate the trigeminovascular system? It has been reported that severe hypertension, induced by experimental head injury, leads to synthesis of bradykinin (Ellis *et al.* 1987) and oxygen-derived free radicals (Wei *et al.* 1985). Bradykinin is a potent stimulus of prostaglandin synthesis within blood vessels (Derian and Moskowitz 1986). Unmyelinated C fibres are depolarized by bradykinin (Armstrong 1970) as well as by potassium (Moskowitz *et al.* 1983). High levels of potassium have been recorded in the extracellular space during seizures (Leniger-Folert 1984). Furthermore, prostaglandins sensitize sensory fibres to the effects of bradykinin (Mikami and Miyasaka 1979; Martin *et al.* 1987). We suggest that one or more of these molecules are mediators of trigeminovascular activation during severe hypertension, seizures and, perhaps, during migraine headaches.

What is the relationship between headache and increases in flow? Interestingly, headache often accompanies severe hypertension or seizures. Should flow increases always accompany headache? This is unlikely because cerebral blood flow is a complex vector that depends on many other neural and metabolic factors. In fact, many of the same molecules that either activate or sensitize pain fibres may also constrict blood vessels (for example, prostaglandins, or serotonin). Furthermore, the trigeminovascular system is not a major mechanism for controlling blood flow. Hence, increases in blood flow need not occur *pari passu* with activation of the trigeminovascular system. For example, blood flow may decrease during a painful condition such as subarachnoid haemorrhage (and perhaps classical migraine), even when the trigeminovascular system is activated. Hence, the relationship between pain and blood flow is necessarily complex.

No doubt, the pain that characterizes vascular headaches (for example, migraine and cluster headaches) develops from molecular mechanisms similar to those briefly described above during hypertension and seizures. The pathophysiological sequence that leads to the synthesis of pain-inducing molecules, however, may be unique to the particular headache type. The studies reported here demonstrate an approach to elucidating the complex role of the sensory fibres in cephalic blood vessels.

Summary

Acute severe hypertension and seizures, two conditions associated with headache, are accompanied by vasodilatation of pial arterioles and dramatic increases in cortical grey matter blood flow. During acute severe hypertension, arteriolar dilatation was reduced on the side of the trigeminal lesion. Similarly, increases in cortical grey matter blood flow were attenuated ipsilaterally by approximately 25–30 per cent during hypertension or seizures (bicuculline). These asymmetries were not observed when the same experiments were performed in animals subjected to either sham trigeminal ganglionectomy or trigeminal rhizotomy. Since trigeminal cell bodies and peripheral axons are destroyed or degenerate following ganglionectomy but not following trigeminal rhizotomy, local axonal mechanisms mediate a novel regulation of cerebral blood flow. We infer from these findings that

(1) the trigeminal nerve is activated during severe hypertension and seizures; (2) hypertension-induced blood flow increases are not entirely passive to the perfusion pressure; and (3) that the vasodilatation and increases in brain blood flow reported in some vascular headaches may be mediated, in part, by the trigeminal nerve.

References

Arbab, M.A.-R., Delgado, T., Wiklund, L., and Svendgaard, N.A. (1988). Brain stem terminations of the trigeminal and upper spinal ganglia innervation of the cerebrovascular system: WGA-HRP transganglionic study. *Journal of Cerebral Blood Flow and Metabolism*, **8**, 54–63.

Armstrong, D. (1970). Pain. *Handbook of Experimental Pharmacology*, **25**, 434–80.

Davis, K.D. and Dostrovsky, J.O. (1986). Activation of trigeminal brain-stem nociceptive neurons by dural artery stimulation. *Pain*, **25**, 395–401.

Derian, C. and Moskowitz, M.A. (1986). Polyphosphoinositide hydrolysis in endothelial cells and carotid artery segments. *Journal of Biological Chemistry*, **261**, 3831–6.

Ellis, E., Wei, E.P., Holt, S.A., and Kontos, H. (1987). Evidence that bradykinin stimulates the cyclooxygenase-dependent cerebral arteriolar abnormalities following concussive brain injury. *Federation Proceedings*, **46**, 800.

Heistad, D.D., Marcus, M.L., and Gross, P.M. (1978). Effects of sympathetic nerves on cerebral vessels in dog, cat and monkey. *American Journal of Physiology*, **235**, H544–H552.

Leniger-Folert, E. (1984). Mechanisms of regulation of cerebral microflow during bicuculline induced seizures in anaesthetised cats. *Journal of Cerebral Blood Flow and Metabolism*, **4**, 150–65.

Levasseur, J.E., Wei, E.P., Raper, H.A., Kontos, H.A., and Patterson, J.L. (1975). Detailed description of a pial window technique for acute and chronic experiments. *Stroke*, **6**, 308–17.

Liu-Chen, L.-Y., Han, D.H., and Moskowitz, M.A. (1983*a*). Pia arachnoid contains substance P originating from trigeminal neurons. *Neuroscience*, **9**, 803–8.

Liu-Chen, L.-Y., Mayberg, M.R., and Moskowitz, M.A. (1983*b*). Immunohistochemical evidence for a substance P-containing pathway to pial arteries in cats. *Brain Research*, **268**, 162–6.

Liu-Chen, L.-Y., Norregaard, T.V., and Moskowitz, M.A. (1985). Some cholecystokinin-8 immunoreactive fibers in large pial arterioles originate from trigeminal ganglia. *Brain Research*, **359**, 166–76.

Liu-Chen, L.-Y., Liszczack, T., King, J., and Moskowitz, M.A. (1986). An immunoelectron microscopic study of substance P-containing axons in cerebral arteries. *Brain Research*, **369**, 12–20.

Marcus, M.L., Heistad, D.D., Ehrhardt, J.C., and Abboud, F.M. (1976). Total and regional blood flow measurements with 7-, 10-, 15-, 25-, and 50-μm microspheres. *Journal of Applied Physiology*, **40**, 501–7.

Markowitz, S., Saito, K., and Moskowitz, M.A. (1987). Neurogenically-mediated leakage of plasma protein occurs from blood vessels in dura mater but not brain. *Journal of Neuroscience*, **7**, 4129–36.

Martin, H.A., Basbaum, A.I., Kwiat, G.C., Goetzl, E.J., and Levine, J.D. (1987). Leukotriene and prostaglandin sensitization of cutaneous high-threshold C- and

A-delta mechanonociceptors in the hairy skin of rat hindlimbs. *Neuroscience*, **22**, 651–9.

McCulloch, J., Uddman, R., Kingman, T.A., and Edvinsson, L. (1986). Calcitonin gene-related peptide: functional role in cerebrovascular regulation. *Proceedings of the National Academy of Sciences USA*, **83**, 5731–5.

Mikami, T. and Miyasaka, K. (1979). Potentiating effects of prostaglandins on bradykinin-induced pain and the effects of various analgesic drugs on prostaglandin E_1 potentiated pain in rats. *Journal of Pharmacy and Pharmacology*, **31**, 856–7.

Moskowitz, M.A. (1984). The neurobiology of vascular headache. *Annals of Neurology*, **16**, 157–68.

Moskowitz, M.A., Reinhard, J.F., Romero, J., Melamed, E., and Pettibone, D.J. (1979). Neurotransmitters and the fifth cranial nerve: Is there a relationship to the headache phase of migraine? *Lancet*, **ii**, 883–5.

Moskowitz, M.A., Brody, M., and Liu-Chen, L.-Y. (1983). In vitro release of immunoreactive substance P from putative afferent nerve endings in bovine pia arachnoid. *Neuroscience*, **9**, 809–14.

Moskowitz, M.A., Wei, E.P., Saito, K., and Kontos, H. (1988). Trigeminalectomy modifies pial arteriolar responses to hypertension or norepinephrine. *American Journal of Physiology*, **255**, H1-H6.

Norregaard, T.V. and Moskowitz, M.A. (1985). Substance P and the sensory innervation of intra- and extracranial feline cephalic arteries: Implications for vascular pain mechanism in man. *Brain*, **108**, 517–33.

O'Connor, T.P. and van der Kooy, D. (1988). Enrichment of a vasoactive neuropeptide (calcitonin gene related peptide) in the trigeminal sensory projection to the intracranial arteries. *Journal of Neuroscience*, **8**, 2468–76.

Saito, K., Greenberg, S., and Moskowitz, M.A. (1987). Trigeminal origin of beta-preprotachykinin in feline pial blood vessels. *Neuroscience Letters*, **76**, 69–73.

Sakas, D.E., Moskowitz, M.A., Wei, E.P., Kontos, H.A., Kano, M., and Ogilvy, C. (1989). Trigeminovascular fibers increase blood flow in cortical grey matter by axon-dependent mechanisms during acute severe hypertension and seizures. *Proceedings of National Academy of Sciences USA*, **86**, 1401–5.

Strassman, A., Mason, P., Moskowitz, M.A., and Maciewitz, R. (1986). Response of brainstem trigeminal neurons to electrical stimulation of the dura. *Brain Research*, **379**, 242–50.

Uddman, R., Edvinsson, L., Ekblad, E., Hakanson, R., and Sundler, F. (1986). Calcitonin gene-related peptide: perivascular distribution and vasodilatory effects. *Regulatory Peptides*, **15**, 1–23.

Wei, E.P., Kontos, H.A., Christman, C.W., DeWitt, D.S., and Povlishock, J.T. (1985). Superoxide generation and reversal of acetylcholine-induced cerebral arteriolar dilatation after acute hypertension. *Circulation Research*, **57**, 781–7.

Yarowsky, P.J. and Ingvar, D.H. (1981). Symposium summary. Neuronal activity and energy metabolism. *Federation Proceedings*, **40**, 2353–62.

Discussion

GRYGLEWSKI: In your 'pial window' models, have you used substance P locally in hypertensive and normotensive animals?

MOSKOWITZ: No, we have not, because the cat is not a very good model for examining the pial responses to substance P. In cats, substance P is not a very potent vasodilator in the pial circulation. However, calcitonin gene-related peptide (CGRP) in the cat is likely to be a mediator. In the dog, substance P appears to be more potent.

SCHWARTZ: Mast cells are believed to be involved in axon reflexes in peripheral tissues. It is now apparent that substance P fibres in various tissues, including the brain, are closely associated with mast cells. Could the changes that you see in cerebral blood flow be effected by mediators released by these mast cells?

MOSKOWITZ: We ourselves have tried to implicate the mast cell in the pathogenesis of neurogenic inflammation in the dura mater of the rat (Markowitz *et al.* 1989). There are some interesting ultrastructural data that show a relationship between the sensory fibre and the mast cell (Skofitsch *et al.* 1985). But our results were compellingly negative. We used a number of pharmacological and electrical manipulations but could not implicate mast cell degranulation. This result surprised us because dural blood vessels contain an abundance of mast cells. Perhaps degranulation is not sensitive enough. The population of mast cells is quite sparse in pial vessels. We have not looked at the mast cell activity in the pial circulation, as such, but our results from the dural circulation discourage us from pursuing this.

WELCH: When you cut the sensory nerve supply to the trigeminal vascular system on one side you saw less protein extravasation on that deafferented side. Suppose you assume that the protein extravasation is a purely mechanical effect relating to endothelial dilatation. After a trigeminal vascular nerve ablation there is less flow increase on that side. Can you really say that the extravasation is related to decreased neurogenic input?

MOSKOWITZ: That is a good point. Some of the changes in permeability can be flow-related. We have been hoping to study this phenomenon of the albumin leakage in more detail, perhaps with the aid of differential isotopes. We would like to know whether the flow alone can account for the permeability, or whether a permeability-promoting molecule is involved. At present, all we can say is that there is a change in the amount of oedema in the brain.

WELCH: Are you assuming, in your axon reflex hypothesis, that the local reflex releases pain-sensitizing substances?

MOSKOWITZ: Not necessarily. When the sensory fibre depolarizes and the neurotransmitter has been released, the 'pain' has already been experienced because the depolarization wave has passed to central structures. The molecules substance P, neurokinin A, CGRP, and so on, are not themselves pain-inducing, but are released in *response* to pain, and the dilatation and the permeability changes are then seen. I have sometimes been misinterpreted because the subtlety of that important distinction has not been appreciated. These are not nociceptive molecules like bradykinin or, perhaps, prostaglandins. Nevertheless, some investigators have suggested that antidromic mechanisms are important in the sensitization phenomenon (Fitzgerald 1979).

WELCH: The point of my question is to ask whether you would concede that a wave of depolarization could involve the sensory fibres?

MOSKOWITZ: We had, over the years, come to consider the sensory fibre as a passive partner. The extracellular concentration of potassium in spreading depression has been measured at levels of 25–30 mM, which will surely depolarize adjacent nerve fibres.

WELCH: So why does pain not develop immediately, with the aura?

MOSKOWITZ: The only brain blood vessels that are pain-sensitive to mechanical disruption or electrical stimulation are at the base of the brain. The vessels over the convexity receive a much less dense sensory innervation, as assessed by peptide levels, or by immunohistochemistry. So my simple-minded notion is that the wave of depolarization starts in the occipital cortex and moves at a rate of 2–6 mm min^{-1} until it reaches the ventral fibres 20–30 minutes later, where it passively depolarizes perivascular fibres and gives rise to the headache. This model is the best I can put forward. By the way, explaining the phenomenon of pain on the contralateral side of the brain has been easy (because it is based on the general organization of the brain). The interesting question is how to explain the pain on the ipsilateral side (see discussion after Peatfield, p. 266).

LANCE: A point from our work on the extracranial circulation supports what you are saying. If we stimulate the Gasserian ganglion or the trigeminal nerve, we see an increase in extracranial blood flow (Lambert *et al.* 1984). If we cut the trigeminal root, as you did, or cut the facial nerve 80 per cent of that increase disappears; hence the term trigeminovascular reflex. On the other hand, 20 per cent of the increased extracranial blood flow persists, and the only explanation for this is the antidromic release of vasodilator peptides, as you mentioned. This has been supported by work in the human patient by Peter Goadsby, collaborating with Lars Edvinsson (Goadsby *et al.* 1988). They have found, in patients who undergo thermocoagulation of the trigeminal ganglion for *tic douloureux* (trigeminal neuralgia), that CGRP and substance P concentrations increase in the external jugular blood, as we mentioned earlier (p. 36). We have also done parallel work in the cat, showing that stimulation of the trigeminal ganglion will evoke an increase in substance P and CGRP concentration in the external carotid artery. Curiously, we do not see an increase in vasoactive intestinal peptide (VIP), which is surprising because of the data I presented earlier on extracranial dilatation produced reflexly by stimulation of brainstem structures, a phenomenon that appears to depend on the release of VIP.

MOSKOWITZ: The half-life of substance P in plasma is extremely small, and for CGRP it is about seven minutes. But what is the half-life of VIP in plasma?

EDVINSSON: It is similar to that for substance P. The trick that we are using in these studies that Professor Lance has mentioned is to collect the blood in the jugular vein and analyse it immediately. This is the reason why we can see the changes, while others have failed to detect them (Schon *et al.* 1987).

MOSKOWITZ: If the trigeminal nerve does increase blood flow as I have shown you, and if it does promote the permeability of blood vessels in specified conditions (not to mention its role in pain transmission), then it would seem to be an obvious target for pharmacological manipulations that are intended to increase flow and permeability, and to decrease pain.

OLESEN: If substance P, neurokinin A, and calcitonin gene-related peptide are not directly painful and do not induce pain, what *are* the mechanisms of pain induced by the trigeminal vascular system? Is it a long-lasting process with neurogenic inflammation?

MOSKOWITZ: The first problem is: what is activating the pain system? My paper was not about migraine headache, as such, because it is unclear what a migraine headache is. However, certain conditions associated with headache — severe hypertension, seizures, and certain types of stroke — are easier to study. Before we can attempt to pin-point the mechanism of pain generation in migraine, we need to clarify the mechanism in conditions that we *know* to be painful. Kontos and Povlishock (1986) observed that the severe hypertension associated with head injury (and, indeed, hypertension by itself) is associated with significant endothelial changes and blood vessel damage. One can block some of that damage in the head injury model, for example, by bradykinin antagonists (Ellis *et al.* 1989). Some, perhaps minor, injury to the vessel wall (for example, severe hypertension) sets up the synthesis of bradykinin, and the subsequent generation of prostaglandins and free radicals; all three of these can have an effect on primary nociceptors. In the seizure model, the extracellular levels of K^+, measured in the cerebrospinal fluid, are high enough to depolarize sensory fibres, and may thus cause headaches. Ultimately, chemical signals and transduction mechanisms must be implicated. We shall have to explain how drugs work by classical neurophysiological and neurochemical approaches to the study of pain. Migraine is, after all, a pain syndrome.

PEATFIELD: Are you ruling out any trigeminal nerve firing as the factor that *initiates* migraine?

MOSKOWITZ: No. There is the potential for viral infections to affect the trigeminal vascular system; and there is a potential for mechanisms that are related to the central terminations, although the evidence for that is weak (Moskowitz *et al.* 1988*a, b*).

PEATFIELD: You are talking about how one can *feel* that the migraine is hurting. The question that Jes Olesen is asking is: what starts off the pain of a spontaneous migraine attack? If we assume that in common migraine (without aura) the pain is of central origin, is it a message going down the trigeminal system, or is it going down one of the other pathways that Professor Lance has spoken about?

MOSKOWITZ: Well, Harold Wolff and Bronson Ray (Ray and Wolff 1940) made one fundamental error in their otherwise admirable series of studies on mapping the pain-sensitive structrues in the cranium. They listed three 'pain-sensitive' structures: the proximal vessels of the circle of Willis, the venous sinuses, and the dural arteries. They forgot the sensory nerves themselves. I would not rule out the possibility that some sort of pathological condition could be intrinsic to the nerve fibre itself, but no-one yet has evidence for it.

EDVINSSON: McCulloch's group (see McCulloch and Reid 1986) gave capsaicin to deplete the trigeminal system, and they did not see any change in the blood–brain barrier.

MOSKOWITZ: That is what one would predict. What I said was that in order to see the trigeminal effects one has to disrupt the blood–brain barrier. In 1925, Florey wrote a paper in *Brain* which discouraged people from studying the axon reflex. He systematically applied a wide range· of irritants to the cortex of the brain. His results showed unequivocally, by the methods of that time, that there was no axon reflex in the brain. Of course, that conclusion was incorrect. We ourselves applied xylene to the surface of the brain to see if we could get increased leakage of Evans blue and we did not (unpublished results). The trick was, however, to disrupt the blood–brain barrier first, as with severe hypertension. The trigeminal vascular system does not, by itself, disrupt the blood–brain barrier. Something else is needed, before the full expression of the axon reflex is possible. That is why I am not surprised by Florey's results.

References

Ellis, E.F., Holt, S.A., Wei, E.P., and Kontos, H.A. (1989). Kinins induce abnormal vascular reactivity. *American Journal of Physiology*, in press.
Fitzgerald, M. (1979). The spread of sensitization of polymodal nociceptors in the

rabbit from nearby injury and by antidromic nervous stimulation. *Journal of Physiology (London)*, **297**, 207–16.

Florey, J. (1925). Microscopical observations on the circulation of the blood in cerebral cortex. *Brain*, **48**, 43–64.

Goadsby, P.J., Edvinsson, L., and Ekman, R. (1988). Release of vasoactive peptides in the extracerebral circulation of humans and the cat during activation of the trigeminovascular system. *Annals of Neurology*, **23**, 193–6.

Kontos, H.A. and Povlishock, J.T. (1986). Oxygen radicals in brain injury. *Central nervous system trauma*, **3**, 257–63.

Lambert, G.A., Bogduk, N., Goadsby, P.J., Duckworth, J.W., and Lance, J.W. (1984). Decreased carotid arterial resistance in cats in response to trigeminal stimulation. *Journal of Neurosurgery*, **61**, 307–15.

Markowitz, S., Saito, K., Buzzi, M.G., and Moskowitz, M.A. (1989). The development of neurogenic plasma extravasation does not depend upon the degranulation of mast cells in the rat dura mater. *Brain Research*, **477**, 157–65.

McCulloch, J. and Reid, J. (1986). The effect of capsaicin on blood-brain barrier permeability in the rat. *Journal of Physiology (London)*, **374**, 208.

Moskowitz, M.A., Henrikson, B.M., Markowitz, S., and Saito, K. (1988a). Intra- and extracranial nociceptive mechanisms and the pathogenesis of head pain. In *Basic mechanisms of headache*, (ed. J. Olesen and L. Edvinsson), pp. 429–35. Elsevier, Amsterdam.

Moskowitz, M.A., Saito, K., Sakas, D., and Markowitz, S. (1988b). The trigemino-vascular system and pain mechanisms from cephalic blood vessels. In *Proceedings of the fifth world congress of pain*, (ed. R. Dubner, G.F. Gebhart, and M.R. Bond), pp. 177–85. Elsevier, Amsterdam.

Ray, B.S. and Wolff, H.G. (1940). Experimental studies on headache: pain-sensitive structures of the head and their significance in headache. *Archives of Surgery*, **41**, 813–56.

Schon, F., Thomas, D.T., Jewkes, D.A., Ghatei, M.A., Muldery, P.K., and Bloom, S.R. (1987). Failure to detect plasma neuropeptide release during trigeminal thermocoagulation. *Journal of Neurology, Neurosurgery and Psychiatry*, **50**, 642–3.

Scofitsch, G., Savitt, J.M., and Jacobowitz, D.M. (1985). Suggestive evidence of a functional unit between mast cells and substance P fibers in the rat diaphragm and mesentery. *Histochemistry*, **82**, 5–88.

8. Regional cerebral blood flow in migraine

Jes Olesen, Tom Skyhøj Olsen, and Lars Friberg

Introduction

Until recently, both migraine with aura (classical migraine) and migraine without aura (common migraine) had been considered as clinical variants of the same underlying pathophysiological process, that is, a reduction of cerebral blood flow (CBF) followed by a hyperaemic phase during which the headache occurred (Wolff 1963).

This concept was questioned by Olesen *et al.* (1981*a*). According to their experience, migraine with aura was associated with alterations in regional cerebral blood flow (rCBF), while migraine without aura was associated with normal CBF. Hyperaemia has, however, been observed quite commonly by other investigators during attacks of migraine without aura. On the other hand, virtually all observers agree that rCBF is reduced during attacks of migraine with aura. Even if the concept of Olesen and co-workers may undergo modifications in the future, the available scientific data make it imperative to study migraine with aura and migraine without aura separately in the future, especially when CBF is concerned. This has also been acknowledged in the new international headache classification (Headache Classification Committee 1988).

Several methods for measuring rCBF are now available (Lassen and Friberg 1988). Each method and equipment has its own advantages and drawbacks. The xenon-133 (^{133}Xe) inhalation or injection techniques and the recording of rCBF with systems of stationary or rotating γ-radiation detectors have, until now, been the most useful methods for studying migraine patients. With these methods it is possible to repeat measurements before, during, and after a migraine attack in the same patient and, thereby, to elucidate the course of dynamic rCBF changes. Almost all the rCBF studies referred to below were done with the ^{133}Xe technique.

Migraine with aura (classical migraine)

CBF during migraine attacks with aura was measured quantitatively for the first time by Skinhøj and Paulson (1969) and Skinhøj (1973). Since then, and particularly during recent years, significant new knowledge has accumulated, and a fairly detailed picture has been established. Nevertheless, the basic findings of Skinhøj and Paulson still seem to hold true: the aura symptoms are associated with a reduction of rCBF. This is followed by increased rCBF and, finally, normalization. Although the neurological symptoms of the aura can be explained by cortical neuronal dysfunction in the low-flow area, the link between rCBF changes and headache is still unknown.

rCBF in the aura phase

Type, location and extent of rCBF changes   Studies of rCBF during the aura phase have all shown a reduction (Skinhøj and Paulson 1969; O'Brien 1971; Skinhøj 1973; Simard and Paulson 1973; Norris *et al.* 1975; Mathew *et al.* 1976; Edmeads 1977; Hachinski *et al.* 1977; Sakai and Meyer 1978; Juge and Gauthier 1980; Olesen *et al.* 1981*a*; Staehelin Jensen *et al.* 1981; Lauritzen *et al.* 1983*a*; Lauritzen and Olesen 1984; Herold *et al.* 1985; Skyhøj Olsen *et al.* 1987). Focal as well as global reductions in rCBF have been reported but investigations that used equipment with a high spatial resolution — for example, the 254 multidetector scintillation camera described by Sveinsdottir *et al.* (1977) — have all shown a focal start for the reduction in rCBF.

This was first made clear in the study of Olesen *et al.* (1981*a*) and was confirmed by Lauritzen *et al.* (1983*a*) and Skyhøj Olsen *et al.* (1987). Each of the 254 detectors in this camera measures rCBF in an area of approximately 1 cm^2 of the cortical mantle of the brain. It is possible to measure rCBF in the same patient up to ten times at 5–10 minute intervals. Up to now, measurements have been published from 25 patients who were followed from the pre-aura phase, during the aura phase, and into the headache phase (Olesen *et al.* 1981*a*; Lauritzen *et al.* 1983*a*; Skyhøj Olsen *et al.* 1987).

For unknown reasons a carotid angiography seems to provoke an attack of migraine with aura if the patient already suffers from this disease (Janzen *et al.* 1972). The rCBF studies quoted above were all preceded by a carotid arteriography. In most patients with such provoked attacks, aura symptoms occur within 30–60 minutes after puncture of the common carotid artery. This is the reason why it has been possible to measure the rCBF during the whole course of an attack of migraine with aura, including measurements just before the onset of the aura symptoms.

Essentially the same was observed in all 25 patients and the findings have been confirmed in a large unpublished series of studies by the present authors (Plate 8.1). A focal flow reduction first appeared in the posterior regions of the brain. The blood flow reduction gradually enlarged to involve larger and larger areas of the brain and, in some cases, finally involved the entire hemisphere. This explains why earlier investigators sometimes found focal and sometimes global reductions of flow in the aura phase. An attack of migraine with aura is a dynamically changing process, and the extent of hemispheric involvement is strongly time-dependent.

Focal diminution of flow has also been demonstrated in patients investigated with the single-photon-emission computed tomographic (SPECT) technique during spontaneous attacks (Plate 8.2; Lauritzen and Olesen 1984; Andersen et al. 1988). It is almost impossible, however, to demonstrate the initial, gradual enlargement of the low-flow area during spontaneous attacks, since this would require that the study be started before the flow changes were maximal, that is, within 15–30 minutes of onset of the aura symptoms. The spontaneous attacks were studied at an average of three hours after onset, and never earlier than 30 minutes after onset.

The gradual enlargement of the low-flow area — denoted as 'spreading oligaemia' by Olesen et al. (1981a) — reportedly progresses at approximately 2–3 mm min^{-1} in the posterior-to-anterior direction, but this calculated value must be taken with caution (Lauritzen et al. 1983a). A focal low-flow area may, however, also appear in the central part of the frontal region (Lauritzen et al. 1983a). This low-flow area spreads with the same speed in all directions so that nearly all the frontal lobe may be affected by spreading oligaemia. A similar spread of an oligaemic area has been observed after 'Leão's spreading depression' in experimental animals.

The localization and the mode of progression of the reduction in rCBF — which does not respect vascular territories — definitely rules out the possibility that classical migraine can be due to spasm in one or more individual large arteries (Olesen et al. 1981a; Lauritzen et al. 1983a; Skyhøj Olsen et al. 1987). This conclusion accords with findings from most angiograms taken in patients during attacks of migraine with aura. Constriction or occlusion of angiographically visible arteries has only very rarely been observed (Symonds 1952; Connor 1962; Pearce and Foster 1965; Skinhøj 1973; Boisen 1975; Lauritzen et al. 1983a; Skyhøj Olsen et al. 1987). Even in cases where a rCBF study — which documented reduced flow during the aura — was followed by angiography, no occlusions or vasospasms were identified (Skinhøj 1973; Norris et al. 1975; Hachinski et al. 1977). However, the retrograde flow of the contrast agent from the carotid territory into the vertebrobasilar territory has been observed, which indicates an increase of blood pressure in the carotid territory relative to the blood pressure in the vertebrobasilar territory (Skinhøj 1973; Norris et al. 1975; Hachinski et al. 1977). In other words, there is an increased vascular resistance in the carotid territory. Arteriolar vasoconstriction is, therefore, a likely explanation for the observed rCBF reduction.

Olesen et al. (1981a) described a focal hyperaemia, which preceded the focal spreading oligaemia, in three of six patients. This phenomenon had not been observed previously, and has been noted in only one later series

(Friberg *et al.* 1987*a*), which used the same technique. Its significance is therefore uncertain and has to await verification in further studies.

In three patients with a history of migraine with aura, who were investigated with carotid angiography and the ^{133}Xe injection technique, Friberg *et al.* (1987*a*) observed that the attacks were associated with the development of focal hypoperfusion in the frontal lobe. The low-flow areas subsequently enlarged and spread backwards to involve the precentral and postcentral regions. This is the first published report in which spreading oligaemia did not originate in the posterior part of the brain. Interestingly, none of these three patients had visual symptoms during the aura.

Methodological problems in quantifying rCBF reduction with ^{133}Xe *techniques* The degree of the blood-flow reduction in migraine attacks has been the subject of much discussion. The question has been: is the blood-flow reduction of sufficient magnitude to cause ischaemia? Controversies about this are undoubtedly caused by the phenomenon of scattered radiation, also called Compton scatter — an inborn source of error when ^{133}Xe is used for measuring CBF.

Compton scatter involves the interaction between an incident photon and an orbital electron. As a result of the interaction, the photon changes direction (with decreased energy). In practice, this means that part of the radiation emerging from the ^{133}Xe isotope is recorded by detectors at a distance from the place where the γ-radiation originates (scattered radiation; see Fig. 8.1). The detectors placed over a low-flow area, as in migraine with aura, do not only detect radiation from isotope actually deposited (and washed out) in the low-flow area, but it has been estimated that up to 50 per cent of the counts might originate from isotope deposited (and washed out) in areas with a higher flow (Skyhøj Olsen *et al.* 1981). The washout curves obtained from low-flow areas are the result of washout of isotope actually deposited in the low-flow area (and representative of 'true' flow) as well as the result of 'washout' of Compton-scattered radiation from the surroundings, thus causing an overestimation that is proportional to the flow in the surroundings and inversely proportional to the 'true' flow in the low-flow area (Skyhøj Olsen *et al.* 1981).

It follows that determination of the blood-flow reduction in attacks of migraine with aura can only be semiquantitative. The only absolutely certain statement is that CBF in the low-flow area is even lower than the values actually recorded. Thus, if the measured flow is at ischaemic levels, the presence of ischaemia cannot be disputed. This is actually shown in the low-flow regions in Plate 8.1.

The degree of blood flow reduction Until recently, the CBF studies in migraine with aura have had too few patients to allow an evaluation of the

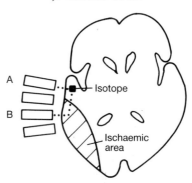

FIG. 8.1. A schematic demonstration of the effect of Compton scatter on rCBF recordings. Isotope from a normally perfused area is recorded by detector A, and the measurement reflects the true blood flow in the area. Scattered radiation from the same area is deflected and recorded by detector B. This Compton scatter is washed out at normal rate, since rCBF is normal at the site of its origin, but it is recorded as if it came from a low-flow area. All detectors receive Compton-scattered radiation. If rCBF beneath detector B was normal, Compton scatter would not significantly influence the wash-out curves recorded by this detector. If, however, true rCBF beneath detector B is focally reduced, as indicated on the figure, the contribution of Compton scatter to the wash-out curve gives rise to an overestimation of rCBF in the low-flow area, because the Compton scatter comes from an area with a higher blood flow and, therefore, also with a higher wash-out rate.

presence or absence of ischaemia in the low-flow areas. Nevertheless, in the reports of Skinhøj and Paulson (1969), Skinhøj (1973), Simard and Paulson (1973), Hachinski et al. (1977), and Olesen et al. (1981a), cases were reported in which rCBF approached ischaemic levels critical for metabolism. Olesen et al. (1981a) investigated six patients, and Lauritzen et al. (1983a) seven patients, with the intracarotid injection technique. rCBF reduction in the low-flow areas averaged 35 per cent and 25 per cent, respectively. With ^{133}Xe inhalation and SPECT, Lauritzen and Olesen (1984), in eight patients, found rCBF reductions averaging 17 per cent. As argued above, the true reductions must have been greater than those directly measured.

Skyhøj Olsen et al. (1987) attempted to estimate the degree of focal blood-flow reduction, when taking the Compton scatter effect into consideration. This was made possible because a relatively large series of CBF studies in patients during migraine with aura was available — that is, 42 individual investigations in 11 patients who developed focal low-flow areas during attacks. The estimated 'true' focal blood-flow reduction averaged 50 per cent or more, corresponding to a level of 20–25 ml 100 g^{-1} min^{-1} (Fig. 8.2).

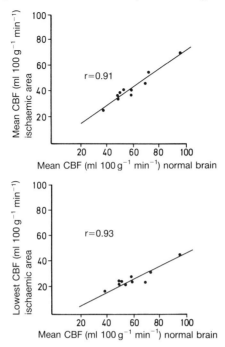

FIG. 8.2. Diagram demonstrating the influence of Compton scatter on rCBF measurements in low-flow areas of patients with classical migraine (with aura). CBF in normally perfused areas of the brain is plotted against CBF in the ischaemic low-flow areas. CBF in the ischaemic low-flow areas is proportional to CBF in the surrounding non-affected brain tissue, as a reflection of the overestimation of CBF in the low-flow areas that is provided by the Compton-scattered radiation. *Top*: Mean CBF values in the low-flow areas. *Below*: The lowest values in the low-flow areas measured farthest away from the normally perfused areas. These values represent the best estimate of CBF in the low-flow areas, as the effect of Compton scatter decreases with increasing distance from the normally perfused areas. Note that rCBF in eight patients is between 16 and 25 ml 100 g^{-1}min^{-1}. (Reproduced from Skyhøj Olsen *et al.* 1984, by courtesy of the editors of *Acta Neurologica Scandinavica*.)

In patients undergoing carotid endarterectomy, the amplitude of electroencephalographic (EEG) waves diminished when rCBF fell below 23 ml 100 g^{-1} min^{-1} (Trojaborg and Boysen 1973). In awake monkeys with experimental occlusion of the middle cerebral artery, neurological deficits appear when flow decreases below 23 ml 100 g^{-1} min^{-1} (Jones *et al.* 1981). Yet, tissue viability is maintained until rCBF falls to less than 10 to 12 ml 100 g^{-1} min^{-1} (Morawetz *et al.* 1978). Below 10 ml 100 g^{-1} min^{-1}, tissue necrosis ensues within 2–3 hours (Morawetz *et al.* 1978). Thus, with flow in the range 10–23 ml 100 g^{-1} min^{-1}, the brain tissue may be structurally intact, although the flow is insufficient for normal cortical activity.

Friberg *et al.* (1987*a*) in their report of 'frontal migraine' observed that the washout curves recorded in the low-flow areas were non-linear in the semi-logarithmic plot. A fluctuating slope indicated severe ischaemia that alternated with short periods of hyperaemia of between 20 and 60 seconds. However, the average flow, calculated on the basis of the slope of the one-minute washout curves, was always reduced. The explanation suggested was a transient constriction of the arterioles that alternated with short episodes of vasodilatation — a state denoted as 'vascular tone instability.' Preliminary statistical analysis of washout curves from patients with 'spreading oligaemia' in the posterior part of the brain also seems to reveal vascular tone instability (Fig. 8.3; Friberg and Skyhøj Olsen 1989). The pathophysiological significance of this phenomenon is unknown. It is not seen between attacks or in non-affected areas during attacks. It may be a primary pathophysiological mechanism or it may be secondary to another pathophysiological event such as 'Leão's spreading depression' or a primary arteriolar vasoconstriction.

It is our opinion that rCBF is reduced to ischaemic levels during most attacks. This does not necessarily mean, however, that the blood supply is insufficient for metabolic demands since cerebral metabolism may also be depressed. Further studies of metabolism and blood flow with positron emission tomography (PET) are necessary to answer this question. Owing to the transient nature of the symptoms of migraine with aura, in relation to the long time needed for recording the complex PET measurements, the technique has not yet been used to study the onset of an attack. Herold *et al.* (1985) used PET measurements to study a patient with classical migraine during the headache phase, 2.5 hours after onset of the aura while the patient was still experiencing left-sided neurological deficits. CBF was reduced in the temporo-occipital region, but the oxygen extraction was correspondingly increased and balanced the CBF reduction. Hence, CMR_{O_2} (i.e. oxygen metabolism) was normal and neither *metabolic depression* nor *ischaemia* was found. The measurements could, thus, not explain why the patient had neurological deficits. Different results might have been obtained earlier in the attack.

Sachs *et al.* (1986) studied regional cerebral glucose metabolism ($rCMR_{glu}$) in five patients with common or classical migraine during headaches induced by reserpine. They found a decrease in $rCMR_{glu}$ of between 10 and 30 per cent in both types of patient. Surprisingly, and in contradiction to studies with ^{133}Xe and above PET study by Herold *et al.* (1985) no laterality was apparent. The cause of the reduced glucose metabolism — whether ischaemia or metabolic depression — was not found.

Flow 1

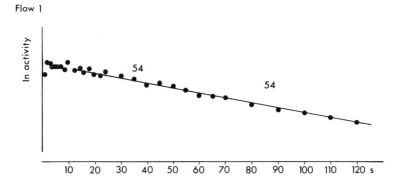

Flow 4

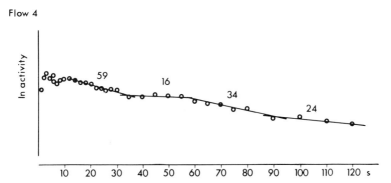

FIG. 8.3. Logarithmically transformed clearance curves from a patient with an attack of migraine with aura. Both recordings were done with the same posteriorly situated detector. *Upper plot*: shows the linear wash-out rate during the first flow measurement at a time when there was a normal rCBF distribution and no symptoms. *Lower plot*: shows the unstable clearance curve when a low-flow region and aura symptoms developed at the time of the fourth measurement. Figures above each part of the suggested linear components indicate the blood-flow value calculated from that component. The figure illustrates the phenomenon of 'cerebrovascular tone instability' in the low-flow region. It is seen that blood flow for short intervals is reduced to very low values–even lower than the calculated mean blood flow values as they appear on the rCBF pictures (Plate 8.1).

Although it remains uncertain whether a metabolic depression or an arteriolar constriction is the primary event, it is obvious that cerebral cortical function is disturbed. This was also shown by two EEG studies performed simultaneously with CBF measurements during attacks of migraine with aura (M. Lauritzen, B. Stigsby and T. Skyhøj Olsen, unpublished observations). Both studies revealed the development of focal, slow-frequency activity corresponding to the low-flow areas.

A delay of 5–10 minutes between the appearance of low flow and the occurrence of symptoms was taken as an argument against flow reduction being the cause of the aura symptoms (Lauritzen *et al.* 1983*a*). However, the CBF reduction usually originates in posterior temporoparietal regions where cortical dysfunction may be undetectable clinically if the symptoms (such as aphasia, apraxia, agnosia, and dysfunction of other higher cortical functions) are mild. Furthermore, the severity of the neurological deficits parallels the CBF reduction when CBF falls below 23 ml 100 g^{-1} min^{-1} (Jones *et al.* 1981). If rCBF during an attack of migraine with aura falls to 23 ml 100 g^{-1} min^{-1}, or slightly lower, the deficits would be mild and, therefore, hard to detect.

Vascular reactivity   Vascular responses to different agents are important therapeutically and may elucidate the basic mechanisms underlying migraine with aura. Thus, the finding of a normal vascular reactivity (the responses to changes of Pa_{CO_2} and blood pressure) in a low-flow area indicates that the vessels are unaffected by the disease process. If vascular reactivity, on the other hand, is impaired or abolished, this speaks in favour of vascular mechanisms being behind the attack.

There is no consensus in published work about vascular reactivity in the low-flow areas. Simard and Paulson (1973) investigated one patient with the intra-arterial injection method during an attack of migraine with aura. rCBF did not react to changes of Pa_{CO_2}. (Flow was globally reduced in this patient so that Compton scatter could not influence the measurement.) Unfortunately, autoregulation was not studied. Sakai and Meyer (1979) found an impaired response to Pa_{CO_2} as well as to changes of systemic blood pressure in patients investigated with the ^{133}Xe inhalation technique and with stationary detectors. Lauritzen *et al.* (1983*b*) concluded from their studies with the ^{133}Xe intracarotid injection technique that autoregulation was normal while the Pa_{CO_2} response was reduced but not abolished (Tables 8.1 and 8.2). This was taken to indicate that the vessels were not primarily affected by the disease process. It is questionable, however, whether it is possible to use ^{133}Xe techniques to measure cerebrovascular reactivity in attacks of migraine with aura. Skyhøj Olsen *et al.* (1986) re-evaluated the results of Lauritzen *et al.* (1983*b*), by taking Compton scatter into account. CBF in the low-flow areas did not change after blood pressure was increased by about 20 mmHg. This, however, does not necessarily mean that autoregulation was normal. It has recently been calculated that if true flow in the low-flow area is in the range 20–25 ml 100 g^{-1} min^{-1}, with the normal flow being about 50 ml 100 g^{-1} min^{-1}, then even a fairly large hypocapnia-induced blood-flow reduction in the low-flow area cannot be detected at all (T. Skyhøj Olsen and N.A. Lassen, unpublished observation). It is therefore not possible, with the available techniques, to determine whether vascular

TABLE 8.1. *Regional cerebral blood flow during classical migraine attacks: effect of hypertension**

Patient no.	Mean arterial blood pressure (mmHg)			CBF in hypoperfused area (ml 100 g^{-1} min^{-1})		CBF in normally perfused area (ml 100 g^{-1} min^{-1})		$P_{A\,CO_2}$ (mmHg)	
	Rest	Test	Change	Rest	Test	Rest	Test	Rest	Test
384	128	140	12	34	34	53	51	45	44
449	113	142	29	39	34	55	49	44	41
450	113	150	37	35	36	51	54	43	43
452	88	111	23	37	40	58	64	37	37
457	100	125	25	33	35	55	56	40	40
470	105	135	30	30	38	50	54	46	47
Mean ± standard deviation			24 ± 7						

*Hypertension was induced by intravenous infusion of angiotensin. CBF, cerebral blood flow; $P_{A\,CO_2}$, arterial carbon dioxide tension. (Reproduced from Lauritzen *et al.* 1983b, by courtesy of the editors of *Annals of Neurology*.)

TABLE 8.2. *Regional cerebral blood flow during classical migraine attacks: effect of hyperventilation*

Patient no.	$P_{A_{CO_2}}$ (mmHg)			CBF in hypoperfused area (ml 100 g^{-1} min^{-1})					CBF in normally perfused area (ml 100 g^{-1} min^{-1})					Mean cerebral blood pressure (mmHg)	
	Rest	Test	Change	Rest	Test	Change	k	Reactivity (%)	Rest	Test	Change	k	Reactivity (%)	Rest	Test
384	44	39	5	34	29	5	0.032	3.3	53	36	17	0.077	8.0	128	110
449	42	27	15	34	24	10	0.022	2.2	49	28	21	0.038	3.9	113	106
	41	27	14	35	23	12	0.030	3.0	49	25	24	0.048	4.9	113	119
450	42	34	8	37	28	9	0.035	3.5	56	34	22	0.062	6.4	113	120
452	38	26	12	34	26	8	0.022	2.2	53	27	26	0.056	5.8	88	100
457	40	25	15	33	20	13	0.033	3.4	56	24	32	0.056	5.8	20	100
470	46	39	7	30	28	2	0.001	1.0	50	37	13	0.043	4.4	110	110
Mean ± standard deviation			14 ± 1					2.7 ± 0.93					5.6 ± 1.37		

k, slope of the natural logarithm CBF:$P_{A_{CO_2}}$ relationship; other abbreviations as in Table 1.
(Reproduced from Lauritzen *et al.* 1983*a*, by courtesy of the editors of *Annals of Neurology*.)

reactivity (autoregulation as well as Pa_{CO_2} response) is preserved, impaired, or abolished.

Functional tests like speech, reading, listening, and armwork elicit increased CBF in specific areas of the brain. During attacks of migraine with aura these activation procedures were not accompanied by the usual increase of CBF in the low-flow areas, whereas a normal, focal CBF increase was observed in the non-affected parts of the brain (Olesen *et al.* 1981*a*; Lauritzen *et al.* 1983*b*). Whether this is caused by a primary arteriolar vasoconstriction or a metabolic depression of the brain in the low-flow areas remains to be settled.

rCBF in the headache phase

Since Wolff forwarded the theory of migraine as a cerebrovascular disorder, a hyperaemic phase that follows the ischaemic phase has been accepted as the cause of the headache. Several investigators have demonstrated focal or global hyperaemia in the headache phase of patients having migraine with aura — a finding considered to confirm Wolff's vascular hypothesis (Skinhøj 1973; Norris *et al.* 1976; Sakai and Meyer 1978). The concept was challenged first by Olesen *et al.* (1981*a*) and later by Lauritzen *et al.* (1983*a*), Lauritzen and Olesen (1984) and Skyhøj Olsen *et al.* (1987*a*). They reported a large number of patients who had headache, nausea, and even vomiting, while CBF remained depressed. Hyperaemia was not observed, particularly not at the onset of the headache. Lauritzen and Olesen (1984) followed patients from the end of the aura phase and 4–6 hours into the headache phase, but they observed hyperaemia in only two of 10 patients. Two patients studied with PET during the headache phase had no hyperaemia (Herold *et al.* 1985).

The 'missing link' between the conflicting observation of hyperaemia by the early investigators and the observations of our research group in Copenhagen seems now to be found. Gullichsen and Enevoldsen (1984) studied CBF in three patients during migraine with aura, 24 hours after its onset, with the ^{133}Xe inhalation method and with 32 stationary detectors. A focal hyperaemia was found the day after the attack in these three patients. One patient was even seen in the aura phase, where a focal blood-flow reduction occurred. Fifteen hours later, a pronounced hyperaemia was seen in the very same area. Andersen *et al.* (1988) followed seven patients by ^{133}Xe inhalation and SPECT methods, from the end of the aura phase (30 minutes to three hours after its onset) into the headache phase (after 3–5 hours and 6–8 hours) and in the post-headache phase (after 20–24 hours). Initially a focal low-flow area was present posteriorly in the relevant hemisphere. After 3–5 hours, three patients had developed hyperaemia in the previous low-flow area. Two patients still had a pronounced low-flow area but at examination after 6–8 hours, these two patients had also developed hyperaemia in the previously oligaemic area. After 20–24 hours, CBF had normalized in three patients while three others still showed a slight focal hyperaemia. CBF was normal in all after one week. This study clearly shows that timing is crucial to demonstrating hyperaemia during attacks of migraine with aura. Headache began during the low-flow period, and hyperaemia often persisted after the headache had subsided. A relationship between the severity of the aura symptoms, severity of ischaemia, and degree as well as duration of hyperaemia was indicated.

Andersen et al. (1988) suggested that hyperaemia may reflect previous arteriolar vasoconstriction (reactive hyperaemia). It remains to be studied whether hyperaemia is associated with subclinical cortical dysfunction (for example, low-frequency activity on EEG) and why it is so long-lasting.

Migraine aura without headache

Patients sometimes experience aura symptoms that are not followed by headache. If these symptoms are typical (for example, migrainous scintillations and paraesthesias), and if they gradually spread and disappear, and last 15–30 minutes, the clinical diagnosis is easy. In patients without a history of migraine or if the aura symptoms present atypically (for example, suddenly), the episodes may mimic transient ischaemic attacks (TIA) or minor strokes. It is, of course, important to distinguish thromboembolic TIA/stroke, from migrainous TIA/stroke because the treatment, prophylaxis and prognosis are completely different. In a report of 120 cases with 'late-life migraine accompaniments as a cause of unexplained transient ischemic attacks', Fisher (1980) has penetratingly discussed these clinical problems. Friberg et al. (1987b) reported the development of flow changes typical for migraine with aura during rCBF measurements with the ^{133}Xe intracarotid injection method in six patients admitted to hospital with a diagnosis of TIA or minor strokes. In association with the rCBF changes, they developed symptoms mimicking the TIAs or aggravation of minor stroke symptoms. All patients recovered completely. None of the patients developed headache. This finding may indicate that the strokes/TIA of these patients who had no history of migraine, nevertheless were migrainous or, alternatively, that angiography and rCBF investigation may provoke 'spreading oligaemia' in susceptible persons. Perhaps part of the normal population has a lower threshold for developing 'spreading oligaemia', including some individuals without classical migraine and even without a family history of it.

Migrainous infarction

Migraine auras may occasionally be permanent (Connor 1962; Pearce and Foster 1965; Boisen 1975; Bousser et al. 1980; Bickerstaff 1982; Bartleson 1984; Skjeldal et al. 1986; Skyhøj Olsen et al. 1987). Focal low-frequency activity on EEG, and CT-verified cerebral infarcts have been reported in such patients (Slatter 1968; Bousser *et al.* 1980; Bickerstaff 1982; Bartleson 1984; Skyhøj Olsen *et al.* 1987). Such deficits and lesions may be caused by severe ischaemia, itself caused by the spreading migrainous oligaemia. The rCBF, in patients with cerebral infarcts that developed during attacks of migraine with aura, does not differ from the rCBF in patients with thromboembolic stroke: that is, there is ischaemic low flow in the infarcted area with decreased CMR_{O_2} and decreased oxygen extraction (Bousser *et al.* 1980; Skjeldal *et al.* 1986).

Migraine without aura (common migraine)

While there seems to be general agreement concerning rCBF changes during migraine attacks with aura, this is certainly not true for migraine without aura. Our research group in Copenhagen has found normal CBF and an absence of focal abnormalities, but other investigators have described cerebral hyperaemia — focal as well as global.

Olesen *et al.* (1981*b*) studied rCBF in eight patients in whom migraine without aura was induced by ingestion of red wine. Three were studied with the ^{133}Xe inhalation method and with 16 stationary detectors, four were studied with single photon tomography (SPECT), and one patient with the intracarotid injection technique. CBF was studied in the resting, headache-free state before and after ingestion of red wine, at the very onset of the attacks and during the fully developed attacks. A slight global increase in the observed CBF was not significant. It was suggested that migraine with aura and migraine without aura might be two different diseases, and should be considered separately, particularly in regard to CBF. Lauritzen and Olesen (1984) confirmed these findings by studying, with SPECT, 12 patients during spontaneous attacks of migraine without aura. The measurements were taken at an average of seven hours (range 3–20 hours) after onset of the attacks. In none of these patients were focal or global CBF changes observed. Again, the CBF was globally but non-significantly increased in the headache phase. Herold *et al.* (1985) studied one patient with PET, three hours after onset of a migraine without aura. CBF and metabolism were normal, and no difference between the two hemispheres was observed.

Skinhøj (1973) studied four patients whose type of migraine was not clearly described with the intracarotid ^{133}Xe injection method. No focal abnormalities were observed, but three of the patients exhibited global hyperaemia during the attack. Sakai and Meyer (1978) studied rCBF with ^{133}Xe inhalation and found that the CBF increased for up to 48 hours. In headache-free periods the CBF was normal, as also reported by Olesen *et al.* (1981*b*) and Lauritzen and Olesen (1984). Juge and Gauthier (1980) studied 23 patients, within 48 hours of their attacks, with ^{133}Xe inhalation and stationary detectors. Compared to a control group, the CBF was increased during the attacks of migraine without aura.

It should be kept in mind that the presence of increased CBF during an attack does not necessarily indicate that hyperaemia is involved in the pathophysiological process that leads to headache. In fact, hyperaemia has definitely been ruled out as the cause of headache in migraine with aura, as discussed above, because the headache always starts in the low-flow period, hours before the hyperaemia, and the hyperaemia may be present when the headache is over. Hyperaemia during attacks of migraine without aura may well be secondary to pain, arousal, and discomfort during the investigation (Ingvar *et al.* 1975). Whether migraine without aura is associated with and/or caused by cerebral hyperaemia could perhaps be clarified by comparing the CBF during attacks with that during other painful events.

Gelmers (1982) reported a focal CBF reduction in two patients during attacks of migraine without aura. Both studies were performed with the intracarotid injection technique and a 254-detector camera. In both patients, the low-flow areas appeared in the posterior part of the hemisphere, but without the gradual spread that is usually seen in classical migraine with aura. One patient was a known sufferer from common migraine, while the other had never had migraine. This is the only known report of focal low-flow areas developing during attacks of migraine without aura. In one patient the low-flow area was, indeed, very small, and considerably smaller than those seen by our research group. The other patient had a large low-flow area, but the rCBF was apparently reduced by only about 10 per cent. It is a matter of definition whether this should be considered abnormally low. CBF in the posterior parts of the brain is usually about 10 per cent below the mean CBF (Larsen *et al.* 1978).

Vascular reactivity during attacks of migraine without aura has been evaluated only by Sakai and Meyer (1978, 1979), who used ^{133}Xe inhalation and stationary detectors. The response to arterial P_{CO_2} was reduced during headache but no side-to-side differences were found. By 48 hours or more after the attacks, the response to hypercapnia was excessive while the response to hypocapnia was normal. Autoregulation was normal in the two patients.

References

Andersen, A.R., Friberg, L., Skyhøj Olsen, T., and Olsen, J. (1988). SPECT demonstration of delayed hyperemia following hypoperfusion in classic migraine. *Archives of Neurology*, **45**, 154–9.

Bartleson, J.D. (1984). Transient and persistent neurological manifestations of migraine. *Stroke*, **15**, 383–6.

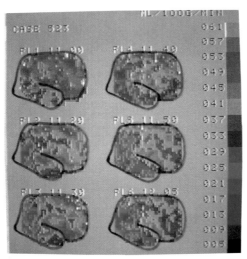

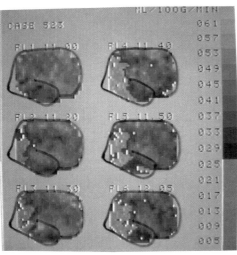

PLATE 8.1 One patient (case 523) studied with the intracarotid ^{133}Xe injection technique, and with 254 stationary detectors.

Upper picture. On the scale to the right, blood flow values in ml per 100 g of brain tissue per minute are translated into colours. Blue represents a low flow; red represents a high flow; yellow and green are intermediate. Regional cerebral blood flow (rCBF) was measured six times at 10–20 minute intervals; the actual time of the measurement is indicated above each figure. The first rCBF study is shown at the top left, and the last at the bottom right. Note the blue colour (low flow) beginning posteriorly and spreading anteriorly. A hypoperfusion developed in the posterior part of the brain during a classical migraine attack.

Lower picture. Same as above, except that for illustrative reasons the colour scale has been changed to a grey tone, and the regions with a flow of less than 25 ml per 100 g per minute appear pink. In the pink areas, the rCBF is, without doubt, around or below the ischaemic threshold.

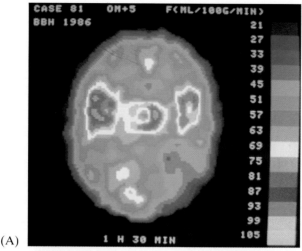

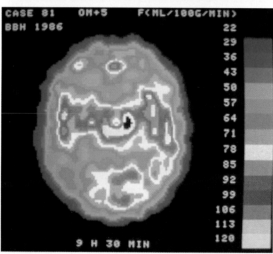

PLATE 8.2 Regional cerebral blood flow (rCBF) tomograms obtained with ^{133}Xe inhalation and single-photon-emission computed tomography (SPECT). rCBF values are translated into colours on the scale to the right. Blue represents a low flow; red/white represent a high flow; green and yellow are intermediate. Horizontal sections are shown, 5 cm above the orbitomeatal line. The frontal lobes are at the top, and the occipital lobes at the bottom of each illustration; the right side is shown on the right (that is, the brain is viewed from above). The blue rim surrounding the coloured area is outside the brain. Illustrations A–C are from one patient (case 81) and illustration D is from another patient (case 35). (A) First rCBF measurement, obtained 1.5 hours after appearance of first aura symptoms during a spontaneous classical migraine attack (case 81). During this measurement there were left-sided neurological symptoms: homonymous scotoma, numbness, and paraesthesia of the left hand and the left side of the tongue. These symptoms were in regression, and a right-sided throbbing headache gradually developed, accompanied by nausea and

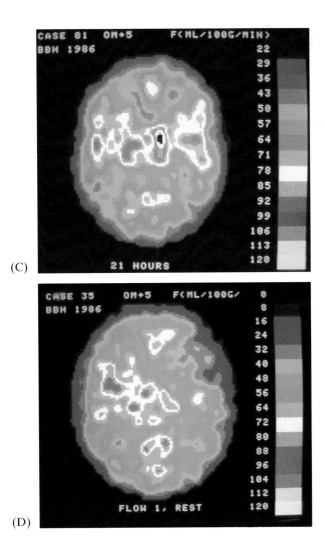

(C)

(D)

vomiting. The rCBF measurement showed severe hypoperfusion of the posterior part of the right hemisphere. (B) Second measurement, 9.5 hours after the start of the symptoms. At the time of measurement the severe, throbbing headache had disappeared, leaving a mild, right-sided, residual headache. The rCBF picture showed that the region previously hypoperfused was now replaced by a focal hyperaemia (tardive hyperaemia). (C) Third measurement, 21 hours after the start of the symptoms. All symptoms were gone, and the patient was feeling well. A normal rCBF picture was now restored. (D) This illustration was obtained from a stroke patient (case 35) with CT-verified infarction in the right frontal lobe, due to thrombo-embolic vascular occlusion. It is included in order to illustrate the difficulty in estimating the exact flow in regions of low or nil flow with the ^{133}Xe SPECT method. A comparison with illustration A shows that it is not possible to distinguish between a low, focal flow in an infarct region and a hypoperfusion that appears transiently during a (classical) migraine attack with aura.

Bickerstaff, E.R. (1982). Complicated migraine. The 1982 Sandoz Foundation Lecture. In *Progress in migraine research 2*, (ed. F. Clifford Rose), pp. 83–101. Pitman, London.

Boisen, E. (1975). Strokes in migraine: Report on seven strokes associated with severe migraine attacks. *Danish Medical Bulletin*, **22**, 100–6.

Bousser, M.G., Baron, J.C., Iba-Zizen, M.T., Comar, D., Cabanis, E., and Castaigne, P. (1980). Migrainous cerebral infarction: A tomographic study of cerebral blood flow and oxygen extraction fraction with the oxygen-15 inhalation technique. *Stroke*, **11**, 145–8.

Connor, R.C.R. (1962). Complicated migraine: A study of permanent neurological and visual defects caused by migraine. *Lancet*, **ii**, 1072–5.

Edmeads, J. (1977). Cerebral blood flow in migraine. *Headache*, **17**, 148–52.

Fisher, C.M. (1980). Late-life migraine accompaniments as a cause of unexplained transient ischemic attacks. *Canadian Journal of Neurological Sciences*, **7**, 9–17.

Friberg, L. and Skyhøj Olsen, T. (1989). Rapid extreme oscillations of focal cerebral blood flow during the aura phase of migraine. In *Further advances in headache research*, (ed. F. Clifford Rose), pp. 163–8. Smith-Gordon, London.

Friberg, L., Skyhøj Olsen, T., Roland, P.E., and Lassen, N.A. (1987*a*). Focal ischemia caused by instability of cerebrovascular tone during attacks of hemiplegic migraine. *Brain*, **110**, 917–34.

Friberg, L., Skyhøj Olsen, T., and Lassen, N.A. (1987*b*). Cerebrovascular tone instability causing focal ischemia in TIA and stroke patients. In *Controversies in EIAB for cerebral ischemia*, (ed. R. Gagliardi and L. Benvenuti), pp. 87–93. Monduzzi Editore, Bologna.

Gelmers, H.J. (1982). Common migraine attacks preceded by focal hyperemia and parietal oligemia in the rCBF pattern. *Cephalalgia*, **2**, 29–32.

Gullichsen, G. and Enevoldsen, E. (1984). Prolonged changes in rCBF following attacks of migraine accompagnée. *Acta Neurologica Scandinavica*, **69** (Suppl. 98), 270–1.

Hachinski, V.C., Olesen, J., Norris, J.W., Larsen, B., Enevoldsen, E., and Lassen, N.A. (1977). Cerebral hemodynamics in migraine. *Canadian Journal of Neurological Sciences*, **4**, 245–9.

Headache Classification Committee of the International Headache Society (Jes Olesen, chairman). (1988). Classification and diagnostic criteria for headache disorders, cranial neuralgias and facial pain. *Cephalalgia*, **8**, Suppl. 7, 1–96.

Herold, S., Gibbs, J.M., Jones, A.K.P., Brooks, D.J., Frackowiak, R.S.J., and Legg, N.J. (1985). Oxygen metabolism in migraine. *Journal of Cerebral Blood Flow and Metabolism*, **5**, Suppl. 1, 445–6.

Ingvar, D.H., Rosen, I., and Elmqvist, D. (1975). Effects of somatosensory stimulation upon rCBF. In *Blood flow and metabolism in the brain*, (ed. A.M. Harper, W.B. Jennett, J.D. Miller, and J.O. Rowan) pp. 14.29–14.32. Churchill Livingstone, Edinburgh.

Janzen, R., Tanzer, A., Zschocke, S., and Dieckmann, H. (1972). Postangiographische Spätreaktionen der Hirngefässe bei Migräne-Kranken. *Zeitschrift fuer Neurologie*, **201**, 24–42.

Jones, T.H. *et al.* (1981). Thresholds of focal cerebral ischemia in awake monkeys. *Journal of Neurosurgery*, **54**, 773–82.

Juge, O. and Gauthier, G. (1980). Mésures de debit sanguin cérébral régional (DSCR) par inhalation de Xenon 133: applications cliniques. *Bulletin der Schweizerischen Akademie der Medizinischen Wissenschaften*, **36**, 101–15.

Larsen, B., Skinhøj, E., and Lassen, N.A. (1978). Variations in regional cortical blood flow in the right and left hemisphere during automatic speech. *Brain*, **101**, 193–202.

Lassen, N.A. and Friberg, L. (1988). Methods for measurement of regional cerebral blood flow. In *Basic mechanisms of headache*, (ed. J. Olesen and L. Edvinsson) pp. 61–8. Elsevier, Amsterdam.

Lauritzen, M. and Olesen, J. (1984). Regional cerebral blood flow during migraine attacks by Xenon-133 inhalation and emission tomography. *Brain*, **107**, 447–61.

Lauritzen, M., Skyhøj Olsen, T., Lassen, N.A., and Paulson, O.B. (1983*a*). The changes of regional cerebral blood flow during the course of classical migraine attacks. *Annals of Neurology*, **13**, 633–41.

Lauritzen, M., Skyhøj Olsen, T., Lassen, N.A., and Paulson, O.B. (1983*b*). The regulation of regional cerebral blood flow during and between migraine attacks. *Annals of Neurology*, **14**, 569–72.

Mathew, N.T., Hrastnik, F., and Meyer, J.S. (1976). Regional cerebral blood flow in the diagnosing of vascular headache. *Headache*, **15**, 252–60.

Morawetz, R.B., DeGirolami, U., Ojemann, R.G., Marcoux, F.W., and Crowell, R.M. (1978). Cerebral blood flow determined by hydrogen clearance during middle cerebral artery occlusion in unanesthetized monkeys. *Stroke*, **9**, 143–9.

Norris, J.W., Hachinski, V.C., and Cooper, P.W. (1975). Changes in cerebral blood flow during a migraine attack. *British Medical Journal*, **3**, 676–7.

Norris, J.W., Hachinski, V.C., and Cooper, P.W. (1976). Cerebral blood flow changes in cluster headache. *Acta Neurologica Scandinavica*, **54**, 371–4.

O'Brien, M.D. (1971). Cerebral blood changes in migraine. *Headache*, **10**, 139–43.

Olesen, J., Larsen, B., and Lauritzen, M. (1981*a*). Focal hyperemia followed by spreading oligemia and impaired activation of rCBF in classic migraine. *Annals of Neurology*, **9**, 344–52.

Olesen, J., Tfelt-Hansen, P., Henriksen, L., and Larsen, B. (1981*b*). The common migraine attack may not be initiated by cerebral ischemia. *Lancet*, **ii**, 438–40.

Pearce, J.M.S., Foster, J.B. (1965). An investigation of complicated migraine. *Neurology*, **15**, 323–40.

Sachs, H., Wolf, A., Russell, J.A.G., and Christman, D.R. (1986). Effect of reserpine on regional cerebral glucose metabolism in control and migraine subjects. *Archives of Neurology*, **43**, 1117–23.

Sakai, F. and Meyer, J.S. (1978). Regional cerebral hemodynamics during migraine and cluster headache measured by the 133-Xe inhalation method. *Headache*, **18**, 122–32.

Sakai, F. and Meyer, J.S. (1979). Abnormal cerebrovascular reactivity in patients with migraine and cluster headache. *Headache*, **19**, 257–66.

Simard, D. and Paulson, O.B. (1973). Cerebral vasomotor paralysis during migraine attack. *Archives of Neurology*, **29**, 207–9.

Skinhøj, E. (1973). Hemodynamic studies within the brain during migraine. *Archives of Neurology*, **29**, 95–8.

Skinhøj, E. and Paulson, O.B. (1969). Regional cerebral blood flow in internal carotid distribution during migraine attack. *British Medical Journal*, **3**, 569–70.

Skjeldal, O.H., Russell, D., Gjerstad, L., Nyberg-Hansen, E., and Rottwelt, K. (1986). Complicated migraine: CT, angiographic and cerebral blood flow findings. *Uppsala Journal of Medical Sciences*, Suppl. **43**, 86 (abstract).

Skyhøj Olsen, T., Larsen, B., Bech Skriver, E., Enevoldsen, E., and Lassen, N.A.

(1981). Focal cerebral ischemia measured by the intra-arterial 133-Xenon method. Limitations of 2-dimensional blood flow measurements. *Stroke*, **12**, 736–44.

Skyhøj Olsen, T., Lauritzen, M., and Lassen, N.A. (1984). Focal ischemia during migraine attacks in patients with classical migraine. *Acta Neurologica Scandinavica*, **69**, (Suppl. 98), 258–9.

Skyhøj Olsen, T., Friberg, L., and Rønager, J. (1986). Cerebral autoregulation and CO_2-reactivity are completely abolished during attacks of classic migraine. Further support of the vasospastic theory. *Uppsala Journal of Medical Sciences*, Suppl. **43**, 87 (abstract).

Skyhøj Olsen, T., Friberg, L., and Lassen, N.A. (1987) Ischemia may be the primary cause of the neurological deficits in classic migraine. *Archives of Neurology*, **44**, 156–61.

Slatter, K.H. (1968). Some clinical and EEG findings in patients with migraine. *Brain*, **91**, 85–98.

Staehelin Jensen, T., Voldby, B., Olivarius, B.F., and Jensen, F.T. (1981). Cerebral hemodynamics in familial hemiplegic migraine. *Cephalalgia*, **1**, 121–5.

Sveinsdottir, E., Larsen, B., Rommer, P., and Lassen, N.A. (1977). A multidetector scintillation camera with 254 channels. *Journal of Nuclear Medicine*, **18**, 168–74.

Symonds, C. (1952). Migrainous variants. *Transactions of the Medical Society of London*, **67**, 237–50.

Trojaborg, W. and Boysen, G. (1973). Relation between EEG, regional cerebral blood flow and internal carotid artery pressure during carotid endarterectomy. *Electroencephalography and Clinical Neurophysiology*, **34**, 61–9.

Wolff, H.G. (1963). Headache and other head pain. (2nd edn), Oxford University Press, New York.

Discussion

WELCH: Are your blood flow values corrected to allow for Compton scattering?

OLESEN: No, they are not corrected. There are many parallels between blood flow changes and Leão's spreading depression. The main thing that arguably could be against it is the marked blood flow reduction during migraine. Our measurements strongly suggest Leão's spreading depression, and the big challenge at the moment is to fit that with arteriolar vasoconstriction, which is also present.

WELCH: Dr Gardner-Medwin has also studied spreading depression and I should like to ask him what the latency period is for initiation of spreading depression in the cortex. Is the latency period shorter in primates than in the rat?

GARDNER-MEDWIN: With most of the techniques for eliciting spreading depression in animals, the latent period in the immediate locality is very short: it is of the order of 10 seconds. However, if the recording is being made some distance away, or if one requires it to affect a substantial zone of tissue, it will be longer.

WELCH: So could a stimulus fire off spreading depression every 10 seconds?

GARDNER-MEDWIN: No; there is a refractory period afterwards of the order of two or three minutes in rats and rabbits, and a longer one in cats and macaque monkeys (Van Harreveld *et al.* 1956).

WELCH: It is possible, then, for several waves of spreading depression to be distributed over the cortex?

GARDNER-MEDWIN: Yes. In the work of Bureš *et al.* (1974) with conscious rats, for example, unilateral cortical dysfunction lasts for several hours, with repeated waves of spreading depression propagating from a site of continuous application of potassium chloride. It is also possible in special circumstances to elicit waves that recirculate without a continuous stimulus. After asphyxia in the rat, a brief eliciting stimulus may also evoke several waves of spreading depression (Bureš and Burešová 1960).

BLAU: In Leão's (1944a) paper, he illustrates a band of electrical silence migrating across the cortex over a period of minutes. I do not think, Professor Olesen, that you have shown that there is such a band; your results, instead, show a spreading depression that persists for hours. In addition, you have not shown electrical silence. Leão (1944b) also showed that following the band of pallor is an area of hyperaemia which is so intense that there is arterialization of the venous circulation. Yet you had to look hard to find this hyperaemia. Further, there was no correlation between the neurological symptoms and blood flow reduction: your photographs show that four hours after the onset there was still reduced blood supply in the occipital cortex; it is highly unlikely that a visual aura would still be present then, yet your theory would suggest that there should be. Similarly with parietal hypoperfusion, patients would be expected to have hemianaesthesia, and with temporal lobe involvement there should be dysphasia. Nevertheless, the rate of progression of the wave in mm per minute is important, because that does provide a correlation between your blood flow observations and Leão's spreading depression.

OLESEN: Spreading depression is like a very narrow band (only about 3 mm wide) that moves across the cortex. At the frontier the neurones fire intensively, and blood flow is increased, followed by a rapid recovery. We cannot measure this band for two reasons: it is not broad enough; and, secondly, it moves. We have seen an initial hyperaemia in a very few patients, and it may be due to the angulated clearance curves.

With our spreading depression model, we are not measuring brain blood flow within the frontier that is moving across the brain, but within the depression that follows in the wake of this frontier. Lauritzen et al. (1982) have shown that blood flow remains depressed, after experimentally induced spreading depression, for as long as one hour in the rat, even if the brain recovers its electrical activity more quickly. I do not know how that can be explained. There is no other known phenomenon in the brain that gradually moves across the cortex like this in a contiguous manner. So, despite species differences, we know the main characteristics of this phenomenon, and can see that something similar is going on in the human brain.

MOSKOWITZ: Surely spreading depression is an electrophysiological phenomenon, and not primarily a blood-flow phenomenon? If possible, we should try to evaluate its presence or absence by electrophysiological techniques. In a sense, examining flow is the equivalent of looking at an electrocardiogram in order to determine the diameter of the coronary vessels! It stretches the limits of the methods and, although useful, it is not the most appropriate technique to characterize the electrophysiological changes.

GARDNER-MEDWIN: Are the regions of very low blood flow restricted to the regions where one could attribute symptoms of the aura? Or have you seen this oligaemia in regions where you have not been able to identify focal symptoms related to that zone?

OLESEN: Large areas of the human cortex are so-called silent areas, so it is difficult to answer your question precisely. Over the years, however, we have found quite a good relationship between the symptomatology and the extent of the oligaemia.

GARDNER-MEDWIN: I should have restricted the question to the regions known not to be silent, such as the visual cortex and the somatosensory areas. For example, do you ever find oligaemia in the occipital zone without detecting visual symptoms?

OLESEN: No.

VANE: In your coloured photographs of hyperaemia, when you see a white area or a red area, how much of that is the expected variation from day to day in a normal brain?

OLESEN: The variation in the mean flow over the whole hemisphere is 5 per cent between days 1 and 2 and 10 per cent between days 1 and 3. The virtue of these methods lies mostly in their regionality. One can obtain a good reproducibility by using a right/left index in various areas. In those cases we see less than 5 per cent variability in regions covering 20 per cent of a hemisphere (Vorstrup 1988).

VANE: You very nicely showed that the aura was not associated only with vasoconstriction; the blood flow was down after the aura was over. Yet you and others have been saying that headaches can be pulsating, which suggests that there is a vascular component. The observation that going up and down stairs may increase the headache also suggests a movement element to it. The change of blood flow that you are measuring in the microcirculation may not be the relevant change. Perhaps it is a change of pulsation in the macrovessels that is relevant.

OLESEN: That may very well be so.

WELCH: In the illustrations you have shown, it seemed that the oligaemia stopped at the great fissures.

OLESEN: Yes. We have seen that repeatedly. There is something about the somatosensory cortex that is resistant to this phenomenon.

WELCH: Are the great fissures places where spreading depression may stop?

GARDNER-MEDWIN: Yes. Failure of propagation is common at sulci and at some architectonic boundaries (see Bureš *et al.* 1974; and also Marshall 1959).

References

Bureš, J. and Burešová, O. (1960). Activation of latent foci of cortical spreading depression in rats. *Journal of Neurophysiology*, **23**, 225–36.

Bureš, J., Burešová, O., and Krivánek, J. (1974). *The mechanism and applications of Leão's spreading depression of electroencephalographic activity.* Academic Press, New York.

Lauritzen, M., Balslev Jorgensen, M., Diemer, N.H., Gjedde, A., and Hansen, A.J. (1982). Persistent oligemia of rat cerebral cortex in the wake of spreading depression. *Annals of Neurology*, **12**, 469–74.

Leão, A.A.P. (1944a). Spreading depression of activity in cerebral cortex. *Journal of Neurophysiology*, **7**, 359–90.

Leão, A.A.P. (1944b). Pial circulation and spreading depression of activity in the cerebral cortex. *Journal of Neurophysiology*, **7**, 391–6.

Marshall, W.H. (1959). Spreading depression of Leão. *Physiological Reviews*, **39**, 236–64.

Van Harreveld, A., Stamm, J.S., and Christensen, E. (1956). Spreading depression in rabbit, cat and monkey. *American Journal of Physiology*, **184**, 312–20.

Vorstrup, S. (1988). Tomographic cerebral blood flow measurements in patients with ischemic cerebrovascular disease. *Acta Neurologica Scandinavica*, **77**, Suppl. 114, 1–48.

9. Migraine pathogenesis examined with contemporary techniques for analysing brain function

K.M.A. Welch

Introduction

Progress in the understanding of migraine pathogenesis has been hampered by the unavailability of animal models for this disorder. Thus, we have been limited to the study of the human condition itself. Until recently, direct examination of brain function could not be performed without hazard to the patient. Now, with techniques such as positron emission tomography, nuclear magnetic resonance spectroscopy, ^{133}Xe-inhalation cerebral blood flow (CBF) and magnetoencephalography we can derive insights into central mechanisms of the attack. In this paper I shall review the evidence obtained by these non-invasive techniques in the context of a conceptual mechanism for migraine — that is, that the attack is due to an abnormality of the normally finely tuned interaction between neuronal and vascular elements of the central nervous system (CNS).

The concept of threshold

A CNS threshold for the migraine attack has been proposed (Welch 1987) which, when exceeded, sets into motion the mechanism of the attack. This threshold can be potentiated by a number of factors: for example, endocrine status, chronic stress, and psychological and genetic make-up. Once the threshold is primed the factors that activate migraine — for example, glare, diet, and acute stress — can take effect. Results from non-invasive measurements of CBF and metabolism have supported the concept of a migraine threshold by yielding evidence of variable brain function in between attacks. For example, Levine *et al.* (1987) studied regional CBF (rCBF) asymmetries in controls and migraine patients with or without neurological aura. The results indicated a difference in rCBF patterns in the headache-free migraine patients, as well as revealing posterior asymmetries of flow that were consistent with the site of activation of migraine attacks. These findings are entirely compatible with labile control of the cerebral circulation and a shifting threshold for a migraine attack. The results have been substantiated

TABLE 9.1. *Brain energy ratios and pH during and between migraine attacks*

Measurement	Control subjects $n = 27$	Migraine subjects	
		Interictal $n = 9$	Attack $n = 11$
PCr/Pi ratio	2.07 ± 0.51	1.75 ± 0.56 (>0.23)	1.56 ± 0.55 (<0.02)
PCr/TP ratio	0.12 ± 0.01	0.12 ± 0.02 (>0.97)	0.11 ± 0.01 (<0.02)
Pi/TP ratio	0.06 ± 0.02	0.08 ± 0.02 (<0.05)	0.08 ± 0.02 (<0.03)
pH	6.99 ± 0.09	6.98 ± 0.05 (>0.87)	6.97 ± 0.06 (>0.77)

All results are taken from combined cortical regions.
( ), p-value from analysis of covariance, to compare the specified group with the controls, with adjustment for age and sex.
±, standard deviation.
n, number studied.
TP, total phosphate; Pi, inorganic phosphate; PCr, phosphocreatine.

in a larger series of cases (Robertson *et al.* 1989), in which a slower rate of CBF decline with age was found in migraine patients as well as lower CBF values in young and middle-aged sufferers. This study is of particular interest, not only because it is further evidence of altered cerebrovascular resistance between attacks, but also because the brain is more susceptible to spreading depression at lower CBF values (Lauritzen 1987).

We have derived similar evidence of altered cerebral function from the measurement of brain phosphate energy metabolism in a preliminary cross-sectional study of patients with classical and common migraine. For this study we used *in vivo* ^{31}P-nuclear magnetic resonance (NMR) spectroscopy (Welch *et al.* 1989). We found that brain metabolism differed from normal between attacks in that the cellular inorganic phosphate (Pi) levels were elevated (Table 9.1). A decreased ratio of phosphocreatine (PCr) to Pi, an index of energy status, was also observed in anterior cerebral cortex (Table 9.2). Alteration of brain energy phosphate metabolism might, therefore, be a feature of a migraine-susceptible brain, perhaps by reflecting a greater energy consumption, itself caused by increased neuronal activity. The findings in regions of the anterior brain are of interest in view of our

TABLE 9.2. *Regional difference in brain energy ratios during and between migraine attacks*

	Phosphate ratio	Control subjects n = 24	Migraine subjects	
			Interictal n = 7	Attack n = 9
Anterior cerebrum	PCr/Pi	2.09 ± 0.49	1.52 ± 0.63 (<0.02)	1.58 ± 0.56 (<0.02)
	PCr/TP	0.12 ± 0.01	0.11 ± 0.02 (>0.52)	0.11 ± 0.01 (<0.04)
	Pi/TP	0.06 ± 0.02	0.08 ± 0.03 (>0.05)	0.08 ± 0.03 (<0.04)
		n = 17	n = 4	n = 5
Posterior cerebrum	PCr/Pi	2.09 ± 0.53	1.98 ± 0.81 (>0.29)	1.62 ± 0.70 (>0.12)
	PCr/TP	0.13 ± 0.02	0.14 ± 0.02 (>0.88)	0.11 ± 0.03 (<0.04)
	Pi/TP	0.07 ± 0.01	0.08 ± 0.03 (>0.07)	0.07 ± 0.02 (>0.44)

( ), p value from analysis of covariance, to compare the specified group with the controls, with adjustment for age and sex.
±, standard deviation.
n, number studied.
TP, total phosphate; Pi, inorganic phosphate; PCr, phosphocreatine.

postulated concept that the orbitofrontal cortex is involved in activation of a migraine attack (Welch 1987).

To pursue the possibility that these high energy phosphate changes could be due to instability of neuronal membranes, we also examined phospholipid turnover by using ^{31}P-NMR in the same patients. The ratio of phosphomonoesters to phosphodiesters, both measurable in the ^{31}P spectrum, provides an approximate index of phospholipid turnover. The ratio was, however, unaltered in migraine patients between attacks.

The magnesium ion (Mg^{2+}) plays an important role in membrane stability. Cellular free Mg^{2+} (expressed as pMg^{2+}: the higher the pMg^{2+} the less the free Mg^{2+}) can also be measured from the ^{31}P spectrum by examining the chemical shift properties of ATP. Preliminary results obtained from the same patients described above, in between their migraine attacks, revealed no significant differences in free cellular Mg^{2+} compared to controls (Table 9.3).

TABLE 9.3. *Brain magnesium in control subjects and migraine patients*

Comparison	n	Mean pMg^{2+}	s.d.	p value
Controls	25	3.52	0.07	>0.05
All migraine	19	3.57	0.10	
Controls	25	3.52	0.07	<0.02
During attacks	10	3.61	0.12	
Controls	25	3.52	0.07	>0.57
Between attacks	9	3.54	0.06	

p-value from two-tailed *t*-test.
s.d., standard deviation.

The mechanisms of a migraine attack

Positive visual phenomena, followed by negative phenomena such as scotoma or hemianopia, account for well over half the transient neurological manifestations of the classical migraine attack. The characteristically slow progression of this symptom complex suggests that the migraine attack originates in the CNS with a burst followed by depression of neuronal activity. Olesen *et al.* (1981), from their observations of spreading oligaemia in migraine attacks, have suggested that spreading depression of Leão can account for the clinical and cerebral blood flow findings. However, on reconsidering these findings, Skyhøj-Olsen *et al.* (1987) suggested that low flow areas had been missed in these patients owing to overestimation of flows because of the problem of scattered radiation in the ^{133}Xe technique. Skyhøj-Olsen *et al.* (1987) themselves demonstrated ischaemic foci during a classical migraine attack. Their evidence, together with PET findings of increased cerebral oxygen extraction (Sigrid *et al.* 1985), has reintroduced the notion of a primary vascular cause for the migraine attack. The controversy may be reconciled by the concept that there is a spontaneous depolarization of intrinsic neurones, which also supply intraparenchymal resistance microvessels. This process would lead to vasoconstriction and to a consequent flow reduction below the threshold for K$^+$ release from the neurone. Increased extracellular K$^+$ then might precipitate depolarization of contiguous cortical neurones. Thus, a low flow in major intracerebral vessels may be caused by an increased downstream resistance, and therefore not by vasospasm (Welch 1987).

Positron emission tomography studies have added little to resolve the controversy of whether ischaemia or neuronal depression is responsible for the low CBF state. Sachs *et al.* (1986) studied regional cerebral glucose consumption in a small number of patients with common or classical mig-

TABLE 9.4. *Brain phospholipid metabolism during migraine*

Subjects	PME/TP	PDE/TP	p value*
Control subjects (n = 27)	0.09 ± 0.01	0.30 ± 0.01	
All migraine (n = 11)	0.10 ± 0.02	0.30 ± 0.02	0.05, 0.53
Classical migraine (n = 5)	0.10 ± 0.01	0.30 ± 0.02	0.05, 0.89

*p-values represent significance for controls.
PME, phosphomonoesters; PDE, phosphodiesters; TP, total phosphate.

raine, during headaches induced by reserpine. The regional cerebral glucose consumption fell by between 10 and 30 per cent. The reduction, however, was generalized to the whole brain cortex, unlike the laterality of the cerebral blood flow abnormality. It is uncertain whether the measured changes in regional cerebral glucose consumption are artefactual ones, caused by problems with reproducibility of the technique. Even if these results reflect a biological phenomenon they do not resolve the issue of the attack mechanism.

In a further attempt to resolve the blood flow controversy with a metabolic measurement, we studied *in vivo* ^{31}P-NMR spectroscopy in patients during an attack. A decrease of PCr and an increase of Pi was observed (Welch *et al.* 1989) in classical but not in common migraine. Although similar changes in these substances can be found in both spreading depression and ischaemia, the pattern of change favoured the former (Table 9.2). The anterior cortical location of the PCr/Pi reduction and the Pi increase during an attack could reflect the progression of spreading depression anteriorly by the time the patients were available for study, because a residual decrease of PCr was still present in posterior brain regions.

Intracellular pH was also measured in the same studies (Table 9.1). There was no evidence of a pH shift during a migraine headache (Welch *et al.* 1988). Thus, the long-standing hypothesis that the headache of migraine is due to cerebral vasodilatation, as a residuum of cerebral ischaemic acidosis, remains unproven. Finally there was an increased mole percentage of phosphomonoesters during an attack in patients with classical migraine (Table 9.4). The phosphomonoester peak contains phospholipids essential for membrane function and, thus, these results provide indirect evidence for a disturbance of brain cellular membrane function during an attack.

Stronger evidence for a cellular membrane abnormality *during* a migraine attack was obtained from free Mg^{2+} studies. When pMg^{2+}, calculated from ^{31}P-NMR spectra, was compared to normal controls (Table 9.3) it was

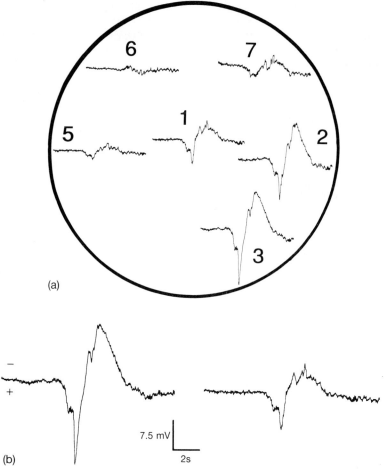

FIG. 9.1. Magnetoencephalographic recording from the left occipital cortex of a patient vulnerable to effort-induced migraine. The traces were recorded 20 min after exercise. Although no migraine attack ensued, note the spontaneous onset of slow magnetic wave shifts of different amplitude, depending on the site of recording. (a) shows the placement of the seven separate recording devices (single quantum interference devices, SQUIDS) over the occipital cortex (SQUID 4 failed for technical reasons). (b) shows detail from two of the SQUIDS in (a) with scale bars for voltage and duration of the recordings.

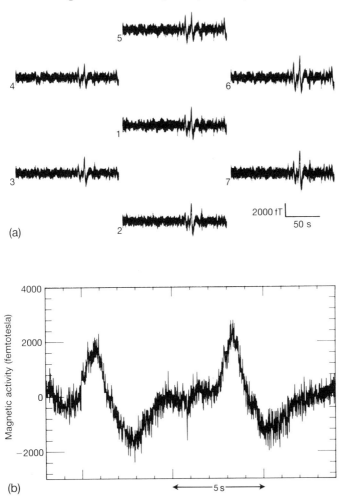

FIG. 9.2. Magnetoencephalographic recording obtained from the right occipital cortex of a 27-year-old male during an episode of migraine headache with inferior quadrantanopsia and left cheiro-oral spreading dysaesthesia. A two-minute epoch of recording from 7 separate SQUIDS is shown in (a). Note slow magnetic shifts of different amplitude at separate recording sites. The slow magnetic shifts were frequently multiple (see (b) for detail) and occurred intermittently throughout the recording, subsiding as the headache and neurological deficit subsided. fT = femtotesla.

significantly ($p < 0.02$) higher in the migraine patients. Of relevance is that experimental spreading depression can be abolished by Mg^{2+} application. Thus, a decreased free Mg^{2+} may be involved in the susceptibility of a migrainous brain to spreading depression. Alternatively, the low Mg^{2+} could be secondary to a functional disturbance during the migraine attack.

Results from the non-invasive techniques of brain function are, so far, compatible with the migraine attack originating in the CNS and with a threshold for the event. It has been argued that the attack is initiated by a burst of neuronal activity that results in a slow neuronal depolarization which may spread into contiguous brain regions in a manner that resembles spreading depression. To date, slow, direct current (DC) potential shifts have not been seen in human brain because of the unavailability of electrophysiological techniques that can detect such phenomena. Recently, Okada *et al.* (1988) have measured slowly varying magnetic fields during spreading depression in the isolated turtle cerebellum, by using magnetoencephalography (MEG). We can now report some MEG findings in migraine patients. Figure 9.1 shows a slowly varying magnetic field obtained by MEG in a patient with effort-induced migraine who unsuccessfully attempted to precipitate an attack by exercising. Nevertheless MEG findings similar to those of the spreading depolarization recorded in animal brain were recorded from the occipital cortex of this patient. Figure 9.2 shows similar, slow magnetic field shifts obtained from the occipital cortex of a migraine patient. The recordings were made during an attack of migraine headache accompanied by left inferior quadrantanopsia and left-sided numbness. Such activity was recorded frequently throughout a 30-min. period of study. We have now examined three migraine patients with MEG under conditions that would normally precipitate their migraine attacks. Although in each case an attack was not precipitated, nevertheless slow magnetic field shifts were seen in two of the three. No such phenomena have been observed in a larger series ($n = 8$) of controls. Indeed, such findings have never been reported in normal human subjects.

In summation, the development of non-invasive techniques for measuring brain blood flow, and metabolic and neuronal function have substantiated the concept of a CNS origin for migraine. Variability in brain function between attacks indicates a threshold for migraine susceptibility. The initiation of a migraine attack appears to be a primary neuronal phenomenon with cerebrovascular and metabolic consequences.

References

Lauritzen, M. (1987). Regional cerebral blood flow during cortical spreading depression in rat brain increased reactive hyperperfusion in low flow states. *Acta Neurologica Scandinavica*, **75**, 1–8.

Levine, S.R., Welch, K.M.A., Ewing, J.R., Joseph, R., and D'Andrea, G. (1987). Cerebral blood flow asymmetries in headache-free migraineurs. *Stroke*, **18**, 1164–5.

Okada, Y.C., Lauritzen, M., and Nicholson, C. (1988). Magnetic field associated with spreading depression; a model for the detection of migraine. *Brain Research*, **442**, 185–90.

Olesen, J., Larsen, B., and Lauritzen, M. (1981). Focal hyperemia followed by spreading oligemia and impaired activation of rCBF in classic migraine. *Annals of Neurology*, **9**, 344–52.

Robertson, W.M., Welch, K.M.A., Levine, S.R., and Schultz, L. (1989). The effects of aging on cerebral blood flow in migraine. *Neurology*, **39**, 947–51.

Sachs, H., Wolf, A., Russell, J.A.G., and Christman, D.R. (1986). Effect of reserpine on regional cerebral glucose metabolism in control and migraine subjects. *Archives of Neurology*, **43**, 1117–23.

Sigrid, H. *et al.* (1985). Oxygen metabolism in migraine. *Journal of Cerebral Blood Flow and Metabolism*, **4**, S445–S456.

Skyhøj-Olsen, T.S., Friberg, L., and Lassen, N.A. (1987). Ischemia may be the primary cause of the neurologic deficits in classic migraine. *Archives of Neurology*, **44**, 156–61.

Welch, K.M.A. (1987). Migraine: a biobehavioral disorder. *Archives of Neurology*, **44**, 323–6.

Welch, K.M.A., Levine, S.R., D'Andrea, G., and Helpern, J.A. (1988). Brain pH during migraine studied by in-vivo 31-Phosphorus NMR spectroscopy. *Cephalalgia*, **8**, 273–7.

Welch, K.M.A., Levine, S.R., Helpern, J.A., and D'Andrea, G. (1989). Preliminary observations on brain energy metabolism in migraine studied by in vivo 31-Phosphorus NMR spectroscopy. *Neurology*, **39**, 538–41.

Discussion

VANE: What does your Figure 9.1 represent?

WELCH: This magnetoencephalography (MEG) is a new technique, and we would be glad to have some critical appraisal of it during this discussion. Figure 9.1 represents the spontaneous, slowly varying magnetic field emanating from the head. In different regions of the occipital cortex, we obtained waves of different amplitude and duration. With this technique we have examined three patients, two with classical migraine and one with common migraine. Each of these patients is known to have migraine precipitated by certain stimuli. The common migraine patient and one of the classical migraine patients have shown this phenomenon. We have compared them with one patient with severe headache from an Arnold-Chiari malformation, which did not show anything. Eight control patients have been shown to have no such wave abnormality whatsoever. The only other (unpublished) report of slow-wave shifts that I have is from Germany, which showed slow-wave shifts in patients with epilepsy. We do not yet know whether these waves occur during all migraine attacks. Recently we tested a fourth migraine patient with a left quadrantanopsia and left-sided numbness, which was persisting through a very severe headache; this was a 'classical' migraine. Figure 9.2a in my paper displays slow magnetic field shifts every three or four minutes for about 30 minutes. Each trace represents a recording from a different site on the right occipital cortex. Figure 9.2b showed a similar trace from the same patient, but magnified. Between 30 and 60 minutes into the recording, his headache subsided, and so too did these slowly varying magnetic fields. Similar waves have been seen in the turtle (Okada *et al.* 1988), and more animal studies are needed for comparison with our results on humans. We need to find out what it is we are measuring. These slow potential shifts in the brain may have some relevance to the acute migraine attack. We have observed them in migraine patients who are not going through an attack. These depolarizing waves may involve the microvasculature, and changes in blood flow. We could speculate that the threshold for these waves may be modulated by the ascending noradrenergic and serotoninergic systems. If anyone can throw light on what it is we are recording, we would be glad to know. Perhaps it is artefact. We simply believe that these waves look very like the magnetic waves that one sees with the DC (direct current) potential shifts in animal brain (Okada *et al.* 1988).

VANE: Are you postulating that upwards in Figure 9.1 is depolarization and downwards is polarization?

WELCH: We do not know. Conduction of an impulse in a neurone sets up a magnetic field. We can record the magnetic activity when the recording is made perpendicular to the direction of conduction of the neurone, but not otherwise.

PEATFIELD: Are those magnetic flux changes (in Fig. 9.2) moving across the cortical surface?

WELCH: We cannot tell. We would not expect to see spreading depression because as the neurone conducts it sets up a sequence of magnetic fields, which may tend to cancel each other. However, if there is a sudden onset of depolarization one might see spreading depression when that depolarization terminates. The waveform has different amplitudes and durations in different places, but they might be coalescing from different foci in the occipital cortex, rather than spreading in a wave. Perhaps, in spreading depression, there are *repeated* depolarizing events going on.

PEATFIELD: Did your patients have a typical migraine aura during the examination?

WELCH: The patient with inferior quadrantanopsia (Fig. 9.2) had a 'classical' migraine aura with scintillating phenomena at the edges of his visual field.

GLOVER: Have any of your control (non-migraine) patients been examined after exercise?

WELCH: No. But exercise is not the only precipitant we have attempted to use to trigger attacks before examination by MEG. A woman whose classical migraine was usually produced by aspartame did not have one of her typical classical migraines after taking the aspartame prior to examination. For another patient, the precipitant we tried was macaroni and cheese which normally gave him a common migraine, but unfortunately failed to do so before examination. But these are very early data.

SANDLER: You mentioned a subject who often has migraine attacks after aspartame. Yet this phenomenon has been hotly denied recently (Schiffmann *et al.* 1987).

WELCH: This subject usually develops quite a florid, classical migraine attack within half an hour of taking a diet-drink that contains aspartame. No other sweeteners cause her to develop migraine. When we examined her by MEG, on this one occasion, however, she did not have migraine, nor did she have any migranous visual aura.

BLAU: One of the intriguing things about migraine is that it often occurs *after* a stimulus such as a period of tension, but not *during* the period of tension. In a similar way, the stiffness of muscle after unaccustomed exercise tends to occur the morning afterwards. Positron emission tomography (PET) techniques can be used to examine muscle state. It would be intriguing to use PET techniques to compare the two delayed effects — muscle stiffness and migraine — to see if one could throw some light on the other. Have you observed any changes in muscle that could indicate precisely what causes the muscle stiffness?

WELCH: I have not yet looked at the changes in magnesium content of muscle after exercise. We have some ^{31}P spectroscopy data from muscle, showing altered energy metabolism.

GARDNER-MEDWIN: Marcussen and Wolff (1950) showed that carbon dioxide inhalation can abort the aura of a migraine attack, and I showed that it can stop the propagation of spreading depression, within about a minute (Gardner-Medwin 1981). It would be very interesting to observe the effect of CO_2 inhalation on these patterns of magnetic flux density that you have described.

WELCH: That is a good idea. We would also be interested to try the effects of β-blockers on these prolonged events.

VANE: How do your results compare with putting the magnetometer over a nerve fibre and tracking the movement of an action potential?

WELCH: We cannot do that. It is not sensitive enough to look at a single nerve fibre. We are also interested in measuring the magnetic activity from the fetus in late pregnancy.

VANE: The sciatic nerve, for example, is surely large enough for you to be able to detect a synchronous nerve action potential running down it, especially if you are able to record this *asynchronous* activity in the brain?

WELCH: We could certainly try sciatic nerve stimulation in an animal preparation.

SCHWARTZ: Have you any idea about the depths at which the events you register are taking place?

WELCH: No. We know that the MEG goes 5 cm deep, because it can be used clinically to localize deep epileptogenic bursts from the temporal lobe, as an alternative to using deep electrodes during open operation, when one is looking for epileptogenic foci prior to topectomy for chronic temporal lobe seizures (Sutherling *et al.* 1987).

SCHWARTZ: I am asking about the depth of recording because of the possible influence of noradrenergic fibres. In the cerebral cortex the noradrenergic axons arrive vertically and cross the various layers towards the cortical surface up to the last layer, and then they turn horizontally, running parallel to the pial surface and displaying extensive arborization; the innervation of the molecular layer is extremely abundant.

WELCH: The results we have recorded in migraine subjects are not at all like those we have so far looked at in patients with epilepsy, who show epileptogenic 'spikes' that are more rapid and of smaller amplitude than magnetic waves.

GLOVER: Have you tried to induce similar magnetic waves with any serotoninergic or noradrenergic preparations?

WELCH: That is obviously what we have to do. With a brain as small as that of the cat we could use our magnetometer to study all areas of the brain in response to such types of stimuli. Because we have only seven single-quantum interference devices, this limits the total area of the human cortex that we can study at any one time, but it is an expensive technique already. We hope to do some work on the cat brain.

GARDNER-MEDWIN: It might be helpful at this stage to stress a few points that have emerged from animal experiments on spreading depression. I should like to dispel two ideas about spreading depression that are sometimes found in the published work on migraine: (1) the idea that spreading depression *is* spreading oligaemia; and (2) the idea that the depression of neuronal activity during spreading depression results in reduced metabolic activity and perfusion. Both ideas are wrong.

First, it is clear that the mechanisms of spreading depression do not involve the circulation. This is most plainly shown in work on the chick retina (Martins Ferreira and de Oliveira-Castro 1966). This is an avascular tissue, which exhibits spreading depression that is very similar to that in the mammalian cortex. You can initiate spreading depression with a pinprick and see its progress in this retina very clearly, as an advancing whitish band. This is a sign of the ionic disturbance, not of ischaemia or hypoxia. When spreading depression occurs in vascular tissue, then the circulation is affected. The spreading oligaemia demonstrated by Olesen and his colleagues in classical migraine has, as Professor Olesen has described in this volume, many characteristics suggesting that it may be caused by spreading depression. If so, it is a phenomenon occurring in the wake of the spreading depression, like inflammation caused by injury.

The local neural dysfunction during an episode of spreading depression is very profound, and probably total. This is easily understood from the fact that the extracellular potassium and calcium concentrations rise or fall, respectively, by factors of ten or more (Nicholson and Kraig 1980). This acute dysfunction is quite separate from the oligaemia that can occur in the wake of spreading depression. The oligaemia may lead to subtle dysfunctions later on, but it is an incidental phenomenon so far as the spreading depression itself is concerned.

Neuronal activity is depressed in the acute phase of spreading depression. Metabolic activity, on the other hand, is markedly enhanced at about this time. The neurones do not fire action potentials, but they are metabolizing hard to restore normal ionic balance and transmitter stores. There are rises in temperature, blood flow, and lactate production and falls in P_{O_2} and glycogen (see Bureš *et al.* 1974 for review). The effect is dramatically evident in infrared thermographic pictures from the work of Shevelev *et al.* (1986), which show a propagating rise of temperature of about 1°C on the rat skull during spreading depression. From the metabolic point of view, spreading depression is really 'spreading activation'. The extra metabolic stress may represent a risk to the tissue when there are conditions of marginal metabolic sufficiency such as those that occur in neurosurgery (Gardner-Medwin and Mutch 1984).

MOSKOWITZ: What causes the change in appearance of the chick retina during spreading depression?

GARDNER-MEDWIN: This is probably due to cell swelling associated with increases in membrane permeability and flux of Na^+ and Cl^- ions into cells (Martins Ferreira and de Oliveira-Castro 1966). There is a consequent change in light scattering. It could be important to try to relate this phenomenon to the rare patients who have retinal migraine. Retinal disturbances suggestive of oedema have been visible in this condition without obvious vasoconstriction (Wolter and Burchfield 1971).

BLAU: What is the highest mammal in which spreading depression has been demonstrated?

GARDNER-MEDWIN: It has been demonstrated in macaque and squirrel monkeys (see Bureš *et al.* 1974) and in the caudate nucleus and hippocampus in humans, deliberately elicited during stereotaxic surgery (Sramka *et al.* 1977). Harris *et al.* (1981) have, in baboons, also seen ionic changes that appear identical to spreading depression, though the disturbance appears not to have spread very far from the initiating site. We know that in primates spreading depression is harder to elicit, and more prone to failure of propagation. In these species it may occur only in tissue that is already somewhat abnormal (Marshall 1959).

BLAU: Gloor (1986), who has done extensive electrocorticography on epileptic patients in Montreal, has published a letter to say that his group has never seen spreading depression, in nearly 1000 patients. Furthermore, Professor Lindsay Symon's neurosurgical group at the National Hospital, Queen Square, London, have looked for spreading depression in monkeys and not seen it. Is the evidence for it very strong?

PEATFIELD: Only a small number of people in the population have classical migraine. There is probably an inherent tendency to have it, which may not have been present in Professor Symon's patients.

GARDNER-MEDWIN: I would put it more strongly than that. In patients with classical migraine, we know that the profound disturbance during the aura fails to propagate beyond what is usually quite a small region of the brain. Otherwise, those with classical migraine would each show the whole galaxy of sensory and motor syndromes, referrable to different parts of the brain, that are occasionally seen separately in different patients. Even in migraine-susceptible patients, one would need during neurosurgery to be looking in the right part of the brain, for a negative result to carry much weight.

BLAU: Spreading depression protagonists have always said that the sulci stop the spreading. But I should like to see some evidence for this notion.

MOSKOWITZ: I agree that we have to (almost) re-invent the wheel with regard to spreading depression, and ask whether it occurs in the human brain under different conditions.

BLAU: However, one must make an important, positive point. The concept of spreading depression provides a helpful model to account for this slow spread of the visual aura and perhaps hypoperfusion. If the chick retina model helps to give a lead, or is a suitable basis for neurochemists to work on, then the ideas we are debating could be fruitful.

VANE: I am confused by spreading depression. Is there a tenuous link between a reaction to an insult, such as a pinprick on a chick's retina, and migraine? If there is a link, would you please tell me what it is?

GARDNER-MEDWIN: The chick retina is only one of many tissues that shows spreading depression. It is a good preparation for studying the phenomenon in isolation. Spreading depression seems to be a common reaction of synaptic neuropile to a variety of insults. The link to the migraine aura is at present only circumstantial: the two phenomena have very many features in common (see Gardner-Medwin 1981). Michael Welch's recent magnetic data suggest additional similarities. Even if spreading depression occurs in the migraine aura, we do not know whether it is instrumental in causing other aspects of the migraine syndrome, for example the headache. There are, however, mechanisms — for example, the substantial release of potassium and neurotransmitters — through which spreading depression might have prolonged and widespread effects on the brain, the vasculature, and the meninges.

WELCH: In three patients who have not had an attack and in one patient who *has* had an attack, there are slow magnetic wave shifts in the cortex of the brain. Whether or not that is spreading depression, or whether it is a sudden burst of spreading depolarization, and where it is coming from I cannot answer, because I do not have the evidence. The time-course of some of these waves is 15 seconds, or more, which is a long time for an event in the human brain. I cannot say for sure that it is the same as spreading depression.

References

Bureš, J., Burešová, O., and Křivánek, J. (1974). *The mechanism and applications of Leão's spreading depression of electroencephalographic activity.* Academic Press, New York.

Gardner-Medwin, A.R. (1981). Possible roles of vertebrate neuroglia in potassium dynamics, spreading depression and migraine. *Journal of Experimental Biology*, **95**, 111–27.

Gardner-Medwin, A.R. and Mutch, W.A.C. (1984). Experiments on spreading depression in relation to migraine and neurosurgery. *Anais da Academia Brasileira de Ciencias*, **56**, 423–30.

Gloor, P. (1986). Migraine and cerebral blood flow. *Trends in Neurosciences*, **9**, 21.

Harris, R.J., Symon, L., Branston, N.M., and Bayhan, M. (1981). Changes in extracellular calcium activity in cerebral ischemia. *Journal of Cerebral Blood Flow and Metabolism*, **1**, 203–9.

Marcussen, R.M. and Wolff, H.G. (1950). Studies on headache: effects of CO_2-O_2 mixtures given during preheadache phase of the migraine attack. *Archives of Neurology and Psychiatry (Chicago)*, **63**, 42–51.

Marshall, W.H. (1959). Spreading cortical depression of Leão. *Physiological Reviews*, **39**, 239–79.

Martins Ferreira, H. and de Oliveira-Castro, G. (1966). Light scattering changes accompanying spreading depression in isolated retina. *Journal of Neurophysiology*, **29**, 715–26.

Nicholson, C. and Kraig, R.P. (1980). The behaviour of extracellular ions during spreading depression. In *The application of ion-selective microelectrodes*, (ed. T. Zeuthen), pp. 217–38. Elsevier, Amsterdam.

Okada, Y.C., Lauritzen M., and Nicholson, C. (1988). Magnetic fields associated with spreading depression; a model for the detection of migraine. *Brain Research*, **442**, 185–90.

Schiffman, S.S., *et al.* (1987). Aspartame and susceptibility to headache. *New England Journal of Medicine*, **317**, 1181–5.

Shevelev, I.A. *et al.* (1986). Dynamic thermal mapping of rat brain during sensory stimulation and spreading depression. *Neurophysiology*, **18**, 18–25.

Sramka, M., Brozek, G., Bureš, J., and Nadvornik, P. (1977). Functional ablation by spreading depression: possible use in human stereotaxic surgery. *Applied Neurophysiology*, **40**, 48–61.

Sutherling, W.W., Crandall, P.H., Engel, J., Darcey, T.M., Cahan, L.D., and Barth, D.S. (1987). The magnetic field of complex partial seizures agrees with intracranial localizations. *Annals of Neurology*, **21**, 548–58.

Wolter, J.R. and Burchfield, W.J. (1971). Ocular migraine in a young man resulting in unilateral transient blindness. *Journal of Pediatric Ophthalmology*, **8**, 173–6.

10. The superior pericarotid cavernous sinus plexus and cluster headaches

Michael A. Moskowitz and M. Gabriella Buzzi

Introduction

Little is known about the aetiology or pathology of cluster headache, and even less is known about its possible anatomical origins. In the complete form of cluster headache, patients experience pain referred to the first and second division of the trigeminal nerve, ocular sympathetic dysfunction (Horner's syndrome), forehead and facial sweating due to stimulation of superior cervical ganglia projections, and parasympathetic activation which manifests as lachrymation, conjunctival injection, nasal congestion, and rhinorrhoea. Some severely affected patients are successfully treated with chemical- or heat-induced trigeminal lesions, whereas others benefit from the injection of local anaesthetics into the sphenopalatine fossa or from the removal of the sphenopalatine ganglion. We believe that if a single 'lesion' does exist to explain all these symptoms and treatments, it must be small, and must reside within a remote region of the nervous system to escape detection by presently available diagnostic techniques. Recent anatomical data in primates suggest that such a disturbance may be localized to the superior aspect of the pericarotid cavernous sinus plexus.

Anatomical and functional considerations

The pericarotid cavernous sinus plexus (Ruskell and Simons 1987) provides a locus for convergence of both afferent and autonomic fibres (Fig. 10.1). The ophthalmic trigeminal division sends small branches within the cavernous sinus to innervate the circle of Willis, as previously proposed (Mayberg *et al.* 1984). The maxillary nerve sends recurrent branches as part of the orbitociliary nerve. This nerve reaches the orbit, after traversing the sphenopalatine fossa, close to the sphenopalatine ganglion and provides sensory fibres to the ciliary ganglia and other structures within the orbit. Small filaments (recurrent branches) enter the cranial cavity via the medial infraorbital fissure and join the superior segment of the cavernous sinus plexus that surrounds the distal carotid artery. Sympathetic fibres supplying the plexus project via the internal carotid nerve, and course from proximal to distal

A INTRACAVERNOUS CAROTID ARTERY

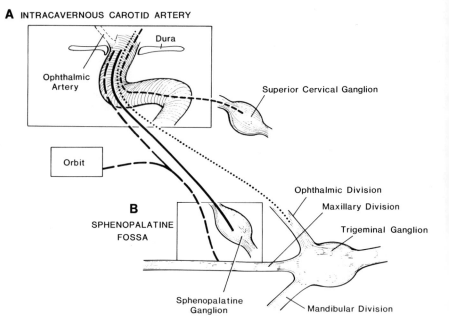

FIG. 10.1. The pericarotid cavernous sinus plexus (after Ruskell and Simons 1987), a possible site of single lesion to explain the cluster headache syndrome.

segments of the cavernous carotid artery to supply the eye and the circle of Willis (Arnold 1851). Sphenopalatine parasympathetic contributions reach the plexus via rami orbitales, as originally described by Ruskell (1970) and may project to the circle of Willis. Hence, the proximal cavernous sinus plexus is supplied predominantly by autonomic fibres, whereas the distal segment contains sensory and autonomic axons (Fig. 10.1). From this plexus, fibres are distributed to the circle of Willis, to orbital structures, and probably to dura mater as well (Ruskell and Simons 1987).

Carotid narrowing within the adjacent carotid canal, as demonstrated by arteriography (Ekbom and Greitz 1970), and occlusion within the cavernous sinus, as detected by orbital phlebography (Hannerz *et al.* 1987), both provide indirect support for the proposed site of lesion in patients with the complete cluster headache syndrome. Carotid narrowing, a reversible lesion, might reflect activation of trigeminovascular fibres and may result in neurogenic inflammation and attendant oedema. Neurogenic inflammation was recently produced experimentally in the dura mater after electrical stimulation of trigeminal fibres (Markowitz *et al.* 1987), and it can be blocked by ergot alkaloids (Markowitz *et al.* 1988; Saito *et al.* 1988). From this, we may make the highly speculative inference (at the moment) that hypothalamic dysfunction (for example, biological rhythm disturbance) described in some patients (Waldenlind 1987) may develop from involvement of that portion of the hypothalamic blood supply provided by arterial branches from the cavernous portion of the carotid artery, and that this involvement could contribute to the periodicity of this disease.

From the above anatomical scheme, we may expect that pain transmission by orbitociliary nerves would be reduced by surgical lesioning within the sphenopalatine fossa or by the application of local anaesthetics to that area (Meyer *et al.* 1970; Kittrelle *et al.* 1985; Hardebo and Elner 1987). Such procedures might also interrupt parasympathetic activity mediated by the sphenopalatine ganglion. Hence, the possibility of relief from headache in selected patients. However, relief may be incomplete or temporary because the plexus is only partially deafferented, and pain would be conveyed by first-division trigeminovascular fibres. Similarly, continued pain after surgical or chemical trigeminal lesioning might reflect incomplete deafferentation of the cavernous sinus plexus (Maxwell 1982; Waltz *et al.* 1985; Onofrio and Campbell 1986; Ekbom *et al.* 1987).

Of course, the above analysis assumes that the cluster headache syndrome develops from a single focus, and that the human anatomy resembles that of the primate. In the incomplete form of cluster headache, a lesion close to the sphenopalatine ganglia, or involving both rami orbitales and orbitociliary nerves, might induce orbital pain and predominantly unilateral parasympathetic activation. In this instance, a Horner's-like syndrome would not develop, and the 'vascular component', including the responsiveness to ergotamine compounds and calcium channel blockers, would probably not occur. Local orbital pathology, particularly within the posterior aspect, might also cause the constellation of symptoms and signs described above, but the lesion would be large. The cavernous sinus remains a most attractive locus because it is situated near the midline and because it possesses bilateral vascular connections — two features that may help to explain the infrequent development of the cluster syndrome, contralaterally. The cavernous sinus is an attractive region for headache development (and for potential drug delivery to convergent sensory axons from the trigeminovascular system) since it contains a unique juxtaposition of vascular and neural structures (carotid artery–neural plexus–venous channels draining facial tissues). As presently conceived, cluster headaches share certain anatomical features in common with Raeder's syndrome (see Mokri 1982; Vijayan and Watson 1986) and with the Tolosa–Hunt syndrome (see Hannerz 1985; Bruyn and Hoes 1986).

In a few patients with a cluster-like headache, lesions have been demonstrated close to the cavernous sinus or middle cranial fossa. For example, pituitary gland tumours have been reported by Tfelt-Hansen *et al.* (1982) and by Greve and Mai (1988). Aneurysms of the anterior communicating artery have been reported by Greve and Mai (1988) and by Sjaastad *et al.* (1988), as was a case of arteriovenous malformation of the left temporal lobe, described by Mokri in 1982. The characteristics of the cluster-like symptoms were uneven. All patients complained of peri-orbital or retro-orbital pain, but only four had lachrymation, two had conjunctival injection, one had nasal congestion and one had rhinorrhoea. Only one patient had ptosis and miosis, and one showed increased forehead sweating during an attack. The clustering pattern was absent in most.

The anatomical evidence described above suggests the need to study this region in cases of cluster headache, particularly in patients who are refractory to medical therapy. If this formulation can be confirmed by imaging studies as well as by *post mortem* examination of the cavernous sinus plexus, treatment strategies can be developed and targeted specifically to cluster headache pathophysiology.

Acknowledgement

This work was supported by a grant from the National Institute of Neurological and Communicative Disorders and Stroke (NS 26361).

References

Arnold, F. (1851). *Handbuch der Anatomie der Menschen*, Vol 2. Breisgau, Freiburg.
Bruyn, G.W. and Hoes, M.J.A.J.M. (1986). The Tolosa-Hunt syndrome. In *Handbook of clinical neurology*, (ed. F. Clifford Rose), Vol. 4, Headache, pp. 291–307. Elsevier, Amsterdam.
Ekbom, K. and Greitz, T. (1970). Carotid angiography in cluster headache. *Acta Radiologica Diagnosis* **10**, 177–86.
Ekbom, K., Lindgren, L., Nilsson, B.Y., Hardebo, J.E., and Waldenlind E. (1987). Retro-Gasserian glycerol injection in the treatment of chronic cluster headache. *Cephalalgia*, **7**, 21–7.
Greve, E. and Mai, J. (1988). Cluster headache-like headaches: a symptomatic feature? *Cephalagia*, **8**, 79–82.
Hannerz, J. (1985). Pain characteristics of painful ophthalmoplegia (the Tolosa-Hunt syndrome). *Cephalalgia*, **5**, 103–6.
Hannerz, J., Ericson, K., and Bergstrand, G. (1987). Chronic paroxysmal hemicrania: orbital phlebography and steroid treatment. *Cephalalgia*, **7**, 189–92.
Hardebo, J.E. and Elner, A. (1987). Nerves and vessels in the pterygopalatine fossa and symptoms of cluster headache. *Headache*, **27**, 528–32.
Kittrelle, J.P., Grouse, D.S., and Seybold, M.E. (1985). Cluster headache. Local anesthetic abortive agents. *Archives of Neurology*, **42**, 496–8.
Markowitz, S., Saito, K., and Moskowitz, M.A. (1987). Neurogenically mediated leakage of plasma protein occurs from blood vessels in dura mater but not in brain. *Journal of Neuroscience* **7**, 4129–36.
Markowitz, S., Saito, K., and Moskowitz, M.A. (1988). Neurogenically mediated plasma extravasation in dura mater: effect of ergot-alkaloids. A possible mechanism of action in vascular headache. *Cephalalgia*, **8**, 83–91.
Maxwell, R.E. (1982). Surgical control of chronic migrainous neuralgia by trigeminal ganglio-rhizolysis. *Journal of Neurosurgery*, **57**, 459–66.

Mayberg, M.R., Zervas, N.T., and Moskowitz, M.A. (1984). Trigeminal projections to supratentorial pial and dural blood vessels in cats demonstrated by horseradish peroxidase. *Journal of Comparative Neurology*, **223**, 46–56.

Meyer, J.S., Binns, P.M., Ericsson, A.D., and Vulpe, M. (1970). Sphenopalatine ganglionectomy for cluster headache. *Archives of Otolaryngology* **92**, 474–84.

Mokri, B. (1982). Raeder's paratrigeminal syndrome. Original concept and subsequent deviations. *Archives of Neurology* **39**, 395–9.

Onofrio, B.M. and Campbell, J.K. (1986). Surgical treatment of chronic cluster headache. *Mayo Clinic Proceedings* **61**, 537–44.

Ruskell, G.L. (1970). The orbital branches of the pterygopalatine ganglion and their relationship with internal carotid nerve branches in primates. *Journal of Anatomy*, **106**, 323–39.

Ruskell, G.L. and Simons, T. (1987). Trigeminal nerve pathways to the cerebral arteries in monkeys. *Journal of Anatomy*, **155**, 23–37.

Saito, K., Markowitz, S., and Moskowitz, M.A. (1988). Ergot alkaloids block neurogenic extravasation in dura mater: proposed mechanism of action in vascular headache. *Annals of Neurology*, **24**, 732–7.

Sjaastad, O. *et al.* (1988). Cluster headache-like headache, Hageman trait deficiency, retrobulbar neuritis, and giant aneurysm. *Cephalalgia* **8**, 111–20.

Tfelt-Hansen, P., Paulson, O.B., and Krabbe, A.E. (1982). Invasive adenoma of the pituitary gland and chronic migrainous neuralgia. A rare coincidence or a causal relationship? *Cephalalgia*, **2**, 25–8.

Vijayan, N. and Watson, C. (1986). Raeder's syndrome, pericarotid syndrome and carotidynia. In *Handbook of clinical neurology*, (ed. F. Clifford Rose), Vol. 4, Headache, pp. 329–41. Elsevier, Amsterdam.

Waldenlind, E. (1987). *Cluster headache: studies on monoaminergic platelet functions and endocrine rhythms*. Repro Print AB, Stockholm.

Waltz, T.A., Dalessio, D.J., Ott, K.H., Copeland, B., and Abbott, G. (1985). Trigeminal cistern glycerol injections for facial pain. *Headache*, **25**, 354–7.

Discussion

SANDLER: You failed to mention that cluster headache predominantly affects men. Some extreme treatments for the condition involve the administration of anti-androgens (Sicuteri 1988). Following on from that, could there not be a humoral component in cluster headache, to account for the lachrymation, rhinorrhoea, and puffy eyes, by analogy with the rare condition of bronchial carcinoid syndrome (Sandler 1968)? In this latter disease, the symptoms of salivation, lachrymation, and rhinorrhoea are believed to be due to a peptide such as bombesin or caerulein, produced by the highly localized carcinoid tumour.

MOSKOWITZ: Those symptoms of lachrymation and rhinorrhoea are, surely, parasympathetically mediated, and I do not believe that they are initiated humorally via the blood since they are predominantly unilateral. They might be related to the greater superficial petrosal pathway that Professor Lance has been studying. The anatomical arrangement that I have described would, nevertheless, be ideally suited to respond to humoral influences. In the superior pericarotid cavernous sinus is a unique juxtaposition of an artery, surrounded by venous blood, divided by trabeculae, within which will course the sensory nerves of the cavernous sinus plexus. One could speculate that if there are humoral influences, they may depend on this very anatomical arrangement to gain access both to nerves and to the two circulations.

LANCE: I agree that these autonomic symptoms are mediated by the greater superficial petrosal nerve. Gardner *et al.* (1947) showed a long time ago that section of the greater superficial petrosal nerve would eliminate autonomic symptoms completely, but patients still experienced pain. The autonomic system is therefore not the primary cause of the pain. Peter Drummond (1988) has suggested that not only does the discharge in the greater superficial petrosal through the sphenopalatine ganglion account for vasodilatation in the external carotid circulation, but also that fibres which loop back from the ganglion to the internal carotid siphon may cause vasodilatation of the *vasa vasorum* and, thus, swelling of the carotid wall. This swelling, in turn, compromises the third neurone of the sympathetic in that area.

MOSKOWITZ: I would expect that if swelling is present, it is due primarily to neurogenic inflammation and to the discharge from sensory rather than from parasympathetic fibres.

LANCE: The problem of pain in cluster headache is that it involves not only the first division of the trigeminal nerve but it may also involve the second and even the third divisions in some patients.

MOSKOWITZ: That is probably because at least two of the trigeminal divisions innervate the carotid in this region. I have been attempting to focus here on the orbitociliary branch of the maxillary nerve that innervates the cavernous sinus. There may be more central organizational mechanisms associated with the spread of pain from the ophthalmic and maxillary receptive fields, as shown by Sessle *et al.* (1986).

LANCE: Yet pain may spread right down over the face.

MOSKOWITZ: But that is unusual, and may be linked with a different phenomenon; electrodes placed in the first division of the trigeminal dermatome can activate, by intense stimulation, caudalis neurones associated with the mandibular division. Thus, there is something about intense stimulation that in some way 'disobeys' the organization of the nervous system that we traditionally accept. I would suggest that the pain in the neck, the jaw, and so on, is explained by such a mechanism. The first and second division fibres innervate the area of putative pathology, nevertheless.

LANCE: There must still be some central lesion to initiate the whole cluster phenomenon. Very often, these greater superficial petrosal symptoms — the eye redness, watering, and blockage of the nostril — occur in severe migraine as well. People who have not seen many patients clinically often confuse migraine with cluster headache, because severe migraine may be associated with precisely the same outflow along the greater superficial petrosal nerve and sometimes, with ptosis and miosis as well. I would regard the greater superficial petrosal symptoms as separate phenomena that may be associated with the severe pain of cluster headache or, much less commonly, with the severe pain of migraine.

MOSKOWITZ: I disagree. One need not postulate a central lesion. The trigger might be a centrally or peripherally mediated event that occurs in normal individuals but does not cause pain if a vascular lesion is not present. The parasympathetic system is so intimately involved in cluster headache that I have difficulty in believing that it is a remote effect; its expression is present more often than not. That is not true for classical migraine or common migraine.

LANCE: Discharge of trigeminal neurones could induce activity in the greater superficial petrosal nerve which then causes the sympathetic deficit by swelling in the wall of the carotid siphon.

MOSKOWITZ: It is possible, but not probable here. If ptosis and miosis occur with sparing of forehead sweating, one has to propose a focus in the internal carotid artery. The brainstem need not contain a lesion. Why propose two sites when one will suffice?

LANCE: We are agreed on the internal carotid arterial wall as the site of origin of sympathetic involvement.

BLAU: It may be helpful here to describe the pattern of cluster headache. The condition typically occurs in middle-aged men, who have annual attacks that last from six to twelve weeks. In these cluster periods they are woken by pain in the early morning ('alarm-clock' headache) or within an hour of going to sleep. The pain builds up over five to 10 minutes and lasts, typically, from 40 to 60 minutes. Any theory about cluster headache needs to explain not only the site of the lesion but also this temporal pattern of symptoms. A vascular origin for cluster headache is supported by the observation that one can induce an attack within 20 to 30 minutes by giving alcohol in such a high proportion of patients that they already know they need to avoid alcohol before it has even been mentioned by a doctor.

MOSKOWITZ: I have noticed that an antecedent history of head injury in men with cluster headache has sometimes been described.

BLAU: I have not observed any evidence for a relationship to head injury.

LANCE: Neither has Kudrow (1980) in a series of over 400 patients. I have noticed an association in individual cases between the site of head trauma and the later development of cluster headache affecting the same area.

OLESEN: Thinking about the symptoms of cluster headache, and where we can put it in our classification (Headache Classification Committee of the International Headache Society 1988), I have a difficulty with the peculiar blend of hyperactivity and hypo-activity of the autonomic nervous system at the same time. The sympathetic system can be both hypo-active and hyperactive, for example, miosis and increased sweating.

MOSKOWITZ: I am suggesting that the fibres going to the eye are being destroyed selectively perhaps because the lesion here is very close to the convergence of oculosympathetic fibres at the point that sympathetic fibres join the supraorbital nerve and ophthalmic artery. Hence, oculosympathetics do not respond to activation of the superior cervical ganglia as do sweat fibres of the face.

OLESEN: So two things are going on at the same time.

MOSKOWITZ: I am suggesting that the constellation of pain (activation of pain fibres) as well as activation of the sphenopalatine and superior cervical ganglia relates to their presence (for example, termination sites) within a unique, pathophysiological pericarotid focus. The fact that only the above pathways are activated relates to the anatomy of this region. Sympathetic (superior cervical ganglion) and parasympathetic (sphenopalatine ganglion) activation may arise by one or more mechanisms. Since trigeminalectomy blocks both pain and autonomic symptoms and signs, the more likely mechanism relates to central transmission via the trigeminovascular fibres. Then, via polysynaptic brainstem and spinal cord pathways, the superior cervical and sphenopalatine ganglia are activated. A second possible mechanism relates to retrograde activation via autonomic termination sites surrounding the carotid artery. It is important to remember, though, that the specificity of autonomic activation relates to the presence of specific termination sites within the perivascular region under consideration. In my paper, I have proposed the minimum lesion that can account for the syndrome expressed in its complete form. More extensive carotid involvement cannot be excluded in proximal segments such as within the carotid canal or distally, either as part of the above formulation, or when the syndrome is expressed in less than its entirely.

PEATFIELD: If something goes wrong within the cavernous sinus, the swelling of the arterial wall could irritate all the nerves that pass through the bony canal at that point. Therefore we must invoke activation of nerves further down the artery to explain the selective sensory and autonomic involvement without ophthalmoplegia. We need to find out which of those nerves is supplying the blood vessel at that level. If we are to hunt for the pathogenesis of this illness, we have to find out what causes the artery to swell.

MOSKOWITZ: I agree, but we do not yet know whether the vessel wall is swollen. If it is, it may be caused by the neurogenic inflammation, or by a herpes infection, for example.

PEATFIELD: Perhaps the way forward is to ask ourselves what *sort* of physiological or pathological process could be taking place in the arterial wall at that point.

ROSE: At this stage Dr Moskowitz is simply discussing the anatomy. Sometimes the symptoms of rhinorrhoea and lachrymation come some time after the start of a cluster headache. Can your anatomical considerations explain that?

MOSKOWITZ: An incomplete expression of the cluster syndrome may be explained by a lesion elsewhere than in the superior aspect of the cavernous carotid. The origin of the pain and the parasympathetic activation may be in the sphenopalatine fossa, but one would not expect to see the Horner's-like syndrome. The lesion could be large and within the orbit, but that might not explain responses to ergot alkaloids. It seems likely that a remote area, with convergence of fibres close to the midline, is the source for the cluster headache. Yet, if more than one lesion were to be involved we would need to rethink this hypothesis.

WELCH: There is evidence of post-junctional supersensitivity affecting the sympathetic system in cluster headache patients (Fanciullacci 1979). Do you know of any similar evidence that suggests a persistent post-junctional supersensitivity in the cholinergic system?

MOSKOWITZ: I do not know of anybody who has addressed the question.

LANCE: Neither do I. The post-junctional supersensitivity in the sympathetic system is one of the reasons why I think the third sympathetic neurone is involved.

MOSKOWITZ: The pathophysiology could be related to a virus infection, or to an infarct in the vessel wall. There are many possibilities, and they now require investigation.

PEATFIELD: Perhaps *post-mortem* examination of this piece of artery could be done *in vitro*, with the techniques that Dr Edvinsson has been using.

EDVINSSON: We have not studied cluster headache patients, but I know of one study where Hardebo *et al.* (1980) reported that the human temporal artery was more sensitive to histamine than arteries from control subjects. Further studies of different peptides and amines are needed in this field.

MOSKOWITZ: Imaging techniques should allow a closer examination of the trigeminal ganglion and its connections to the carotid artery. Magnetic resonance can give information about the calibre and diameter of vessels much smaller than the carotid artery.

WELCH: A lesion at that site might also imply some persistent neurological deficit in the first division, but one never sees that.

MOSKOWITZ: No, because the trigeminovascular fibres do not have a cutaneous branch, and neither do the maxillary fibres that innervate intracranial vessels. We showed that trigeminal fibres that innervate intracranial blood vessels project from a population separate from those that innervate cutaneous structures (Borges and Moskowitz 1983; McMahon *et al.* 1985).

References

Borges, L.F. and Moskowitz, M.A. (1983). Do intracranial trigeminal afferents represent divergent axon collaterals? *Neuroscience Letters*, **35**, 265–70.

Drummond, P.D. (1988). Autonomic disturbances in cluster headache. *Brain*, **111**, 1199–209.

Fanciullacci, M. (1979). Iris adrenergic impairment in idiopathic headache. *Headache*, **19**, 8–13.

Gardner, W.J., Stowell, A., and Dutlinger, R. (1947). Resection of the greater superficial nerve in the treatment of unilateral headache. *Journal of Neurosurgery*, **4**, 105–14.

Hardebo, J.E., Aebelholt-Krabbe, A., and Gjerris, F. (1980). Enhanced dilatory response to histamine in large extracranial vessels in chronic cluster headache. *Headache*, **20**, 316–20.

Headache Classification Committee of the International Headache Society. (Jes Olesen, chairman). (1988). Classification and diagnostic criteria for headache disorders, cranial neuralgias and facial pain. *Cephalalgia*, **8**, Suppl. 7, 1–96.

Kudrow, L. (1980). *Cluster headache: mechanisms and management*. Oxford University Press, Oxford.

McMahon, M.D., Norregaard, T.V., Beyerl, B.D., Borges, L.F., and Moskowitz, M.A. (1985). Trigeminal afferents to cerebral arteries and forehead are not divergent axon collaterals. *Neuroscience Letters*, **60**, 63–8.

Sandler, M. (1968). The role of 5-hydroxyindoles in the carcinoid syndrome. In *Advances in Pharmacology*, Vol. 6B, (ed. E. Costa and M. Sandler), pp. 127–42. Academic Press, New York.

Sessle, B.J., Hu, J.W., Amano, N., and Zhong, G. (1986). Convergence of cutaneous tooth pulp, visceral neck and muscle afferents onto nociceptive and non-nociceptive neurones in trigeminal subnucleus caudalis (medullary dorsal horn) and its implications for referred pain. *Pain*, **27**, 219–35.

Sicuteri, F. (1988). Antiandrogenic medication of cluster headache. *International Journal of Clinical Pharmacology Research*, **8**, 21–4.

11. 5-HT in migraine: evidence from 5-HT receptor antagonists for a neuronal aetiology

J.R. Fozard

Introduction

The substantial biochemical, pharmacological, and anatomical evidence which has accumulated in the last 20 years in support of a role for 5-hydroxytryptamine (5-HT) in migraine is summarized in Table 11.1. Unlike many of the concepts and hypotheses in this field, the idea that 5-HT plays a crucial role in migraine has slowly *gained* in credibility, and few would now question the basic premise; it is the precise nature of that role which remains to be defined.

That agents with selective effects on 5-HT mechanisms can alter the course of migraine is perhaps the strongest evidence implicating 5-HT in migraine (Table 11.1). In particular, the fact that antagonists at certain 5-HT receptor subtypes are effective in the prophylaxis or treatment of migraine implicates the endogenous amine in a causal role in the condition. On the basis of the properties and selectivities of such antagonists, I shall discuss the potential significance of $5\text{-}HT_{1C}$, $5\text{-}HT_2$, and $5\text{-}HT_3$ receptors in the initiation, development and symptomatology of migraine. The likely source(s) of the 5-HT needed to stimulate these sites will be considered, and a hypothesis will be proposed to implicate the activity of the 5-HT neurones arising in the mid-brain raphé nuclei in a key rôle in the aetiology of migraine. The ideas discussed here are developments and extensions of those expressed over a number of years in several review articles (Fozard 1975, 1982*a,b*, 1985; Peatfield *et al.* 1986; Fozard 1988) and are by no means unique (see also Moskowitz 1984; Lance 1985; Richardson *et al.* 1986).

'Classical' 5-HT receptor antagonists and prophylaxis

The efficacy of methysergide and pizotifen in the prophylactic treatment of migraine has been repeatedly demonstrated under controlled conditions (see Gelmers 1983). Fewer data are available with cyproheptadine (Peatfield *et al.* 1986) but prophylactic benefit with this agent is generally conceded (Lance 1982; Peatfield 1986). The receptor binding profiles of these agents

TABLE 11.1.   *Evidence supporting a role for 5-HT in migraine*

Biochemical evidence

Platelet 5-HT concentrations fall rapidly at the onset of a migraine attack.

Increased excretion of 5-hydroxyindoleacetic acid in urine is associated with migraine attacks in some patients.

Pharmacological evidence

Attacks can be triggered by the 5-HT-releasing agents, reserpine and fenfluramine, and by 1-(*m*-chlorophenyl) piperazine (*m*-CPP), a 5-HT receptor agonist with selectivity for 5-HT$_{1C}$ sites.

Zimeldine, a selective blocker of 5-HT tissue uptake, initially worsens attacks.

Antagonists of 5-HT$_{1C}$/5-HT$_2$ receptors (methysergide, pizotifen, and cyproheptadine) are effective prophylactic agents.

MDL 72222, a selective 5-HT$_3$ receptor antagonist, is effective in symptomatic treatment.

Anatomical evidence

Cerebral vessels are innervated by 5-HT-containing neurones arising from mid-brain raphé nuclei and the peripheral nervous system.

Localization of 5-HT receptor subtypes is consistent with their pathophysiological role.

For information sources and extensive discussion, see Fozard 1982*a*, 1985; Richardson *et al.* 1986; Brewerton *et al.* 1988.

are presented in Table 11.2. Although these drugs are by no means selective, it is striking that only at the 5-HT$_{1C}$ and 5-HT$_2$ receptor subtypes do *all* the drugs display high, nanomolar affinity. Blockade of histamine H$_1$ or muscarine receptors is not generally recognized as helpful in prophylaxis. Similar activities at 5-HT$_{1C}$ and 5-HT$_2$ sites are perhaps not too surprising since these sites show similarities both with respect to pharmacology and in their link to the phosphatidyl inositol second messenger pathway (Hoyer 1988). However, 5-HT$_{1C}$ and 5-HT$_2$ sites *can* be discriminated pharmacologically (Hoyer *et al.* 1985) and their distribution in animal (Hoyer 1988) and human (Hoyer *et al.* 1986) brains is quite distinct. Thus, each should be considered separately as possible site(s) of action for methysergide, pizotifen, and cyproheptadine, and in their significance to the pathophysiology of migraine.

5-HT$_{1C}$ receptors and migraine

Although 5-HT$_{1C}$ receptors are found in small amounts in a number of human brain areas including frontal cortex and the pyramidal layer of the

TABLE 11.2. *Receptor-binding affinities of 5-HT receptor ligands with beneficial effects in migraine*

		Prophylaxis			Acute treatment
		methysergide	pizotifen	cyproheptadine	MDL 72222
5-HT$_{1A}$		25	630	316	>1000
5-HT$_{1B}$		>1000	>1000	>1000	>1000
5-HT$_{1C}$		3	8	13	>1000
5-HT$_{1D}$		3	>1000	(−)	>1000
5-HT$_2$		3	16	17	>1000
5-HT$_3$		>1000	(−)	263	6
Adrenoceptors	α_1	>1000	120	100	>1000
	α_2	>1000	480	>1000	>1000
	β	>1000	>1000	>1000	>1000
Histamine	H$_1$	>1000	2	3	>1000
Dopamine	D$_1$	200	99	3	>1000
Muscarine		>1000	23	19	>1000

(−) no data. Values are K_D (5-HT receptor subtypes) or K_I in nM from radioligand binding studies using membranes prepared from various regions of pig, calf, rat, or guinea-pig brains, or mouse neuroblastoma cells (5-HT$_3$). Data sources: Fozard 1984a; Hoyer and Neijt 1988; Hoyer 1989.

hippocampus, it is in the choroid plexus where, in common with other species, these sites are spectacularly enriched (Hoyer *et al.* 1986). Other than their being coupled through G proteins to phospholipase C activation (Conn *et al.* 1986; Hoyer 1988, 1989), little is known of the functional significance of these 5-HT$_{1C}$ sites. The main physiological function of the choroid plexus is to control the volume and composition of the cerebrospinal fluid (Dawson 1967). Since the choroid and the ependymal surface of the ventricular system receive a 5-HT neuronal innervation (Richards *et al.* 1980), it is conceptually possible that 5-HT, acting through 5-HT$_{1C}$ receptors, could play a role in the normal or abnormal functioning of the choroid plexus. However, so little is known of this system that detailed speculation in the context of migraine would not be justified.

What *could* be justified is an increasing research effort to elucidate the putative link between 5-HT$_{1C}$ receptors, the choroid plexus and migraine. In this context, Brewerton *et al.* (1988) have recently shown that typical common migraine-like headaches can be triggered by oral administration of 1-(*m*-chlorophenyl)piperazine (*m*-CPP). *m*-CPP has higher affinity for 5-HT$_{1C}$ receptors than 5-HT itself (Hoyer 1989), 65 per cent of the efficacy of 5-HT in stimulating inositol phosphate production in pig choroid plexus (Hoyer and Schoeffter 1989), and meaningful selectivity *vis à vis* other 5-HT receptor subtypes found in humans (Hoyer 1989; Hoyer and

Schoeffter 1989). In behavioural studies in animals, low doses of m-CPP
$(0.1-1\text{mg kg}^{-1})$ appear to activate selectively 5-HT$_{1C}$ receptors to generate
signs of anxiety and behavioural depression (see Curzon *et al*. this volume).
It bears emphasis that cyproheptadine (Hoyer 1988), methysergide, and
pizotifen (D. Hoyer, personal communication) are 5-HT$_{1C}$ receptor *antagonists*; such a mechanism could well be pertinent to their prophylactic
efficacy in migraine.

5-HT$_2$ receptors and migraine

The 5-HT$_2$ receptors have a widespread distribution, being present in vascular and non-vascular smooth muscle, on platelets and in several areas of
the human brain including frontal cortex and hippocampus (Feniuk 1984;
Bradley *et al*. 1986; Hoyer *et al*. 1986). The high affinity of methysergide,
pizotifen and cyproheptadine for 5-HT$_2$ recognition sites (Table 11.2) trans-
lates into powerful *antagonist* effects at functional 5-HT$_2$ receptors (Feniuk
1984; Van Nueten 1984). If such activity is the basis of the therapeutic
efficacy of these agents, it is pertinent to look in detail at those 5-HT$_2$
receptors most likely to be relevant to migraine. Logically these would be
those associated with the cranial vasculature, the platelets, the neurones
involved in perception and processing of pain, and the sites initiating biochemical events that could trigger or sustain an attack.

The response of the cranial vasculature to 5-HT$_2$ receptor activation is
vasoconstriction (see Saxena 1982) and this is consistent with the classic
concept of intracranial vasoconstriction progressing to extracranial vasodilatation, as the basis of migraine (Wolff 1963). However, recent studies
(Olesen and Lauritzen 1984; Lauritzen and Olesen 1984) show that regional
blood flow changes are negligible in common migraine and, although they
are typical and consistent in classical migraine, they have neither the magnitude nor the temporal characteristics to account for either the initiation or
the symptomatology of an attack (Bruyn 1984; Wilkinson and Blau 1985).
Hence it seems unlikely that 5-HT$_2$-receptor-mediated constriction of the
cranial vascular smooth muscle can be critical in the development of migraine. On the other hand, 5-HT$_2$ receptors are also present on endothelial
cells, contraction of which could lead to rapid fluid extravasation and perivascular oedema (Ortmann *et al*. 1982; Fozard and Middlemiss 1983). The
significance of this occurring in elements of the cerebrovascular bed is
obvious, and the point is developed further below. The 5-HT$_2$ receptor of
the platelet mediates aggregation and enhances the aggregatory properties
of other agents (De Clerck and Hermann 1983). Although the platelet
release reaction can occur in migraine (see Peatfield 1986) and there is a
significant (30–40 per cent) loss of the platelet 5-HT content at the onset of
an attack (see Fozard 1982a) the evidence for a *causal* role for either the
platelet, or its 5-HT$_2$ receptor, or the 5-HT it contains is not convincing.

Indeed, both clinical and biochemical evidence can be adduced against the concept (Fozard 1982a, 1988; Peatfield 1986). If the changes in platelet function during migraine are incidental and non-causal, then a key role for the platelet 5-HT$_2$ receptor cannot be entertained.

Sound evidence from animal studies supports a role for central 5-HT neurotransmission in the perception and processing of pain (Yaksh *et al.* 1981; Roberts 1984). Descending 5-HT neurones, originating in the midbrain raphé nuclei, synapse on secondary nociceptive afferents in the dorsal horn; activation of these descending fibres leads to inhibition of the sensory input that results in nociception. 5-HT$_2$ receptors are present on descending 5-HT neurones but the response to their stimulation is neuronal activation (Llewelyn *et al.* 1983). It is, therefore, not surprising that *hyperalgesia* has been reported following administration of 5-HT$_2$ receptor antagonists (Proudfit and Hammond 1981; Berge 1982). It seems unlikely that inappropriate *stimulation* of the 5-HT$_2$ receptor involved in pain processing could be relevant to migraine.

The 5-HT$_2$ receptor which may be particularly relevant to the aetiology of migraine mediates the generation of eicosanoids from arachidonic acid and their release from tissues. This phenomenon, and its exquisite sensitivity to suppression by 5-HT$_{1C}$/5-HT$_2$ receptor antagonists, was first demonstrated on lung tissue by Bakhle and his colleagues (Alabaster and Bakhle 1970; Bakhle and Smith 1974) and subsequently on vascular smooth muscle cells by Coughlin *et al.* (1981, 1984). The generation of eicosanoid products of arachidonic acid metabolism within the key tissues of the head could be the basis of the development of the 'sterile' inflammatory response of migraine; suppression of that mechanism could explain the efficacy of 5-HT$_{1C}$/5-HT$_2$ receptor antagonists in migraine.

5-HT$_3$ receptor antagonists and acute treatment

Published information is available on only one *selective* 5-HT$_3$ receptor antagonist, MDL 72222 (1αH, 3α, 5αH tropan-3-yl 3,5-dichlorobenzoate), in the treatment of migraine. The results are, however, clear; under both open (Fozard *et al.* 1985) and double-blind, placebo-controlled (Loisy *et al.* 1985) conditions, MDL 72222 (10–40 mg, administered intravenously) proved effective for treating the acute attack. Since MDL 72222 is not vasoactive, has no analgesic or anti-inflammatory properties, and was used at precisely the doses that selectively block 5-HT$_3$ receptors in animals (Fozard 1984a) and humans (Orwin and Fozard 1986), the results are consistent with the hypothesis that the pain of migraine stems from activation of 5-HT$_3$ receptors. Several other selective 5-HT$_3$ receptor antagonists are undergoing evaluation in migraine (Fozard 1987) and the results are awaited with interest.

5-HT₃ receptors and migraine

5-HT₃ receptors are widely distributed in the peripheral and central nervous systems of animals (Fozard 1984*b*; Bradley *et al*. 1986; Richardson and Engel 1986; Richardson and Buchheit 1988) and humans (Richardson *et al*. 1985; Orwin and Fozard 1986). Their activation results in neuronal depolarization and the release of transmitters from autonomic, afferent, and enteric neurones (see Richardson and Buchheit 1988). 5-HT₃ receptors have been visualized by autoradiography in the mammalian central nervous system by the use of [³H]ICS 205-930, a highly selective 5-HT₃ receptor ligand (Waeber *et al*. 1988). The highest densities are seen in areas involved in sensory processing such as the substantia gelatinosa of the spinal cord and the nuclei of the trigeminal nerve, vagus nerve and tractus solitarius (Waeber *et al*. 1988; C. Waeber, D. Hoyer and J.M. Palacios, personal communication). Consistent with this, in humans, 5-HT causes pain both by a direct action on sensory afferent fibres (Keele and Armstrong 1964; Greaves and Schuster 1967; Richardson *et al*. 1985) and by sensitizing such fibres to other nociceptive stimuli (Sicuteri *et al*. 1965; Bleehen and Keele 1977; Richardson *et al*. 1985).

Afferent neuronal stimulation by 5-HT acting through 5-HT₃ receptors may also be relevant to the nausea and vomiting that accompany the majority of migraine attacks. Thus, the vomiting induced by certain cancer radiotherapy and chemotherapy regimens is effectively inhibited by low doses of selective 5-HT₃ receptor antagonists in animals and humans (see Fozard, 1989). Vomiting may be triggered by a sudden release of 5-HT from the intestine (Matsuoka *et al*. 1962; Gunning *et al*. 1987) and may involve both 5-HT₃ receptors of the afferent vagus (Andrews *et al*. 1988) and similar sites in the area postrema (Higgins *et al*. 1989). Whilst it is not known whether a similar mechanism underlies the nausea and vomiting of migraine, it is of interest that attacks may be accompanied by large increases in urinary 5-hydroxyindoleacetic acid implying substantial mobilization of endogenous 5-HT (see Fozard 1982*a*). Clearly, data from clinical trials designed to address this question would be of considerable interest.

The pain-producing properties of 5-HT, its putative role in certain types of vomiting, and the key role of 5-HT₃ receptors in these phenomena are clearly of direct relevance to any theory implicating 5-HT in the pathophysiology of migraine.

A hypothesis for a neuronal aetiology

The above considerations suggest an involvement of certain 5-HT receptor subtypes in the aetiology of migraine and the important question arises as to the source of the 5-HT that activates them. For reasons presented previously (Fozard 1982*a*), the platelet cannot be considered as the source of this

5-HT, but a plausible alternative source is the efferent 5-HT-containing neurones that penetrate deep within the cerebral vasculature (Griffith *et al.* 1982; Griffith and Burnstock 1983; Alafaci *et al.* 1986; Cowen *et al.* 1986, 1987; Chang *et al.* 1987).

The 5-HT-containing neurones that innervate the cerebrovascular bed appear to arise from two sources. Some of these neurones have cell bodies in the median and dorsal raphé nuclei (Moskowitz *et al.* 1979; Reinhard *et al.* 1979; Edvinsson *et al.* 1983; Marco *et al.* 1985; Scatton *et al.* 1985; Tsai *et al.* 1985) and they classically provide the widespread 5-HT innervation of many brain structures (Symposium 1984). On the other hand, 5-HT is present in, and co-exists with noradrenaline in cerebrovascular sympathetic nerves that originate primarily in the superior cervical ganglion (Alafaci *et al.* 1986; Cowen *et al.* 1987; Saito and Lee 1987; Chang *et al.* 1988, 1989). Sound evidence exists that 5-HT is not synthesized within the sympathetic neurones but is taken up by an efficient axonal mechanism (Saito and Lee 1987; Chang *et al.* 1989). 5-HT can be released from perivascular neurones and can induce vasoconstriction (Griffith *et al.* 1982; Saito and Lee 1987). Unlike the platelet, which would deposit its 5-HT *outside* the blood–brain barrier, neuronal release of 5-HT would take place beyond the blood–brain barrier and would allow interaction of 5-HT with the structural elements of the cerebral vasculature and with other neurones of the perivascular plexus. Significantly, innervation by the raphé system would provide a direct link with a central neuronal system integrally involved in the reaction of the individual to stress, hunger and fatigue (Symposium 1984); it may not be coincidental that these encompass the major environmental precipitating factors for migraine. Moreover, the 'common denominator' of precipitating factors is generally considered to be stress in one form or another (Peatfield 1986); activation of the sympathetic nervous system is an inevitable accompaniment to acute stress.

On the basis of anatomical considerations and the properties and distribution of the 5-HT receptor subtypes implicated above, the scenario represented diagrammatically in Figure 11.1 could be envisaged. Migraine would be initiated by an increase in activity of the sympathetic nervous system (SCG in Fig. 11.1) coupled with an inappropriately high and/or fluctuating activity in mid-brain efferent monoamine-containing neurones. Activation of both 5-HT-containing neurones (A in Fig. 11.1) and catecholamine-containing neurones (B) could induce complex changes in blood flow in elements of both the intracranial and extracranial vasculature (C; see Lance *et al.* 1983; Goadsby *et al.* 1985*a,b*). More importantly, perhaps, and certainly *independently of the blood flow changes*, there would be several effects which together would provide a rational explanation for the initiation and development of the 'sterile' inflammatory response of migraine (D).

First, and by activation of 5-HT$_2$ receptors, a direct interaction of 5-HT with the smooth muscle cells of the cerebrovascular bed would lead to the

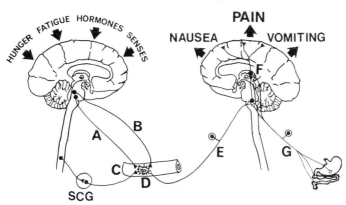

FIG. 11.1. A hypothesis for a neuronal aetiology of migraine based on the properties of 5-HT receptors and their antagonists. Migraine would arise following an inappropriate increase or fluctuation in the activity of monoaminergic neurones in response to a number of environmental (trigger) factors, including stress. Activation of both 5-HT-(A) and noradrenaline-(B) containing neurones arising from nuclei in the brainstem, as well as peripheral sympathetic neurones which store and release both noradrenaline and 5-HT (SCG, superior cervical ganglion), would induce complex blood flow changes in elements of both the intracranial and extracranial vasculature (C). Independently of the vascular changes, the diverse physiological effects of 5-HT mediated through $5-HT_2$, $5-HT_3$ and, possibly, $5-HT_{1C}$ receptors would initiate and sustain the sterile inflammatory response of migraine (D) and would contribute significantly to the generation of pain (E). Nausea and/or vomiting would be triggered by a release of 5-HT within the area postrema or vomiting centre (F) or by an increase in afferent vagal input (G) due to $5-HT_3$ receptor activation by 5-HT mobilized locally within the gastrointestinal tract. The scheme is a development of views expressed in earlier reviews (Fozard 1975, 1982*b*, 1985, 1988) and draws heavily on the ideas of others (Lance 1982, 1985; Moskowitz 1984; Richardson *et al*. 1986). For further details see text.

generation of proinflammatory products of arachidonic acid metabolism (Coughlin *et al.* 1981, 1984; Demolle and Boeynaems 1986; Kokkas and Boeynaems 1988). Second, and also reflecting the activation of $5-HT_2$ receptors, powerful contraction of the endothelial cells could lead to fluid extravasation and perivascular oedema (Ortmann *et al.* 1982; Fozard and Middlemiss 1983). 5-HT released locally within the blood vessels of the head would also, by activating $5-HT_3$ receptors, be expected to interact with elements of the perivascular neural plexus of which the afferent substance P-containing fibres of the trigeminal system (E) are considered of particular relevance to migraine (Moskowitz 1984). This would not only lead to pain (F) but also to exacerbation of inflammation by the local release of substance P both directly or by an axon reflex mechanism (Moskowitz 1984; Orwin and Fozard 1986).

A neurological aetiology based on the overproduction of 5-HT would also allow explanation of the other major symptoms of migraine — nausea and vomiting. Both the area postrema and the elements of the vasomotor centre receive a 5-HT innervation and neurones of the area postrema discharge in response to 5-HT (see Andrews *et al.* 1988). Both the area postrema and the vasomotor centre may also be activated by a $5\text{-}HT_3$ receptor-mediated increase in abdominal vagal afferent neuronal firing in response to an increased release of 5-HT locally in the gut (G in Fig. 11.1; Andrews *et al.* 1988).

Summary and conclusions

The above hypothesis of a neuronal aetiology for migraine assumes a key role for 5-HT, and is based on a variety of biochemical, pharmacological and anatomical evidence (Table 11.1). The distribution and function of $5\text{-}HT_{1C}/5\text{-}HT_2$ and $5\text{-}HT_3$ receptors, at which antagonists show benefits in prophylaxis and acute treatment, respectively, specifically implicate the 5-HT-containing neurones of the mid-brain raphé in a causative role. This concept is attractive because it links a central neuronal system (the raphé), responsive to many environmental factors identified as precipitating factors for migraine, directly to elements of the cerebrovasculature. Migraine would be initiated by an inappropriate increase or fluctuation in the activity of the 5-HT-containing neurones in the cerebrovascular bed. The resulting release of 5-HT within the cerebral vasculature would, by activating $5\text{-}HT_{1C}$ and/or $5\text{-}HT_2$ and $5\text{-}HT_3$ receptors, trigger and sustain the 'sterile' inflammatory response of migraine. Activation of $5\text{-}HT_3$ receptors present on perivascular sensory neurones would produce pain both directly and by sensitization of such fibres to other nociceptive stimuli. Stimulation of $5\text{-}HT_3$ receptors on visceral afferent neurones and/or in the area postrema or vomiting centre could be the basis of the nausea and vomiting of migraine. Although by no means exclusive, the concept does allow credible explanations to be made for: the initiation of migraine by the major trigger factors; the development of the attack; the principal symptoms; and the effects of the major forms of therapy (see Fozard 1985; Richardson *et al.* 1986). To be realistic, however, it would be unwise to assume that any single hormone or transmitter could carry the burden of full responsibility for the aetiology of a multi-faceted condition such as migraine — however plausible the case may be made to appear!

References

Alabaster, V.A. and Bakhle, Y.S. (1970). The release of biologically active substances from isolated lungs by 5-hydroxytryptamine and tryptamine. *British Journal of Pharmacology*, **40**, 528P.

Alafaci, C., Cowen, T., Crockard, II.A., and Burnstock, G. (1986). Cerebral perivascular serotonergic fibres have a peripheral origin in the gerbil. *Brain Research Bulletin*, **16**, 303–4.

Andrews, P.L.R., Rapeport, W.G., and Sanger, G.J. (1988). Neuropharmacology of emesis induced by anti-cancer therapy. *Trends in Pharmacological Science*, **9**, 334–41.

Bakhle, Y.S. and Smith, T.W. (1974). The nature of the tryptamine receptor mediating spasmogen release from rat isolated lungs. *British Journal of Pharmacology*, **50**, 463P.

Berge, O.-G. (1982). Effects of 5-HT receptor agonists and antagonists on a reflex response to radiant heat in normal and spinally transected rats. *Pain*, **13**, 253–66.

Bleehen, T. and Keele, C.A. (1977). Observations on the algogenic actions of adenosine compounds on the human blister base preparation. *Pain*, **3**, 367–77.

Bradley, P.B., Engel, C., Feniuk, W., Fozard J.R., Humphrey, P.P.A., Middlemiss, D.N., Mylecharane, E.J., Richardson, B.P., and Saxena P.R. (1986). Proposals for the classification and nomenclature of functional receptors for 5-hydroxytryptamine. *Neuropharmacology*, **25**, 563–76.

Brewerton, T.D., Murphy, D.L., Mueller, E.A., and Jimerson, D.C. (1988). Induction of migraine-like headaches by the serotonin agonist *m*-chlorophenylpiperazine. *Clinical Pharmacology and Therapeutics*, **43**, 605–9.

Bruyn, G.W. (1984). The pathomechanism of migraine: a clinicians epilogue. In *The pharmacological basis of migraine therapy* (ed. W.K. Amery, J.M. Van Nueten and A. Wauquier), pp. 267–78. Pitman, London.

Chang, J.-Y., Hardebo, J.E., Owman, C., Sahlin, C., and Svendgaard, N.-A. (1987). Nerves containing serotonin, its interaction with noradrenaline and characterization of serotonergic receptors in cerebral arteries of monkey. *Journal of Autonomic Pharmacology*, **7**, 317–29.

Chang, J.-Y., Owman, C., and Steinbusch, H.W.M. (1988). Evidence for coexistence of serotonin and noradrenaline in sympathetic nerves supplying brain vessels of guinea-pig. *Brain Research*, **438**, 237–46.

Chang, J.-Y., Ekblad, E., Kannisto, P., and Owman, C. (1989). Serotonin uptake into cerebrovascular nerve fibres of rat, visualization by immunohistochemistry, disappearance following sympathectomy, and release during electrical stimulation. *Brain Research*, in press.

Conn, P.J., Sanders-Bush, E., Hoffman, B.J., and Hartig, P.R. (1986). A unique serotonin receptor in choroid plexus is linked to phosphatidylinositol turnover. *Proceedings of the National Academy of Sciences USA*, **83**, 4086–8.

Coughlin, S.R., Moskowitz, M.A., Antoniades, H.N., and Levine, L. (1981). Serotonin receptor-mediated stimulation of bovine smooth muscle cell prostacyclin synthesis and its modulation by platelet-derived growth factor. *Proceedings of the National Academy of Sciences USA*, **78**, 7134–8.

Coughlin, S.R. Moskowitz, M.A., and Levine, L. (1984). Identification of a serotonin type 2 receptor linked to prostacyclin synthesis in vascular smooth muscle cells. *Biochemical Pharmacology*, **33**, 692–5.

Cowen, T. Alafaci, C. Crockard, H.A., and Burnstock, G. (1986). 5-HT-containing nerves in major cerebral arteries of gerbil originate in the superior cervical ganglion *Brain Research*, **384**, 51–9.

Cowen, T. Alafaci, C., Crockard, H.A., and Burnstock, G. (1987). Origin and postnatal development of nerves showing 5-hydroxytryptamine-like immunoreactivity supplying major cerebral arteries of the rat. *Neuroscience Letters*, **78**, 121–6.

Dawson, H. (1967). *The physiology of the cerebrospinal fluid*. Little Brown, Boston.

De Clerck, F. and Hermann, A.G. (1983). 5-Hydroxytryptamine and platelet aggregation. *Federation Proceedings*, **42**, 228–32.

Demolle, D. and Boeynaems, J.M. (1986). Prostacyclin production by the bovine aortic smooth muscle. *Prostaglandins*, **32**, 155–9.

Edvinsson, L., Degueurce, A., Duverger, D., MacKenzie, E.T., and Scatton, B. (1983). Central serotonergic nerves project to the pial vessels of the brain. *Nature*, **306**, 55–7.

Feniuk, W. (1984). An analysis of 5-hydroxytryptamine receptors mediating contraction of isolated smooth muscle. *Neuropharmacology*, **23**, 1467–72.

Fozard, J.R. (1975). The animal pharmacology of drugs used in the treatment of migraine. *Journal of Pharmacy and Pharmacology*,**27**, 297–321.

Fozard, J.R. (1982*a*). Serotonin, migraine and platelets. In *Drugs and platelets* (ed. P.A. Van Zwieten and E. Schönbaum), Progress in Pharmacology, Vol. 4, pp. 135–46. Fischer, Stuttgart.

Fozard, J.R. (1982*b*). Basic mechanisms of antimigraine drugs. In *Headache: Physiopathological and clinical concepts*. (ed. M. Critchley, A.P. Friedman, S. Gorini and F. Sicuteri), Advances in Neurology, Vol. 33, pp. 295–307. Raven Press, New York.

Fozard, J.R. (1984*a*). MDL 72222: A potent and highly selective antagonist at neuronal 5-hydroxytryptamine receptors. *Naunyn-Schmiedeberg's Archives of Pharmacology*, **326**, 36–44.

Fozard, J.R. (1984*b*). Neuronal 5-HT receptors in the periphery. *Neuropharmacology*, **23**, 1473–86.

Fozard, J.R. (1985). 5-Hydroxytryptamine in the pathophysiology of migraine. In *Vascular neuroeffector mechanisms*. (ed. J.A. Bevan, T. Godfraind, R.A. Maxwell, J.C. Stoclet and M. Worcel), pp. 321–8. Elsevier, Amsterdam.

Fozard, J.R. (1987). 5-HT: The enigma variations. *Trends in Pharmacological Sciences*, **8**, 501–6.

Fozard, J.R. (1988). The pharmacological basis of migraine treatment. In *Migraine: clinical, therapeutic, conceptual and research aspects*, (ed. J.N. Blau), pp. 165–84. Chapman and Hall, London.

Fozard, J.R. (1989). The development and early clinical evaluation of selective 5-HT$_3$ receptor antagonists. In *The peripheral actions of 5-hydroxytryptamine* (ed. J.R. Fozard), pp. 354–76, Oxford University Press, Oxford.

Fozard, J.R. and Middlemiss D.N. (1983). 5-HT$_2$ receptors mediate the oedematogenic response to 5-hydroxytryptamine in the rat. *Naunyn-Schmiedeberg's Archives of Pharmacology*, **324**, Suppl., R63.

Fozard, J.R., Loisy, C., and Tell, G.J. (1985). Blockade of neuronal 5-hydroxytryptamine receptors with MDL 72222: A novel approach to the symptomatic treatment of migraine. In *Migraine. Proceedings 5th International Migraine Symposium, London, 1984*, (ed. F. Clifford Rose), pp. 264–72. Karger, Basel.

Gelmers, H.J. (1983). Nimodipine, a new calcium antagonist, in the prophylactic treatment of migraine. *Headache*, **23**, 106–9.

Goadsby, P.J., Piper, R.D., Lambert, G.A., and Lance, J.W. (1985*a*). Effect of stimulation of nucleus raphe dorsalis on carotid blood flow. I: The monkey. *American Journal of Physiology*, **248**, R257–62

Goadsby, P.J., Piper, R.D., Lambert, G.A., and Lance, J.W. (1985*b*). Effect of stimulation of nucleus raphe dorsalis on carotid blood flow. II: The cat. *American Journal of Physiology*, **248**, R263–9.

Greaves, M.W. and Schuster, S. (1967). Response of skin blood vessels to bradykinin, histamine and 5-hydroxytryptamine. *Journal of Physiology (London)*, **193**, 255–67.

Griffith, S.G. and Burnstock, G. (1983). Immunohistochemical demonstration of serotonin in nerves supplying human cerebral and mesenteric blood vessels: Some speculations about their involvement in vascular disorders. *Lancet*, **i**, 561–2.

Griffith, S.G., Lincoln, J. and Burnstock, G. (1982). Serotonin as a neurotransmitter in cerebral arteries. *Brain Research*, **247**, 388–92.

Gunning, S.J., Hagan, R.M., and Tyers, M.B. (1987). Cisplatin induces biochemical and histological changes in the small intestine of the ferret. *British Journal of Pharmacology*, **90**, 135P.

Higgins, G.A., Kilpatrick, G.J., Bunce, K.T., Jones B.J., and Tyers, M.B. (1989). 5-HT$_3$ receptors in the area postrema may mediate the anti-emetic effects of 5-HT$_3$ antagonists in the ferret. *British Journal of Pharmacology*, **97**, 247–55.

Hoyer, D. (1988). Molecular pharmacology and biology of 5-HT$_{1C}$ receptors. *Trends in Pharmacological Sciences*, **9**, 89–94.

Hoyer, D. (1989). 5-Hydroxytryptamine receptors and effector mechanisms in peripheral tissues. In *The peripheral actions of 5-hydroxytryptamine*, (ed. J.R. Fozard), pp. 72–99, Oxford University Press, Oxford.

Hoyer, D. and Neijt, H.C. (1988). Identification of serotonin 5-HT$_3$ recognition sites in membranes of N1E-115 neuroblastoma cells by radioligand binding. *Molecular Pharmacology*, **33**, 303–9.

Hoyer, D. and Schoeffter, P. (1989). Are TFMPP, mCPP and CGS 12066 selective for 5-hydroxytryptamine 5-HT$_{1B}$ receptors? *British Journal of Pharmacology*, **96**, 9P.

Hoyer, D., Engel, G., and Kalkmann, H.O. (1985). Molecular pharmacology of 5-HT$_1$ and 5-HT$_2$ recognition sites in rat and pig brain membranes: radioligand binding studies with [^{3}H]5-HT, [^{3}H]8-OH-DPAT, [$(-)^{125}$I] iodocyanopindolol, [^{3}H]mesulergine and [^{3}H]ketanserin. *European Journal of Pharmacology*, **118**, 13–23.

Hoyer, D., Pazos, A. Probst, A., and Palacios, J.M. (1986). Serotonin receptors in the human brain. II: Characterization and autoradiographic localization of 5-HT$_{1C}$ and 5-HT$_2$ recognition sites. *Brain Research*, **376**, 97–107.

Keele, C.A. and Armstrong, D. (1964). *Substances producing pain and itch*. Williams and Wilkins, Baltimore.

Kokkas, B. and Boeynaems, J.-M. (1988). Release of prostacyclin from the dog saphenous vein by 5-hydroxytryptamine. *European Journal of Pharmacology*, **147**, 473–6.

Lance, J.W. (1982). *Mechanism and management of headache* (4th edn) Butterworth, London.

Lance, J.W. (1985). The pathophysiology of migraine. *Annales Academiae Medicae*, **14**, 4–11.

Lance, J.W., Lambert, G.A., Goadsby, P.J., and Duckworth, J.W. (1983). Brainstem influences on the cephalic circulation: experimental data from cat and monkey of relevance to the mechanism of migraine. *Headache*, **23**, 258–65.

Lauritzen, M. and Olesen, J. (1984). Regional cerebral blood flow during migraine attacks by Xenon-133 inhalation and emission tomography. *Brain*, **107**, 447–61.

Llewelyn, M.B., Azami, J., and Roberts, M.H.T. (1983). Effects of 5-hydroxytryptamine applied into nucleus raphé magnus on nociceptive thresholds and neuronal firing rate. *Brain Research*, **258**, 59–68.

Loisy, C., Beorchia, S., Centonze, V., Fozard, J.R., Schechter, P.J., and Tell, G.P. (1985). Effects on migraine headache of MDL 72222 on antagonist at neuronal 5-HT receptors. Double-blind, placebo-controlled study. *Cephalalgia*, **5**, 79–82.

Marco, E.J., Balfagon, G., Salaices, M., Sanchez-Ferrer, C., and Marin, J. (1985). Serotonergic innervation of cat cerebral arteries. *Brain Research*, **338**, 137–9.

Matsuoka, O., Tsuchiya, T., and Furukawa, Y. (1962). The effect of X-irradiation on 5-hydroxytryptamine (serotonin) contents in the small intestines of experimental animals. *Journal of Radiation Research*, **302**, 104–9.

Moskowitz, M.A. (1984). The neurobiology of vascular head pain. *Annals of Neurology*, **6**, 157–68.

Moskowitz, M.A., Liebmann, J.E., Reinhard, J.F. Jr, and Schlosberg, A. (1979). Raphé origin of serotonin-containing neurons within choroid plexus of the rat. *Brain Research*, **169**, 590–4.

Olesen, J. and Lauritzen, M. (1984). The role of vasoconstriction in the pathogenesis of migraine. In *The pharmacological basis of migraine therapy*, (ed. W.K. Amery, J.M. Van Nueten and A. Wauquier), pp. 7–18. Pitman, Bath.

Ortmann, R., Bischoff, S., Radeke, E., Buech, O., and Delina-Stula A. (1982). Correlations between different measures of antiserotonin activity of drugs. Study with neuroleptics and serotonin receptor blockers. *Naunyn-Schmiedeberg's Archives of Pharmacology*, **321**, 265–70.

Orwin, J.M. and Fozard, J.R. (1986). Blockade of the flare response to intradermal 5-hydroxytryptamine in man by MDL 72222, a selective antagonist at neuronal 5-hydroxytryptamine receptors. *European Journal of Clinical Pharmacology*, **30**, 209–12.

Peatfield, R.C. (1986). *Headache*. Springer-Verlag, Berlin.

Peatfield, R.C., Fozard, J.R., and Clifford Rose, F. (1986). Drug treatment of migraine. In *Handbook of Clinical Neurology*, Vol. 4, *Headache*, (ed. F. Clifford Rose), pp. 173–216. Elsevier, Amsterdam.

Proudfit, H.K. and Hammond, D.L. (1981). Alterations in nociceptive threshold and morphine-induced analgesia produced by intrathecally administered amine antagonists. *Brain Research*, **218**, 393–9.

Reinhard, J.F. Jr, Liebman, J.E., Schlosberg, A.T., and Moskowitz, M.A. (1979). Serotonin neurons project to small blood vessels in the brain. *Science*, **206**, 85–7.

Richards, J.G., Lorenz, H.P., Colombo, V.E., Guggenheim, R., and Kiss, D. (1980). Supra-ependymal nerve fibres in human brain: correlative transmission and scanning electron microscopical and fluorescence histochemical studies. *Neuroscience*, **5**, 1489–1502.

Richardson, B.P. and Engel, G. (1986). The pharmacology and function of 5-HT$_3$ receptors. *Trends in Neuroscience*, **9**, 424–8.

Richardson, B.P. and Buchheit, K.-H. (1988). The pharmacology, distribution and function of 5-HT$_3$ receptors. In *Neuronal serotonin*, (ed. N.N. Osborne and M. Hamon), pp. 465–504. Wiley, Chichester.

Richardson, B.P., Engel, G., Donatsch, P., and Stadler, P.A. (1985). Identification of serotonin M-receptor subtypes and their specific blockade by a new class of drugs. *Nature*, **316**, 126–31.

Richardson, B.P. *et al.* (1986). Defective serotoninergic transmission: A possible cause of migraine and a basis for the efficacy of ergot compounds in the treatment of attacks. In *Recent trends in the management of migraine*, (ed. J.W. Lance), pp. 9–21. Editio Cantor, Aulendorf.

Roberts, M.H.T. (1984). 5-hydroxytryptamine and antinociception. *Neuropharmacology*, **23**, 1529–36.

Saito, A. and Lee, T.J.-F. (1987). Serotonin as an alternative transmitter in sympathetic nerves of large cerebral arteries of the rabbit. *Circulation Research*, **60**, 220–8.

Saxena, P.R. (1982). Agonists and antagonists of vascular receptors. In *Headache: Physiopathological and clinical concepts*, Advances in Neurology, Vol. 33, (ed. M. Critchley, A.P. Friedman, S. Gorini and F. Sicuteri), pp. 309–314. Raven Press, New York

Scatton, B. *et al.* (1985). Neurochemical studies on the existence, origin and characteristics of the serotonergic innervation of small pial vessels. *Brain Research*, **345**, 219–29.

Sicuteri, F., Fanciulacci, M., Franchi, G., and Del Bianco, P.L. (1965). Serotonin-bradykinin potentiation on the pain receptors in man. *Life Sciences*, **4**, 309–16.

Symposium (1984). 5-HT, peripheral and central receptors and function. *Neuropharmacology*, **23**, 1511–69.

Tsai, S.H., Lin, S.Z., Wang, S.D., Liu, J.C., and Shih, C.J. (1985). Retrograde localization of the innervation of the middle cerebral artery with horseradish peroxidase in cats. *Neurosurgery*, **16**, 463–7.

Van Nueten, J.M. (1984). Antivasoconstrictor effects of drugs used in migraine therapy. In *The pharmacological basis of migraine therapy*, (ed. W.K. Amery, J.M. Van Nueten and A. Wauquier), pp. 19–35. Pitman, Bath.

Waeber, C., Dixon, K., Hoyer, D., and Palacios, J.M. (1988). Localisation by autoradiography of neuronal 5-HT$_3$ receptors in the mouse CNS. *European Journal of Pharmacology*, **151**, 351–2.

Wilkinson, M. and Blau, J.N. (1985). Are classical and common migraine different entities? *Headache*, **25**, 211–2.

Wolff, H.G. (1963). *Headache and other head pain* (2nd edn). Oxford University Press, New York.

Yaksh, T.L., Hammond, D.L., and Tyce, G.M. (1981). Functional aspects of bulbospinal monoaminergic projections in modulating processing of somatosensory information. *Federation Proceedings*, **40**, 2786–94.

Discussion

SANDLER: I was a reluctant convert to any interpretation of migraine related to 5-hydroxytryptamine (5-HT; serotonin). When Gerald Curzon and I were measuring 5-hydroxyindoleacetic acid in the urine of migraine patients in the late 1960s, we could not find any significant increase. I was never impressed by the findings about reserpine which, as you say, is a 'dirty' drug and does not produce a real migraine headache as far as I know. Fenfluramine, which is analogous to tyramine, and tyramine itself, are themselves dirty drugs, in the sense that they have multiple actions. We know that tyramine not only liberates noradrenaline; amongst its other actions it probably liberates neuropeptide Y (Cheng and Shen 1986). But can I now ask, again, Pramod Saxena's question of 20 years ago? Is it too much or too little 5-HT that promotes migraine?

FOZARD: The migraine attack is a consequence of too much 5-HT, in my opinion. I do not support the depletion hypothesis. Incidentally, surely the idea that tyramine can trigger a migraine is no longer taken seriously?

SANDLER: Yes, although some people would still believe it, I suspect.

FOZARD: So if tyramine does not trigger a migraine, and if it is indeed a dirty drug, the observations with fenfluramine become more significant!

HUMPHREY: It is important for us all to consider the evidence that you have put forward. But I do not believe there *is* any sound proof that 5-HT is involved in the pathogenesis of migraine. There is no correlation between 5-HT plasma levels and the migraine headache; when the platelet level falls, the associated headache later goes, but the platelet 5-HT level continues to remain low. Neither can a raised 5-HT level be involved because in carcinoid syndrome there are no migraine-like headaches, or any form of headache. James Lance's group (Anthony *et al.* 1967) showed that when a migraine-like headache is treated with an intravenous injection of 5-HT, the headache goes, but then other vasoconstrictors are also effective. All the evidence for an involvement of 5-HT seems to me to be circumstantial. In my own paper (this volume) I have tabulated the evidence for and against, and reached the opposite conclusion from you, whilst using the same data.

FOZARD: Clearly, there is something different about a migraine patient compared with a normal individual. That may be why carcinoid patients do not show headache. Furthermore, platelet 5-HT is not necessarily important to my argument. 5-HT released from platelets will be around in the plasma for only a very short time. One passage through the lungs, for example, and 95 per cent of it is gone (Thomas and Vane 1967). So your reference to 5-HT changes in the plasma does not negate my hypothesis. Endogenous 5-HT release, however, as I have tried to describe, does seem to trigger an attack.

HUMPHREY: I understood that it is not a migraine attack that is triggered, but a headache. Good evidence for the involvement of 5-HT is still required, in my opinion.

SANDLER: About 10 per cent of carcinoid patients, incidentally, *do* have a headache.

SAXENA: Also, 10 per cent of the normal population might have a headache at any one time! Dr Fozard, you said that 5-HT_2 antagonists are very good antimigraine drugs, and that methysergide is active in migraine by blocking 5-HT_2 receptors. However, for methysergide one can argue the other way round, because it seems to be a partial agonist at the 5-HT_1 receptors involved in the constriction of cephalic arteries and arteriovenous anastomoses (Saxena and Verdouw 1984; Humphrey *et al.* 1989).

FOZARD: I think not; at least not at the doses in question, which are 2–4 mg per patient, orally. This dose level is much lower than would be required to activate 5-HT_1 receptors.

SAXENA: There is a heterogeneity in the 5-HT_1-like receptors, and it seems to me that the doses of methysergide are sufficient to activate the specific 5-HT_1-like receptor subtype.

FOZARD: But you saw the binding data that I showed; methysergide is at least 300-fold less active at other 5-HT_1 receptor subtypes than at 5-HT_2 or 5-HT_{1C} receptors. These affinity data do have their place in our debate.

SAXENA: It is the functional effects that I am more interested in and, moreover, methysergide can be metabolized to an active metabolite, methylergometrine (Müller-Schweinitzer and Tapparelli 1986). I have another point. The effectiveness of amitriptyline may be related to a blockade of 5-HT uptake, and there are many 5-HT_2 antagonists which are either ineffective (ketanserin) or only a little effective (cyproheptadine, mianserin) in migraine therapy. This is against your thesis that a *high* concentration of 5-HT is associated with the pathophysiology of migraine headache.

FOZARD: At least one controlled study shows mianserin to work (Munro *et al.* 1985), and several studies are available showing that amitriptyline works. Ketanserin, as far as I know, has been tested in a somewhat cursory way, in an open trial.

SAXENA: Your clinical trial reporting the effectiveness of MDL 72222 in acute migraine attacks (Loisy *et al.* 1985) does, I believe, provide evidence about a role for stimulation of 5-HT_3 receptors. However, what worries me is the recent report that another 5-HT_3 receptor antagonist, ICS 205-930 (X.Lataste, Symposium on cardiovascular effects of migraine, Amsterdam, October 1988), does not abort acute migraine attacks. Besides, several other potent and selective 5-HT_3 receptor antagonists have been synthesized but their effects in migraine have not been reported.

FOZARD: The only other compound we yet know about in this context is ICS 205-930, and the results to date have, indeed, not been encouraging.

LANCE: The injection of reserpine in the migrainous patient *does* replicate a typical migrainous headache, to follow up Professor Sandler's initial point in this discussion. If it is given to normal subjects they just get a dull, unpleasant sensation in the head. In a migrainous patient, the headache develops in the falling phase of 5-HT. The 5-HT level then remains low, while patients lose their headache. Indeed, reserpine has been used long-term for the amelioration of migrainous headache. As Pat Humphrey just mentioned, the injection of 5-HT (2.0–7.5 mg) intravenously will stop such an induced headache (Anthony *et al.* 1967). But the platelet content of 5-HT does not vary significantly with the presence or absence of vomiting. We showed (Anthony *et al.* 1969) that when patients vomited there was not a sudden upsurge of 5-HT into the circulation, as one might imagine, but the 5-HT level just recovered slowly with the natural course of the migrainous attack. Another point is that sympathectomy does not affect the natural history of migrainous headache. Therefore I cannot accept that the cervical sympathetic nervous system is directly relevant here. I concede, of course, that the intrinsic autonomic nervous system, arising from locus coeruleus and from the raphé nuclei, *is* playing an important part.

FOZARD: Those observations are interesting. If we accept that migraineurs have a reduced threshold for a migraine attack, relative to normal (non-migrainous) people, they may respond quite differently if their brainstem neurones fire inappropriately.

EDVINSSON: We should try to clear up the question of the 5-HT innervation. 5-HT has two actions: it dilates the small *arterioles* but it constricts large and small arteries. Reinhard *et al.* (1979) took out rat microvessels — arterioles, capillaries and venules — from the brain. We, on the other hand, removed the small pial arterioles on the rat cortex (Edvinsson *et al.* 1983). Others who claim to have found 5-HT in sympathetic nerves have, in principle, worked on the middle cerebral artery or on other arteries of the circle of Willis. An artefact may be operating here: if the animal is sacrificed, and the vessels are removed and examined immunocytochemically, 5-HT is found in the sympathetic fibres. However, if the animal is anaesthetized, perfused with buffer to rinse out the platelets, and then sections are taken for microscopy there is, reportedly, no 5-HT in the sympathetic fibres. We, as well as Reinhard *et al.* (1979), have performed selective raphé lesions, and found that 5-HT levels in pial arterioles or cerebral microvessels are reduced by about half. Sympathectomy in our study did not affect the 5-HT levels. For the small vessels it appears that the raphé system may contribute to the cerebrovascular innervation. This view is supported by the work of Marco et al. (1985) and Scatton et al. (1985). The role of the raphé nucleus merits further study.

FOZARD: There are clear differences in the origin of these vessels, and at least part of the difference in their responses can be explained by their type and size. In the published work of Chang et al. (1987, 1988, 1989) the whole story seems to hang together very well; perhaps their experimental conditions were just right!

OLESEN: You described that the drug, MDL 72222, works on both pain and nausea of a migraine attack. One also reads that ergotamine is one of the few drugs that can affect both of those symptoms. We need to rethink this: the nausea is, surely, in some way a secondary phenomenon to the pain. When patients enter an acute migraine clinic, and are cared for, very often their nausea goes away but their pain does not. Aspirin works highly significantly better than a placebo for the nausea, as well as (obviously) for the pain.

FOZARD: What may be significant with respect to the $5-HT_3$ receptor antagonists is that both in animal experiments and in humans the antagonists are effective against emesis provoked by very severe emetogenic stimuli such as cancer chemotherapy or radiotherapy. There may well be, for both the vomiting of migraine and that produced by cytotoxic drugs or radiation, a common feature in the form of a substantial mobilization of (presumably) intestinal 5-HT (see Fozard 1989).

VANE: If you believe that 5-HT receptor activation releases prostaglandins or prostacyclin, why do we need to use a 5-HT receptor antagonist for treatment? Why can we not just use aspirin, which would act in the same way, or even indomethacin, which gets through the blood–brain barrier better?

FOZARD: Aspirin and indomethacin will take out only a component of the overall inflammatory response; so, too, will a $5-HT_3$ receptor antagonist. I would like to see a trial of a $5-HT_3$ receptor antagonist in patients who are being given indomethacin or aspirin. This could be an interesting combination.

VANE: Has anyone compared indomethacin with aspirin in the treatment of migraine?

PEATFIELD: Indomethacin can *cause* headache, yet all the other non-steroidal agents (for example, naproxen, ibuprofen, mefenamic acid) do not.

VANE: Indomethacin is the only one that gets into the brain.

PEATFIELD: Perhaps the same pathway, when blocked *outside* the central nervous system, prevents headache, while when the pathway is blocked *inside* the central nervous system there may be different actions.

FERREIRA: We should remember, here, that indomethacin gives rise to headache in *arthritic* patients, but not in normal patients. There are no real controls for normal people.

VANE: As for the platelet question, the platelets, I understand, lose around 35 per cent of their 5-HT during a migraine attack (Sjaastad 1975). What else do they lose? Do they lose platelet factor IV, and do they degranulate?

SANDLER: Yes; they lose β-thromboglobulin (Gawel et al. 1979).

VANE: Do the platelets themselves reduce in number?

PEATFIELD: No; the platelet numbers stay much the same (Peatfield et al. 1982).

VANE: But why would one get a platelet release reaction without any aggregation?

FOZARD: There is evidence of an increased number of platelet aggregates associated with the early stages of a migraine attack and there is a platelet release reaction (Hanington 1987).

WELCH: If you study platelets with whole-blood aggregometry, you can see secretion without aggregation (Joseph *et al.* 1989).

SANDLER: Platelet monoamine oxidase certainly becomes decreased at the time of an attack (Sandler *et al.* 1970; Glover *et al.* 1977). Perhaps we have, here, a non-specific platelet-damaging agent.

References

Anthony, M., Hinterberger, H., and Lance, J.W. (1967). Plasma serotonin in migraine and stress. *Archives of Neurology*, **16**, 544–52.

Anthony, M., Hinterberger, H., and Lance, J.W. (1969). The possible relationship of serotonin to the migraine syndrome. *Research and Clinical Studies in Headache*, **2**, 29–59.

Chang, J.Y., Hardebo, J.E., Owman, C., Sahlin, C., and Svengaard, N.A. (1987). Nerves containing serotonin, its interaction with noradrenaline and characterization of serotonergic receptors in cerebral arteries of monkey. *Journal of Autonomic Pharmacology*, **7**, 317–29.

Chang, J.Y., Owman, C., and Steinbusch, H.W.M. (1988). Evidence for coexistence of serotonin and noradrenaline in sympathetic nerves supplying brain vessels of guinea-pig. *Brain Research*, **438**, 237–46.

Chang, J.Y., Ekblad, E., Kannisto, P., and Owman, C. (1989). Serotonin uptake into cerebrovascular nerve fibres of rat, visualization by immunohistochemistry, disappearance following sympathectomy, and release during electrical stimulation. *Brain Research*, in press.

Cheng, J.T. and Shen, C.L. (1986). Tyramine-induced release of neuropeptide Y (NPY) in isolated rabbit intestine. *European Journal of Pharmacology*, **123**, 303–6.

Edvinsson, L., Degueurce, A., Duverger, D., MacKenzie, E.T., and Scatton, B. (1983). Central serotonergic nerves project to the pial vessels of the brain. *Nature*, **306**, 55–7.

Fozard, J.R. (1989). The development and early clinical evaluation of selective 5-HT_3 receptor antagonists. In *The peripheral actions of 5-hydroxytryptamine*, (ed. J.R. Fozard), pp. 354–76. Oxford University Press, Oxford.

Gawel, M.J., Burkitt, M., Rose, F.C. (1979). Platelet release reaction during migraine attacks. *Headache*, **19**, 323–7.

Glover, V. *et al.* (1977). Transitory decrease in platelet monoamine oxidase activity during migraine attacks. *Lancet*, **i**, 391–3.

Hanington, E. (1987). The platelet theory. In *Migraine: clinical, therapeutic, conceptual and research aspects*, (ed. J.N. Blau), pp. 331–53. Chapman and Hall, London.

Humphrey, P.P.A., Feniuk, W., Perren, M.J., Connor, H.E., and Oxford, A.W. 1989. The pharmacology of the novel 5-HT_1-like receptor agonist GR43175. *Cephalalgia*, **9**, Suppl. 9, 23–33.

Joseph, R., D'Andrea, G., Oster, S.B., and Welch, K.M.A. (1989). Whole blood platelet function in acute ischemic stroke. *Stroke*, **20**, 38–44.

Loisy, C., Beorchia, S., Centonze, V., Fozard, J.R., Schechter, P.J., and Tell, G.P. (1985). Effects on migraine headache of MDL 72222, an antagonist at neuronal 5-HT receptors. Double-blind placebo-controlled study. *Cephalalgia*, **5**, 79–82.

Marco, E.J., Balfagon, G., Salaices, M., Sánchez-Ferrer, C.F., and Marin, J. (1985). Serotonergic innervation of cat cerebral arteries. *Brain Research*, **338**, 137–9.

Munro, P., Swade, C., and Coppen, A. (1985). Mianserin in the prophylaxis of migraine: a double-blind study. *Acta Psychiatrica Scandinavica*, **72**, Suppl. 320. 98–103.

Müller-Schweinitzer, E. and Tapparelli, C. (1986). Methylergometrine, an active metabolite of methysergide. *Cephalalgia*, **6**, 35–41.

Peatfield, R.C. *et al.* (1982). Platelet size: no correlation with migraine or monoamine oxidase activity. *Journal of Neurology, Neurosurgery and Psychiatry*, **45**, 826–9.

Reinhard, J.F., Liebmann, J.E. Schlosberg, A.J., and Moskowitz, M.A. (1979). Serotonin neurons project to small blood vessels in the brain. *Science*, **206**, 85–7.

Sandler, M., Youdim, M.B.H., Southgate, J., and Hanington, E. (1970). The role of tyramine in migraine: some possible biochemical mechanisms. In *Background to migraine. Third Migraine Symposium*, (ed. A.L. Cochrane), pp. 103–12. Heinneman, London.

Saxena, P.R. and Verdouw, P.D. (1984). Effects of methysergide and 5-hydroxytryptamine on carotid flood flow distribution in pigs: further evidence for the presence of atypical 5-HT receptors. *British Journal of Pharmacology*, **82**, 817–26.

Scatton, B. *et al.* (1985). Neurochemical studies on the existence, origin and characteristics of the serotonergic innervation of small pial vessels. *Brain Research*, **345**, 219–29.

Sjaastad, O. (1975). The significance of blood serotonin levels in migraine: a critical review. *Acta Neurologica Scandinavica*, **51**, 200–10.

Thomas, D.P. and Vane, J.R. (1967). 5-Hydroxytryptamine in the circulation of the dog. *Nature*, **216**, 335–8.

12. 5-HT in migraine: evidence from 5-HT$_1$-like receptor agonists for a vascular aetiology

P.P.A. Humphrey, W. Feniuk, and M.J. Perren

Early research considerations

In the autumn of 1972 we set out on exploratory work, at Glaxo, aimed at the identification of a novel mechanism for the treatment of migraine. It was clear that migraine is a common disease characterized by debilitating, unilateral headache often associated with nausea, vomiting, and other gastrointestinal dysfunction. However, there were no major clues to its pathogenesis and, despite the spectrum of symptoms the initiating lesion was considered to be vascular in origin. Although the 'vascular' hypothesis, as proposed by Wolff many years ago, has recently been much criticized (Olesen *et al.* 1981), we assumed at the outset of our work that the vascular changes were important. In the very early stages of the project we also, on the basis of experiments by Wolff, assumed that the extracranial, rather than the intracranial, vessels of the head were involved. Thus, Wolff showed experimentally that the migrainous headache could not be relieved by a reduction in cerebrospinal fluid pressure, unlike a histamine-induced headache (see Wolff 1963).

With these considerations in mind, we began to explore the pharmacology of the cephalic extracranial circulation in animals. However, one other major decision was necessary, namely, the choice of the most likely pathological, humoral mediator. At the time, 5-hydroxytryptamine (5-HT; serotonin) and prostaglandins seemed likely candidates and indeed, in 1972, Sandler put forward an attractive hypothesis that involved them both. Thus he speculated that the large amounts of 5-HT released from platelets activated pulmonary 5-HT receptors which mediated the release of prostaglandins from the lung. The concept appealed because prostaglandins E$_1$ and E$_2$, but not I$_2$, are still the only endogenous mediators which have been claimed to initiate migraine-like symptoms in non-migraineurs, following intravenous administration (Carlson *et al.* 1968; Smith 1974; see also Coleman *et al.* 1989). However, the prostaglandin-releasing action of 5-HT, identified in rat and guinea-pig lungs, is very weak and, indeed, later experimenters identified the major cyclo-oxygenase product released as thromboxane A$_2$, and not prostaglandins of the E series (see Coleman *et al.* 1989 for references). In view of such considerations, coupled with the relatively modest efficacy of cyclo-oxygenase inhibitors in the treatment of migraine, we decided, at an early stage in the project, not to pursue the potential involvement of prostaglandins.

Undeniably, however, 5-HT seemed to be important. Thus, Sicuteri's group (Sicuteri *et al.* 1961) had shown the marked increase in excretion of the urinary metabolite of 5-HT, 5-hydroxyindole acetic acid, during a migraine attack. Lance's group have shown that platelet concentrations of 5-HT are markedly depleted during the headache phase and have demonstrated the presence of an endogenous platelet 'releasing-factor' in the blood of migraineurs during an attack (Curran *et al.* 1965). Further strong circumstantial evidence implicating 5-HT was that the majority of drugs used in migraine treatment, such as ergotamine, methysergide, pizotifen, and others, all in some way interact with receptors for 5-HT (Fozard 1975). However, paradoxically some behave as agonists and others as partial agonists or antagonists. Furthermore, even in the early 1970s it was apparent that not all the actions of 5-HT could be explained on the basis of the two known 5-HT receptor types (Gaddum and Picarelli 1957; Drakontides and Gershon 1968; Eyre 1975). We, therefore, set about the characterization of vascular 5-HT receptors (see Apperley *et al.* 1976), in order to gain more much needed key information, whilst we pondered the mysteries of migraine aetiology (see below).

5-Hydroxytryptamine as a putative pathological mediator in migraine

Clearly, there is a large amount of circumstantial evidence linking 5-HT with the pathophysiology of migraine. Thus, for many years it was thought that 5-HT released from platelets causes cerebral vasoconstriction, and in consequence that it causes the prodromal symptoms (various transient neurological deficits such as hemianopia, aphasia, mood changes, or hemiplegia depending on the area of the cortex affected). The subsequent low blood levels of 5-HT were then thought to lead to vasodilatation of the extracranial vessels and headache (see Lance 1973). The evidence for the involvement of 5-HT in these events is summarized in Table 12.1a. However, it is the weight of evidence rather than the quality of evidence which is impressive (see reviews by Anthony *et al.* 1969; Sjaastad 1975; Fozard 1982a). Critical examination of each piece of evidence individually tends to negate the established dogma that release of 5-HT from platelets *per se* is the initiating factor. Indeed it can even be interpreted differently to refute the importance of 5-HT in the pathology of migraine at all (see Table 12.1b). Nevertheless the large number of factors linking 5-HT with migraine is remarkable, and it is still tempting to believe that 5-HT does have a primary role in the

TABLE 12.1a. *Evidence SUGGESTING a causal role for 5-HT in migraine*

Evidence	Comment	References
Platelet 5-HT content falls rapidly by 30–40 per cent at the onset of a migraine attack.	However, 5-HT release from platelets may be a secondary event and not causal. Nevertheless there does appear to be a 5-HT releasing factor which is found only in the blood of migraineurs during an attack (Anthony 1982).	For numerous references, see Fozard 1982*a*.
Increased excretion of 5-hydroxyindole acetic acid in urine during migraine attack.	Suggests that free 5-HT plasma levels are increased.	Sicuteri *et al.* 1961; Curran *et al.* 1965.
Attacks can be triggered (in migraineurs) by the amine-releasing agents reserpine and fenfluramine.	However, reserpine-induced headache is qualitatively different to a migraine attack.	Anthony *et al.* 1967; Carrol and Hilton 1974; Nappi *et al.* 1979; Del Bene *et al.* 1977.
Zimelidine, a selective 5-HT uptake blocker exacerbates the symptoms of migraine.	However, exacerbation of attack may result from the headache-producing action of zimelidine rather than 5-HT uptake blockade *per se*. Long-term treatment with zimelidine actually ameliorates the symptomatology, possibly by increasing the free plasma 5-HT (i.e. 5-HT may relieve and *not* cause migraine).	Syvalahti *et al.* 1979.
Many antimigraine drugs (e.g. methysergide, pizotifen) interact with 5-HT receptors.	However, other 5-HT antagonists with similar anti-5-HT activity are not as effective in migraine. Ergotamine and isometheptene are used in the treatment of acute migraine but at least the latter does not act through 5-HT receptor mechanisms.	Lance *et al.* 1970; Fozard 1975.

TABLE 12.1b.   *Evidence AGAINST a causal role for 5-HT in migraine*

Evidence	Comment	References
Plasma levels of 5-HT do not correlate with onset and severity of headache.	When platelet levels are low migraineurs are frequently refractory to a further attack.	Anthony *et al.* 1967; Sjaastad 1975; Syvalahti *et al.* 1979.
Administration of 5-HT will alleviate rather than cause an attack.	All vasoconstrictors are capable of reversing an attack, providing they are administered quickly enough (Lance 1973).	Kimball *et al.* 1960; Elithorn 1969; Lance 1973; Fozard 1975.
Antimigraine drugs do not all appear to act via blockade of 5-HT receptors (e.g. isometheptene and feverfew).	In contradiction it has been claimed that even drugs like propranolol act through 5-HT$_2$ receptor blockade (Fozard 1982*b*). However, why then is cyproheptadine inferior clinically to methysergide when both are similarly effective as 5-HT$_2$ receptor antagonists?	Lance *et al.* 1970; Fozard 1975; Apperley *et al.* 1976; Johnson *et al.* 1985.
Prostaglandins of the E series produce migraine-like symptoms, but 5-HT does not.	Perhaps 5-HT causes some PGE release but no good evidence in support of this view has been presented since the original proposal by Sandler (Sandler 1972; see this paper).	Carlson *et al.* 1968; Smith 1974.
Carcinoid syndrome is not associated with a marked and obvious increased incidence of migraine.	This observation is consistent with the first two points in this Table.	MacDonald 1956.

pathogenesis of migraine. Others have suggested modifications to the original theory, namely that the 5-HT deficit is in the brain and not in the platelets, and that excessive release of 5-HT from serotoninergic nerves leads to hyperalgesia and the symptoms of migraine (Sicuteri *et al.* 1973; Raskin 1981; Fozard 1982*a*).

The claims that the cerebrovasculature is innervated by serotoninergic nerves from the raphé adds a new dimension to the 'serotonin theory'

(Reinhard *et al.* 1979; Griffith *et al.* 1982; Edvinsson *et al.* 1983). Thus, the primary disorder may reside in these nerves. Hyperactivity in the raphé system, due to stress or other trigger factors, could lead to over-activation of these nerves and a chain reaction of events including vasospasm, hypoxia, sensitization of pain receptors and their subsequent activation by the high local levels of 5-HT. This scenario is an amalgam of a number of hypotheses put forward in recent review articles on a possible central mechanism to explain the aetiology of migraine (Botney 1981; Raskin 1981; Amery 1982; Fozard 1982*b*). Alternatively, it could be hypothesized (controversially) that the serotoninergic nerves control the patency of arteriovenous anastomoses in the carotid circulation. On this basis, a deficit in 5-HT turnover could result in depletion of the transmitter and the consequent reduction in neuronal control of shunt tone leading to opening of the shunts (and their distension), and leading to hypoperfusion of the capillary beds, hypoxia, and a migraine attack (see Implications for migraine therapy, below). Regardless of the debate over 'vascular' and 'central' hypotheses it remains to be seen whether the key to our understanding of the pathogenesis of migraine does still lie in the biology of 5-HT.

Characterization of vascular 5-HT receptors

Notwithstanding the perplexing problem of the pathogenesis of migraine and the possible validity of the 'vascular' hypothesis, we were impressed with the evidence that vasoconstrictors have been shown to be effective in the treatment of a migraine headache (see Lance 1973). The archetypal vasoconstrictor still used therapeutically is ergotamine, whose pharmacological profile is complex, and which produces a generalized vasoconstriction and other unwanted effects. Of great interest to us was the finding that even noradrenaline and 5-HT administered intravenously would ameliorate a migraine headache, but their other actions make them unacceptable as useful therapeutic interventions (see Lance 1973). Knowing that many of the drugs used in the treatment of migraine interact with 5-HT receptors, and that 5-HT is much implicated in the pathophysiology of the disease, we attempted systematically to characterize and classify vascular 5-HT receptors.

As early as 1977, our work led us to propose that 5-HT receptors which mediate vascular smooth muscle contraction were not homogeneous, and that the dog saphenous vein contains a different type of 5-HT receptor from the 'D' (now called $5\text{-}HT_2$) receptor commonly found in most blood vessels (Apperley *et al.* 1977). Furthermore, on the basis of earlier studies by Saxena in the anaesthetized dog (Saxena 1972, 1974), we speculated that 5-HT receptors like those in the dog saphenous vein predominated in the carotid circulation, and that their selective stimulation would lead to selective vasoconstriction within the carotid bed (Apperley *et al.* 1980). We also observed that methysergide, which has been claimed to be particularly useful prophylactically in the treatment of migraine, was *inter alia* a partial agonist at this receptor (Apperley *et al.* 1980). This led us to the speculation that methysergide was more clinically effective as a prophylactic than the other 5-HT antagonists, because of its agonistic rather than its antagonistic properties. We therefore synthesized compounds closely related chemically to 5-HT in an attempt to identify one that would not only selectively stimulate this particular 5-HT receptor type but which would also behave as a full (higher efficacy) agonist. We predicted that such a compound would have a selective vasoconstrictor action within the carotid bed and would also be effective in treating an acute migraine attack. One of the first compounds we identified was 5-carboxamidotryptamine (5-CT), which appeared to be a very potent and selective agonist for the receptor in the dog saphenous vein (Feniuk *et al.* 1981, 1985), but we subsequently found that it also had marked hypotensive properties *in vivo* owing to an even more potent activation of a 5-HT receptor type which mediated vasodilatation (Feniuk *et al.* 1983, 1984; Trevethick *et al.* 1984, 1986; Dalton *et al.* 1986). A convenient isolated preparation in which this latter 5-HT receptor type can be examined is the cat saphenous vein which, when contracted by a variety of spasmogens, can be relaxed by 5-HT and even more potently by 5-CT (Feniuk *et al.* 1984). Following early publication of our work, the Sandoz group synthesized 5-CT and showed it to be a very potent ligand for the 5-HT$_1$ radioligand binding site (Engel *et al.* 1983). Recently, all the 5-HT receptors that are more sensitive to 5-CT than to 5-HT (whether they mediate smooth muscle relaxation or contraction) have been called *5-HT$_1$-like* receptors (Bradley *et al.* 1986). This is because the two receptors, identified by us as a result of profiling the pharmacology of 5-CT, have obvious similarities with the 5-HT$_1$ binding sites but appear not to be the same as any of them. Hence, the all-embracing term 5-HT$_1$-like, rather than 5-HT$_1$ receptor, seems appropriate and circumspect for the present (Humphrey and Richardson 1989). Notwithstanding these considerations, we continued to make tryptamine analogues in the belief that we might identify a tryptamine agonist which stimulated only one of these 5-HT$_1$-like receptors — the one which mediates the vasoconstrictor action of 5-HT in the dog saphenous vein. Eventually we identified AH25086 and GR43175, which have remarkably selective agonistic actions at this receptor. Their discovery has allowed us to identify other 5-HT$_1$-like receptors of this type elsewhere and to determine their importance *in vivo*.

Pharmacological profile of AH25086 and GR43175

Studies on isolated functional preparations

Substituted tryptamines and related compounds were synthesized and screened at Glaxo for their agonistic potency, in various isolated pharmaco-

TABLE 12.2. *Chemical structures of tryptamine analogues which behave as selective 5-HT receptor agonists*

Compound	Substituent				Receptor selectivity
	R_1	R_2	R_3	R_4	
5-Hydroxytryptamine	OH	H	H	H_2	Non-selective
5-Carboxamidotryptamine	$CONH_2$	H	H	H_2	All 5-HT_1-like sub-types
α-Methyl-5-HT	OH	H	CH_3	H_2	5-HT_2
2-Methyl-5-HT	OH	CH_3	H	H_2	5-HT_3
AH25086	$CH_2CONHCH_3$	H	H	H_2	One 5-HT_1-like sub-type*
GR43175	$CH_2SO_2NHCH_3$	H	H	$(CH_3)_2$	One 5-HT_1-like sub-type*

*Selective for the 5-HT_1-like subtype found in the dog saphenous vein.
See Humphrey 1984; Bradley *et al.* 1986; and Table 12.3.

logical preparations containing different functional 5-HT receptor types, by the use of standard techniques. This finally led to the identification of AH25086 and GR43175, compounds with a distinct profile of selectivity at (and within) 5-HT_1-like receptors compared to that of 5-HT or even 5-CT. Their chemical structures, together with those of some agonists with selectivity for other 5-HT receptor types, are shown in Table 12.2.

From the data in Table 12.3 it can be seen that the contractile actions of AH25086 and GR43175 occur selectively in the dog saphenous vein which contains predominantly 5-HT receptors that appear to be a subtype of the 5-HT_1-like group. Thus, although AH25086 and GR43175 are only four and five times less potent than 5-HT in the dog saphenous vein, respectively, they have little or no activity at 5-HT_1-like receptors which mediate relaxation in the cat saphenous vein, at 5-HT_2 receptors which mediate vascular contraction of rabbit aorta, or at 5-HT_3 receptors which mediate neuronal depolarization in rat vagus nerve. 5-Carboxamidotryptamine displays selectivity as an agonist in both 5-HT_1-like receptor-containing preparations but is more potent at the 5-HT_1-like receptor in cat saphenous vein which mediates relaxation. In contrast, 2-methyl-5-HT behaves as a selective agonist at 5-HT_3 receptors (Humphrey 1984; Richardson *et al.* 1985).

The contractile actions of AH25086 and GR43175 in the dog saphenous

TABLE 12.3. *Relative agonist potencies of some structural analogues of 5-HT in isolated tissue preparations containing different 5-HT receptors*

Analogue	Equipotent molar concentration ratios in			
	Dog saphenous vein (Contraction — $5\text{-}HT_1$-like)	Cat saphenous vein (Relaxation — $5\text{-}HT_1$-like)	Rabbit aorta (Contraction — $5\text{-}HT_2$)	Rat vagus nerve (Depolarization — $5\text{-}HT_3$)
5-Hydroxytryptamine	1	1	1	1
5-Carboxamidotryptamine	0.4	0.02	26	>1000
	(0.1–0.9)	(0.006–0.065)	(14–49)	
AH25086	4.0	>100	>1000	>1000
	(1.5–10.5)			
GR43175	4.6	>100	>1000	>1000
	(2.5–8.2)			
α-Methyl-5-HT	13	571	2.2	>1000
	(5–32)	(128–2562)	(1.1–4.1)	
2-Methyl-5-HT	>240	>100	55	3.9
			(6–104)	(3.0–4.9)

Values are geometric mean and 95 per cent confidence limits of at least four experiments. None of the tryptamine analogues tested, when devoid of agonistic actions, had any significant antagonist activity in concentrations up to 10 μM. Data from Humphrey *et al.* 1988; Humphrey and Feniuk 1989.

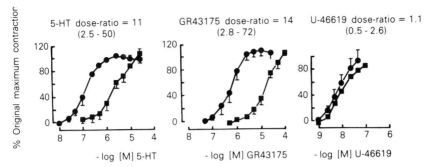

FIG. 12.1. Effect of methiothepin (1×10^{-7} mol 1^{-1}) on contractile effects of 5-HT, GR43175 and the thromboxane A_2 mimetic, U-46619, in dog isolated saphenous vein. Concentration effect curves are shown in the presence of antagonist (■), in comparison with time-matched control responses (●). All values are mean ± s.e.m. from at least four experiments which have been previously published (Humphrey *et al.* 1988). Mean agonist dose ratios (concentration ratios) are shown together with their 95 per cent confidence limits in parentheses. Note that the effects of 5-HT and GR43175, but not U-46619, are antagonized to a similar degree, indicating that GR43175 produces contraction by activation of the same receptor as 5-HT. A comparable profile has been described in similar experiments using AH25086 as the agonist (Humphrey and Feniuk 1989).

vein cannot be antagonized by a variety of antagonists, including phentolamine (1×10^{-6} mol 1^{-1}) and indomethacin (2.8×10^{-6} mol 1^{-1}). These results rule out the involvement of a number of mechanisms, including activation of α-adrenoceptors and prostaglandin release (Humphrey *et al.* 1988; Humphrey and Feniuk 1989). However, the specific antagonism of AH25086 and GR43175 by methiothepin (Humphrey *et al.* 1988; Humphrey and Feniuk 1989; see Fig 12.1) indicates that a 5-HT receptor mechanism is involved. This, together with the lack of antagonism by ketanserin and MDL 72222, suggests that the receptor is not of the $5\text{-}HT_2$ or $5\text{-}HT_3$ type and implicates a $5\text{-}HT_1$-like receptor.

Studies in anaesthetized animals

The haemodynamic profile of AH25086 and GR43175 in anaesthetized dogs and cats is that of a selective carotid vasoconstrictor (Brittain *et al.* 1987; Feniuk *et al.* 1987; Feniuk *et al.* 1989a, and unpublished observations). Thus, in anaesthetized beagle dogs, they each ($1–100\mu g$ kg^{-1} intravenously) have little or no effect on blood pressure or heart rate but markedly reduce blood flow in the carotid arterial bed in a dose-dependent manner (see Fig. 12.2). The cumulative intravenous dose required to produce 50 per cent of maximum vasoconstriction in the carotid arterial bed (maximum normally 80–120 per cent increase in vascular resistance) has been found to be 16 ± 5 and 39 ± 8 μg kg^{-1} for AH25086 and GR43175, respectively (mean ±

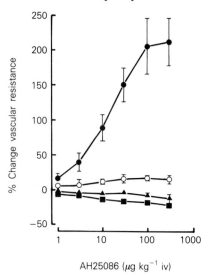

AH25086 (μg kg⁻¹ iv)

FIG. 12.2. Selective carotid arterial vasoconstriction following intravenously administered AH25086 to anaesthetized dogs (previously unpublished observations). Similar findings have been described for GR43175 elsewhere (Feniuk *et al.* 1989*a*). Values are mean ± s.e.m. from four beagle dogs anaesthetized with barbitone (300 mg kg⁻¹ intraperitoneally) and artificially respired. Common carotid arterial blood flow and ascending aortic flow (assumed to be equivalent to cardiac output) were measured with electromagnetic flow probes. Vascular resistance was calculated as 0.33 × arterial pulse pressure + diastolic blood pressure ÷ mean arterial blood flow × 8000 dynes cm⁻⁵ s. All changes are calculated as percentage changes from basal levels prior to drug treatment and measured 15 minutes after cumulative drug administration. Basal values prior to drug treatment, arterial blood pressure (154 ± 12 / 92 ± 10 mmHg); ascending aortic flow (1003 ± 149 ml min⁻¹); common carotid arterial flow (82 ± 10 ml min⁻¹); total peripheral resistance (0.95 ± 0.18 × 10⁴ dynes cm⁻⁵ s; carotid arterial vascular resistance (11.5 ± 1.9 × 10⁴ dynes cm⁻⁵ s). Carotid arterial vascular resistance (●); total peripheral resistance (○); cardiac output (■); diastolic blood pressure (▲).

s.e.m. of four determinations). Measurement of blood flows in other vascular beds of the dog, with electromagnetic flow probes, confirms the selective vasoconstrictor action of AH25086 and GR43175 and that they have little or no effect on total peripheral resistance (Fig. 12.2; Feniuk *et al.* 1989*a*).

The carotid vasoconstrictor action of AH25086 and GR43175 has been further investigated in cats with the aid of radiolabelled microspheres, to determine the effects of these agents on distribution of blood flow within the bed. This is of particular interest because in the anaesthetized cat about 50 per cent of the carotid arterial blood flow bypasses the capillaries and is conveyed back to the venous circulation via arteriovenous anastomoses (or shunts). Furthermore, abnormal vasodilatation of these vessels has been implicated in the aetiology of migraine (Heyck 1969). Both AH25086 and GR43175, as well as ergotamine, potently constrict feline carotid shunt vessels, as shown by the finding that the fraction of microspheres that returns to the venous circulation following administration into the carotid artery is markedly reduced (Fig. 12.3; Feniuk *et al.* 1987; Perren *et al.* 1989). However, in the case of ergotamine, resistance is increased in the whole of the carotid artery bed, vasoconstriction being evident in the capillary as well as in the shunt compartment (Perren *et al.* 1989). In contrast, the increase in total carotid arterial vascular resistance produced by AH25086 and GR43175 can be entirely accounted for by a selective vasoconstriction of shunt vessels. Methysergide, too, has a small but significant vasoconstrictor action localized to the shunt vessels (Fig. 12.3). This is consistent with findings from Saxena's group, and this very small effect presumably relates to the low efficacy of methysergide as an agonist at $5-HT_1$-like receptors such as those in the dog saphenous vein (Spierings and Saxena 1980; Apperley *et al.* 1980).

Interestingly, the prototype 5-HT-like receptor agonist identified at the beginning of our studies, 5-CT, has also been shown to constrict feline carotid shunts, albeit non-selectively. Evidence that this is due to an action at $5-HT_1$-like receptors has been provided by experiments in which the vasoconstrictor action of 5-CT has been effectively antagonized by methiothepin (Saxena and Verdouw 1985). In contrast, the vasoconstrictor action of ergotamine in similar experiments was not antagonized by methiothepin which indicates that, despite the ability of ergotamine to stimulate a variety of receptors for biogenic amines, including $5-HT_2$ receptors, it does not stimulate the $5-HT_1$-like receptor sub-type that occurs in the shunts (Bom *et al.* 1989).

Implications for $5-HT_1$-like receptor classification

In contrast to AH25086 and GR43175, 5-carboxamidotryptamine is a nonselective $5-HT_1$-like agonist and has additional profound vasodilator and hypotensive activity in rats, cats, and dogs. Indeed, 5-CT dilates rather than constricts the total carotid circulation. However, on carotid shunt vessels 5-CT has been shown to produce vasoconstriction like AH25086 and GR43175 (see above), a finding which some might consider paradoxical. Nevertheless, this finding is entirely consistent with our proposal that functional $5-HT_1$-like receptors can be subdivided; and the identification of AH25086 and GR43175 now provides convincing evidence for this claim. Thus, the two agents share the smooth muscle contracting action of 5-HT and 5-CT mediated via the $5-HT_1$-like receptor in the dog saphenous vein, but they do not share the smooth muscle relaxant properties of 5-CT and 5-HT mediated via the other type of $5-HT_1$-like receptor that we first identified, in the cat saphenous vein. The clear differences in potencies of AH25086 and GR43175 compared to 5-CT at $5-HT_1$-like receptors in these two preparations, and the qualitative differences in the responses, seem

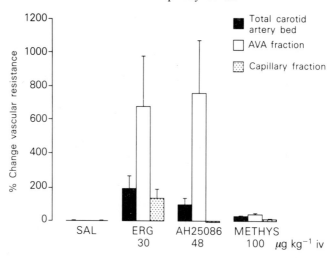

FIG. 12.3. A comparison of the regional changes in carotid arterial vascular resistance following intravenous administration of saline (SAL), ergotamine (ERG 30 μg kg^{-1}), AH25086 (48 μg kg^{-1}), and methysergide (METHYS 100 μg kg^{-1}) in anaesthetized cats (previously unpublished observations). Values shown are mean ± s.e.m. from three–six experiments. Cats weighing 2–3 kg were anaesthetized with chloralose (60 mg kg^{-1} i.p.) and urethane (700 mg kg^{-1} i.p.) and artificially respired. Common carotid arterial blood flow (14.7–44.0 ml min^{-1}) was measured with an electromagnetic flow probe and arterial blood pressure was measured from the aorta via a catheter inserted into a femoral artery. Approximately $1 \times 10^5 - 2 \times 10^6$ radiolabelled 15 μm diameter microspheres (Ce^{141}, Cr^{51}, Nb^{95}, Ru^{103} or Sn^{113}) were injected into the carotid artery via a cannula inserted in the lingual artery. The use of 15 μm diameter microspheres to provide a measure of capillary and arteriovenous anastomotic (AVA; shunt) flow has been discussed extensively by Heymann *et al* (1977). The method described here has been described in detail by Spierings and Saxena (1980). Essentially, 15 μm microspheres, when injected into the carotid circulation, will become trapped in tissue capillaries (diameter, 8 μm) thus providing a measure of capillary blood flow, whilst those escaping entrapment must pass through larger diameter AVAs (diameter >25 μm) to pass eventually into the venous circulation and become trapped in lung capillaries. The radioactivity in the lungs therefore, following the administration of microspheres into the carotid artery, provides a direct measure of AVA flow (shunting) in the carotid circulation. No significant amounts of radioactivity were found in peripheral tissues such as the kidney, which demonstrates the entrapment of microspheres in the lung capillaries. Resistance changes in the total carotid bed as well as metabolic (capillary) and AVA (shunt) fractions of carotid blood flow were calculated as described in Fig. 12.2. Radioactive microspheres were injected prior to drug administration (or saline) and at the peak change in total carotid arterial vascular resistance produced by the drugs.

The increases in total carotid vascular resistance and carotid shunt resistance produced by ergotamine, AH25086, and methysergide were all statistically significant (at p = 0.05). Unlike ergotamine, AH25086 and methysergide had no significant effect on the capillary resistance. The selective effect of AH25086 on shunt resistance was significantly greater than that of methysergide (at p = 0.05). A similar vasoconstrictor profile to that of AH25086 has been described for GR43175 elsewhere (Perren *et al.* 1989).

analogous to the effects of a selective α-adrenoceptor agonist when it is compared to a mixed α- and β-adrenoceptor agonist on smooth muscle. This analogy is reinforced by our finding that the 5-HT_1-like receptor which mediates relaxation of smooth muscle is, like the β-adrenoceptors, linked to adenylate cyclase (Trevethick *et al.* 1984, 1986) and is also evident in cardiac tissue where it mediates tachycardia (Saxena *et al.* 1985; Connor *et al.* 1986). Furthermore, the 5-HT_1-like receptor in dog saphenous vein, like the α_2-adrenoceptor, can mediate both smooth muscle contraction and inhibition of neuronal transmitter release (Watts *et al.* 1981; Humphrey *et al.* 1988).

Neither the 5-HT_1-like receptor which mediates smooth muscle relaxation nor the 5-HT_1-like receptor which mediates smooth muscle contraction can be blocked by ligands such as cyanopindolol, which have high affinity for the 5-HT_{1A} and 5-HT_{1B} sites. Furthermore, since mesulergine does not antagonize contractile or relaxant responses to 5-CT mediated via 5-HT_1-like receptors either, we conclude that neither of these functional receptors corresponds with the 5-HT_{1A}, 5-HT_{1B}, or 5-HT_{1C} sites (Sumner *et al.* 1987; Humphrey *et al.* 1988). It might be that one or the other is equivalent to the 5-HT_{1D} binding site (Heuring and Peroutka 1987) but this does not appear to be the case on the basis of the weak antagonist potency of metergoline (Sumner *et al.* 1987; Humphrey *et al.* 1988). Thus neither of the two functional 5-HT_1-like receptors identified by us seems to be identical to any of the four currently classified 5-HT_1 ligand-binding sites.

Hence, it is clear that the 5-HT_1-like receptor which mediates contraction of the dog saphenous vein and which is relevant to the antimigraine action of GR43175 has yet to be fully characterized and, until the identification of an equivalent radioligand binding site, it will continue to remain without a ready appellation. However, the advent of AH25086 and GR43175 allows the identification of other receptors of this type in other locations.

From such studies it is evident that most peripheral blood vessels do not contain this receptor but, rather, that 5-HT mediates contraction through 5-HT_2 receptors (Humphrey *et al.* 1988). However, blood vessels of intracranial origin do appear to contain 5-HT_1-like receptors, as evidenced by the fact that GR43175 can potently contract the basilar artery from a number of different species including humans (Connor *et al.* 1989; Parsons and Whalley 1989). Clearly, more work is necessary to determine the precise distribution of this receptor throughout the vasculature and, particularly, within the vascular territories of the head.

The clinical profile of 5-HT_1-like receptor agonists as anti-migraine drugs

When it had been shown that AH25086 had such a marked and selective vasoconstrictor action on carotid shunts in animals, AH25086 was tested in patients with acute migraine. After first showing that slow intravenous infusions (over 10–40 minutes) of AH25086 (up to 64 μg kg^{-1} i.v.) were well tolerated in normal human volunteers, the drug was tested in pilot dose-ranging studies in migraineurs before a small placebo-controlled clinical trial was begun (Doenicke *et al.* 1987; Brand *et al.* 1987).

In the controlled study patients (men and women aged 35–70 years), resident for investigation in a migraine clinic, were deprived of their usual medication. When they experienced spontaneous headaches they were treated by intravenous infusion of normal saline or AH25086 at one of three doses (0.05, 0.2, or 0.8 μg kg^{-1} min^{-1}) infused for 30 minutes. Any patients not responding in the placebo and two lower-dose groups then received the highest infusion dose of AH25086 (0.8 μg kg^{-1} min^{-1}) which was usually effective in aborting the attack (Fig. 12.4). It was evident that a total dose of AH25086 of 24 μg kg^{-1} not only abolished or ameliorated the severe headaches but also the accompanying nausea and associated symptoms (Brand *et al.* 1987).

Other laboratory experiments showed that a later compound, GR43175, was more suitable for oral administration. This compound, therefore, progressed into clinical trial, where it displayed a similar profile of activity to that of AH25086 when administered intravenously (Doenicke *et al.* 1988). Excitingly, the more detailed clinical evaluation of GR43175 has shown it to be very effective in aborting an acute migraine attack also when administered subcutaneously and orally (Perrin *et al.* 1989; Doenicke *et al.* 1989; Baar *et al.* 1989).

Implications for migraine therapy

The pharmacology of a potentially new type of drug mechanism for migraine therapy has been reviewed here. AH25086 and GR43175 are evidently selective agonists for 5-HT$_1$-like receptors which mediate vasoconstriction of some blood vessels, notably those in the head (Connor *et al.* 1989; Parsons and Whalley 1989). This specific and selective action at one sub-type of 5-HT receptor will, we hope, provide a novel drug that is safer and clinically more acceptable than agents such as the ergots, which are sometimes used in the treatment of acute migraine and have multiple pharmacological actions (Feniuk *et al.* 1989*b*). However, it remains to be shown whether 5-HT$_1$-like receptor agonists are effective in migraine because they are cranial vasoconstrictors *per se*, or whether the localization of their vasoconstrictor action to certain cranial vessels such as the shunts is important. Heyck (1969) proposed that carotid shunt vessels may be pathologically opened during a migraine attack, thereby depriving capillary beds within the head of essential oxygen. He provided evidence for his claim from limited clinical studies in which he showed that jugular venous blood from migraineurs during an attack had a higher oxygen tension on the side of the headache compared to

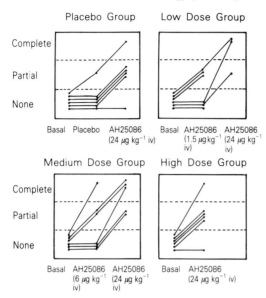

FIG. 12.4. Degree of headache pain relief after initial and further treatment with AH25086. The figure summarizes previously published clinical findings (Brand *et al.* 1987). Similar clinical findings have been described with GR43175 (Perrin *et al.* 1989). Patients with a long history of migraine (5–40 years, and the majority having about four attacks per month) were admitted to the clinic and involved in a placebo-controlled single-blind study during the headache phase of a spontaneous common or classical migraine attack. Twenty-four patients (six male and 18 female caucasians, ranging between 35 and 70 years of age) were treated with either placebo infusion (normal saline) or infusions of low (0.05 μg kg^{-1} min^{-1}), intermediate (0.2 μg kg^{-1} min^{-1}), or high (0.8 μg kg^{-1} min^{-1}) dose AH25086 for 30 minutes. Treatment with AH25086 commenced between 1 and 10 hours after the onset of the headache, the majority of patients being treated four to five hours after the headache started. Eight of the patients had received an alternative treatment for the current attack between 0.75 and 10 hours before administration of AH25086; these various therapies, which were ineffective, included analgesics, metoclopramide and homeopathic remedies, while three patients had taken dihydroergotamine. AH25086 was supplied in 10 ml ampoules as a sterile solution in concentrations of 28, 224 or 1400 μg ml^{-1} and was delivered intravenously (iv) in normal saline via an infusion pump at a rate of 1 ml min^{-1} to produce cumulative doses of either 1.5 μg kg^{-1} (low), 6 μg kg^{-1} (medium) or 24 μg kg^{-1} (high).

The vertical axes show the degree of headache relief as none, partial, or complete. The horizontal axes refer to the position before treatment (basal) or after treatment with placebo or AH25086 at low, intermediate, or high dose infusions. Headache severity was assessed according to an analogue scale where 0 = no headache; 1 = headache but able to work/continue with normal daily activities; 2 = unable to work/continue with daily activities; 3 = severe headache requiring bed-rest. Note the dose-dependent effect of AH25086 in treating the headache.

the contralateral side (Heyck 1969). The decreased arteriovenous oxygen tension difference returned to normal values on cessation of the migraine attack, following dihydroergotamine treatment. Furthermore, Saxena and his group have shown that in anaesthetized cats and pigs large amounts of carotid blood bypass the capillaries via shunt vessels (Saxena 1986). In the cat, these shunts have been shown to be markedly constricted by ergotamine but only poorly by methysergide. However, this concept is extremely controversial because the carotid anatomy of the cat and pig is very different to that in humans, and clinical cerebral blood flow measurements in migraineurs have provided no evidence for the involvement of intracranial shunts in migraine (Clifford Rose 1983). Nevertheless, evidence for the presence of functional carotid arteriovenous anastomoses in human cadavers has been provided (Ogata and Feigin 1972); indeed, their anatomical presence has been demonstrated histologically in human cephalic beds, including those of the face, lips, and dura mater (Rowbotham and Little 1965).

An alternative explanation for the efficacy of vasoconstrictor agents in the treatment of a migraine attack might be that they simply reduce the tensile pressure in the walls of distended pulsating arteries that are sensitized by an acute inflammatory condition. This proposal can be encompassed within the newer, elegant hypothesis that has recently been unfolded for the putative involvement of the trigeminal nerve (fifth cranial) in vascular head pain (see reviews by Moskowitz 1984; Moskowitz and Barley 1985). Thus, Moskowitz and his colleagues have been exploring the concept that the trigeminal nerve that innervates pain-sensitive intracranial vessels such as those of the meninges, as well as the superior sagittal sinus and larger vessels within the circle of Willis, pathologically produces vasodilation and extravasation via the release of substance P, which then leads to a localized painful inflammatory response. This hypothesis, for which there is good experimental evidence in animals, is appealing because it explains the localization of pain to a specific intracranial locus, transmitted via a unique pain pathway which could be consistent with the refractoriness of migrainous pain to traditional analgesic therapy in many cases.

The putative role of the trigeminal nerve pathway in the pathology of migraine is all the more intriguing because of the recent finding that acute ergotamine and chronic methysergide treatment will prevent the cephalic extravasation induced by experimental stimulation of the trigeminal nerve in rats (Markowitz *et al.* 1988). Clearly it is important to confirm this observation and to characterize the mechanism. If a 5-HT$_1$-like receptor like that in the dog saphenous vein were to be involved in the inhibition of substance P release, this would be of great interest. However, even with such considerations, the most simple explanation for the antimigraine action of GR43175 in this scenario is that it acts as a vasoconstrictor on blood vessels within the trigeminal nerve territory, thus offsetting the vasodilatation and extravasation caused by overactivity of the innervating neurones. However, unlike ergotamine and related ergots, GR43175 has a much more selective vaso-constrictor action. Interestingly, the selectivity of action of GR43175 may be further compounded by the fact that this drug does not appear readily to cross the blood–brain barrier (Dallas *et al.* 1989). Thus, one could speculate that its vasoconstrictor action *in vivo* is largely restricted to those cephalic vessels that contain 5-HT$_1$-like receptors *and* which are located extracerebrally. If so, the meningeal vessels might be the target locus for the antimigraine action of GR43175.

Regardless of the above considerations, GR43175 has been shown to be effective when administered subcutaneously and orally as well as when administered intravenously in the treatment of acute migraine (Perrin *et al.* 1989). It is now in phase III clinical trials and promises to provide a major breakthrough in migraine therapy. Importantly, further studies on its clinical mechanism of action are in progress and they will, we hope, be invaluable in elucidating the pathogenesis of migraine and vascular headache.

Acknowledgements

We gratefully acknowledge the contributions of our many colleagues at Glaxo who have had a major involvement in the work which led up to this review. They include Dr A.W. Oxford, Dr D.E. Bays, Dr M.D. Dowle, Dr B. Evans, and Dr C.F. Webb who worked on the chemistry of the indoles synthesized at Ware; Dr G. Dixon and Dr M. Thomas who supervised the early studies in volunteers; and Dr V.L. Perrin who, with Dr M. Hadoke, co-ordinated the early clinical studies. The latter were carried out in Germany by Prof. A. Doenicke in Munchen and by Dr J. Brand in Koenigstein, who have both played an important role in the history of the development of GR43175 to date. We are also extremely grateful to Dr David Jack and Dr Roy Brittain whose idea it was to initiate a project at Ware on migraine.

References

Amery, W.K. (1982). Brain hypoxia: the turning-point in the genesis of the migraine attack? *Cephalalgia*, **2**, 83–109.

Anthony, M. (1982). Serotonin and cyclic nucleotides in migraine. In *Proceedings of headache 1980, International Congress.* (ed. M. Critchley, A.P. Friedman, F. Sicuteri, and S. Gorini), pp. 45–50. Raven Press, New York.

Anthony, M., Hinterberger, H., and Lance, J.W. (1967). Plasma serotonin in migraine and stress. *Archives of Neurology*, **16**, 544–52.

Anthony, M., Hinterberger, H., and Lance, J.W. (1969). The possible relationship of serotonin to the migraine syndrome. *Research and Clinical Studies in Headache*, **2**, 29–59.

Apperley, E., Humphrey, P.P.A., and Levey, G.P. (1976). Receptors for 5-hydroxytryptamine and noradrenaline in rabbit isolated ear artery and aorta. *British Journal of Pharmacology*, **58**, 211–21.

Apperley, E., Humphrey, P.P.A., and Levy, G.P. (1977). Two types of excitatory receptor for 5-hydroxytryptamine in dog vasculature. *British Journal of Pharmacology*, **61**, 465P.

Apperley, E., Feniuk, W., Humphrey, P.P.A., and Levy, G.P. (1980). Evidence for two types of excitatory receptor for 5-hydroxytryptamine in dog isolated vasculature. *British Journal of Pharmacology*, **68**, 215–24.

Baar, H.A., Brand, J., Doenicke, A., Melchart, D., Lüben, V., Tryba, M., and Sahlender, H. (1989). Treatment of acute migraine with subcutaneous GR43175 in West Germany. *Cephalalgia*, **9**, (Suppl. 9), 83–7.

Bom, A.H., Heiligers, J., Saxena P.R., and Verdouw, P.D. (1989). Ergotamine-induced reduction in cephalic arteriovenous shunting is not mediated by 5-HT$_1$-like or 5-HT$_2$ receptors. *British Journal of Pharmacology*, **97**, 383–90.

Botney, M. (1981). An inquiry into the genesis of migraine headache. *Headache*, **21**, 179–85.

Bradley, P.B., Engel, G., Feniuk, W., Fozard, J.R., Humphrey, P.P.A., Middlemiss, D.N., Mylecharane, E.J., Richardson, B.P., and Saxena, P.R. (1986). Proposals for the classification and nomenclature of functional receptors for 5-hydroxytryptamine. *Neuropharmacology*, **25**, 563–76.

Brand, J., Hadoke, M., and Perrin, V.L. (1987). Placebo controlled study of a selective 5-HT$_1$-like agonist, AH25086B, in relief of acute migraine. *Cephalalgia*, **7**, 402–3.

Brittain, R.T., Butina, D., Coates, I.H., Feniuk, W., Humphrey, P.P.A., Jack, D., Oxford, A.W., and Perren, M.J. (1987). GR43175 selectively constricts the canine carotid arterial bed via stimulation of 5-HT$_1$-like receptors. *British Journal of Pharmacology* (Suppl), **92**, 618P.

Carlson, L.A., Ekelund, L.G., and Oro, L. (1968). Clinical and metabolic effects of different doses of prostaglandin E in man. *Acta Medica Scandinavica*, **183**, 423–30.

Carrol, J.D. and Hilton, B.P. (1974). The effects of reserpine injection on methysergide treated control and migrainous subjects. *Headache*, **14**, 149–56.

Clifford Rose, F. (1983). The pathogenesis of the migraine attack. *Trends in Neurosciences*, **6**, 247–8.

Coleman, R.A., Kennedy, I., Humphrey, P.P.A., Bunce, K.T., and Lumley, P. (1989). Prostanoid receptors. In *Comprehensive medicinal chemistry*, Vol. 3. (ed. J.C. Emmett) Chapter 9, Pergamon Press, Oxford, in press.

Connor, H.E., Feniuk, W., Humphrey, P.P.A., and Perren, M.J. (1986). 5-Carboxamido-tryptamine is a selective agonist at 5-HT receptors mediating vasodilation and tachycardia in anaesthetized cats. *British Journal of Pharmacology*, **87**, 417–26.

Connor, H.E., Feniuk, W., and Humphrey, P.P.A. (1989). Characterisation of 5-HT receptors mediating contraction of canine and primate basilar artery by the use of GR43175, a selective 5-HT$_1$-like receptor agonist. *British Journal of Pharmacology*, **96**, 379–87.

Curran, D.A., Hinterberger, H., and Lance, J.W. (1965). Total plasma serotonin, 5-hydroxyindoleacetic acid and p-hydroxy-m-methoxymandelic acid excretion in normal and migrainous subjects. *Brain*, **88**, 997–1007.

Dallas, F.A.A., Dixon, C.M., McCulloch, R.J., and Saynor, D.A. (1989). The kinetics of ^{14}C-GR43175 in rat and dog. *Cephalalgia*, **9**, (Suppl. 9), 53–6.

Dalton, D.W., Feniuk, W., and Humphrey, P.P.A. (1986). An investigation into the mechanisms of the cardiovascular effects of 5-hydroxytryptamine in conscious normotensive and doca-salt hypertensive rats. *Journal of Autonomic Pharmacology*, **6**, 219–28.

Del Bene, E., Anselmi, B., Del Bianco, P.L., Fanciullacci, M., Galli, P., Salmon, S., and Sicuteri, F. (1977). Fenfluramine headache: a biochemical and monoamine receptorial human study. In *Headache: new vistas*, (ed. F. Sicuteri) pp. 101–9. Biomedical Press, Florence.

Doenicke, A., Siegel, E., Hadoke, M., and Perrin, V.L. (1987). Initial clinical study of AH25086B (5-HT$_1$-like agonist) in the acute treatment of migraine. *Cephalalgia*, **7**, 438–9.

Doenicke, A., Brand, J., and Perrin, V.L. (1988). Possible benefit of GR43175, a novel 5-HT$_1$-like receptor agonist, for the acute treatment of severe migraine. *Lancet*, **i**, 1309–11.

Doenicke, A., Melchart, D., and Bayliss, E.M. (1989). Effective improvement of symptoms in patients with acute migraine with GR43175 dispersible tablets. *Cephalalgia*, **9**, (Suppl. 9), 89–92.

Drakontides, A.B. and Gershon, M.D. (1968). 5-Hydroxytryptamine receptors in the mouse duodenum. *British Journal of Pharmacology and Chemotherapy*, **33**, 480–92.

Edvinsson, L., Degueurce, A., Duverger, D., MacKenzie, E.T., and Scatton, B. (1983). Central serotonergic nerves project to the pial vessels of the brain. *Nature*, **306**, 55–7.

Elithorn, A. (1969). Migraine. *British Medical Journal*, **4**, 411–3.

Engel, G., Göthert, M., Müller-Schweinitzer, E., Schlicker, E., Sistonen, L., and Stadler, P.A. (1983). Evidence for common pharmacological properties of [^{3}H]5-hydroxytryptamine binding sites, presynaptic 5-hydroxytryptamine autoreceptors in CNS and inhibitory presynaptic 5-hydroxytryptamine receptors on sympathetic nerves. *Naunyn-Schmiedeberg's Archives of Pharmacology*, **324**, 116–24.

Eyre P. (1975). Atypical tryptamine receptors in sheep pulmonary vein. *British Journal of Pharmacology*, **55**, 329–33.

Feniuk, W., Humphrey, P.P.A., and Watts, A.D. (1981). Modification of the vasomotor actions of methysergide in the femoral arterial bed of the anaesthetized dog by changes in sympathetic nerve activity. *Journal of Autonomic Pharmacology*, **1**, 127–32.

Feniuk, W., Humphrey, P.P.A., and Watts, A.D. (1983). 5-Hydroxytryptamine-induced relaxation of isolated mammalian smooth muscle. *European Journal of Pharmacology*, **96**, 71–8.

Feniuk, W., Humphrey, P.P.A., and Watts, A.D. (1984). 5-Carboxamidotryptamine — a potent agonist at 5-hydroxytryptamine receptors mediating relaxation. *British Journal of Pharmacology*, **86**, 697–704.

Feniuk, W., Humphrey, P.P.A., Perren, M.J., and Watts, A.D. (1985). A comparison of 5-hydroxytryptamine receptors mediating contraction in rabbit aorta and dog saphenous vein. Evidence for different receptor types obtained by use of selective agonists and antagonists. *British Journal Pharmacology*, **86**, 697–704.

Feniuk, W., Humphrey, P.P.A., and Perren, M.J. (1987). Selective vasoconstrictor action of GR43175 on arteriovenous anastomoses (AVAS) in the anaesthetised cat. *British Journal of Pharmacology*, (Suppl), **92**, 756P.

Feniuk, W., Humphrey, P.P.A., and Perren, M.J. (1989*a*). The selective carotid arterial vasoconstrictor action of GR43175 in anaesthetised dogs. *British Journal of Pharmacology*, **96**, 83–90.

Feniuk, W., Humphrey, P.P.A., and Perren, M.J. (1989*b*). GR43175 does not share the complex pharmacology of the ergots. *Cephalalgia*, **9**, (Suppl. 9), 35–9.

Fozard, J.R. (1975). The animal pharmacology of drugs used in the treatment of migraine. *Journal of Pharmacy and Pharmacology*, **27**, 297–321.

Fozard, J.R. (1982*a*). Serotonin, migraine and platelets. *Progress in Pharmacology*, **4/4**, 134–46.

Fozard, J.R. (1982*b*). Basic mechanisms of antimigraine drugs. In *International headache congress, 1980.* (ed. M. Critchley *et al.*), pp. 295–308. Raven Press, New York.

Gaddum, J.H. and Picarelli, Z.P. (1957). Two kinds of tryptamine receptor. *British Journal of Pharmacology and Chemotherapy*, **12**, 323–8.

Griffith, S.G., Lincoln, J., and Burnstock, G. (1982). Serotonin as a neurotransmitter in cerebral arteries. *Brain Research*, **247**, 388–92.

Heuring, R.E. and Peroutka, S.J. (1987). Characterisation of a novel ³H-5-hydroxytryptamine binding site in bovine brain membranes. *Journal of Neuroscience*, **7**, 894–903.

Heyck, H. (1969). Pathogenesis of migraine. *Research and Clinical Studies in Headache*, **2**, 1–28.

Heymann, M.A., Payne, B.D., Hoffman, J.I.E., and Rudolph, A.M. (1977). Blood flow measurements with radionuclide-labelled particles. *Progress in Cardiovascular Diseases*, **20**, 55–79.

Humphrey, P.P.A. (1984). Peripheral 5-hydroxytryptamine receptors and their classification. *Neuropharmacology*, **23**, 1503–10.

Humphrey, P.P.A. and Richardson, B.P. (1989). 5-HT receptor classification: A current view based on a workshop debate. In *Serotonin (Proceedings of the Heron Island Meeting, September 1987)*, (ed. E.J. Mylecharane, J.A. Angus, I.S. de la Lande, and P.P.A. Humphrey), Macmillan Press Limited, England, in press.

Humphrey, P.P.A. and Feniuk, W. (1989). The sub-classification of functional 5-HT₁-like receptors. In *Serotonin (Proceedings of the Heron Island Meeting, September 1987)*, (ed. E.J. Mylecharane, J.A. Angus, I.S. de la Lande, and P.P.A. Humphrey), Macmillan Press Limited, England, in press.

Humphrey, P.P.A., Feniuk, W., Perren, M.J., Connor, H.E., Oxford, A.W., Coates, I.H., and Butina, D. (1988). GR43175, a selective agonist for the 5-HT₁-like receptor in dog isolated saphenous vein. *British Journal of Pharmacology*, **94**, 1123–32.

Johnson, E.S., Kadam, N.P., Hylands, D.M., and Hylands, P.J. (1985). Efficacy of feverfew as a prophylactic treatment of migraine. *British Medical Journal*, **291**, 569–73.

Kimball, R.W., Friedman, A.P., and Valeejo, E. (1960). Effect of serotonin in migraine patients. *Neurology*, **10**, 107–11.

Lance, J.W. (1973). *The mechanism and management of headache*, 2nd edn, Butterworth, London.

Lance, J.W., Anthony, M., and Somerville, B. (1970). Comparative trial of serotonin antagonists in the management of migraine. *British Medical Journal*, **2**, 327–30.

MacDonald, R.A. (1956). A study of 356 carcinoids of the gastrointestinal tract. A report of four new cases of the carcinoid syndrome. *American Journal of Medicine*, **21**, 867–78.

Markowitz, S., Saito, K., and Moskowitz, M.A. (1988). Neurogenically mediated plasma extravasation in dura mater: effect of ergot alkaloids. *Cephalalgia*, **8**, 83–91.

Moskowitz, M.A. (1984). Neurobiology of vascular head pain. *Annals of Neurology*, **16**, 157–68.

Moskowitz, M.A. and Barley, P.A. (1985). The trigeminal system and vascular head pain: a role for substance P. In *Substance P: metabolism and biological actions.* (ed. C. Jordan and P. Oehme), pp 153–63. Taylor and Francis, London.

Nappi, G., Salvoldi, F., Bono, G., and Martignoni, E. (1979). Reserpine-headache and PRL release in migraine. *Headache*, **19**, 273–7.

Ogata, J. and Feigin, I. (1972). Arteriovenous communication in the human brain. *Journal of Neuropathology & Experimental Neurology*, **31**, 519–25.

Olesen, J., Tfelt-Hansen, P., Henriksen, L., and Larsen, B. (1981). The common migraine attack may not be initiated by cerebral ischaemia. *Lancet*, **ii**, 438–40.

Parsons, A.A. and Whalley, E.T. (1989). GR43175 is an agonist at the 5-HT$_1$-like receptor mediating contraction of human isolated basilar artery. *Cephalalgia*, **9**, (Suppl. 9), 47–51.

Perren, M.J., Feniuk, W., and Humphrey, P.P.A. (1989). The selective closure of feline carotid arteriovenous anastomoses by GR43175. *Cephalalgia*, **9**, (Suppl. 9), 41–6.

Perrin, V.L., Farkkila, M., Goasguen, J., Doenicke, A., Brand, J., and Tfelt-Hansen, P. (1989). Overview of initial clinical studies with intravenous and oral GR43175 in acute migraine. *Cephalalgia*, **9**, (Suppl. 9), 63–72.

Raskin, N.H. (1981). Pharmacology of migraine. *Annual Review of Pharmacology and Toxicology*, **21**, 463–78.

Reinhard, J.F., Leibman, J.E., Schlosberg, A.J., and Moskowitz, M.A. (1979). Serotonin neurones project to small blood vessels in the brain. *Science*, **206**, 85–7.

Richardson, B.P., Engel, G., Donatsch, P., and Stadler, P.A. (1985). Identification of serotonin M-receptor subtypes and their specific blockade by a new class of drugs. *Nature*, **316**, 126–31.

Rowbotham, G.F. and Little, E. (1965). New concepts on the aetiology and vascularisation of meningiomata: the mechanism of migraine: the chemical process of cerebrospinal fluid: and the formation of collection of blood or fluid in the subdural space. *British Journal of Surgery*, **52**, 21–4.

Sandler, M. (1972). Migraine: A pulmonary disease? *Lancet*, **i**, 618–9.

Saxena, P.R. (1972). The effects of antimigraine drugs on the vascular responses by 5-hydroxytryptamine and related biogenic substance on the external carotid bed of dogs: possible pharmacological implications to their antimigraine action. *Headache*, **12**, 44–54.

Saxena, P.R. (1974). Selective vasoconstriction in carotid vascular bed by methysergide: Possible relevance to its antimigraine effect. *European Journal of Pharmacology*, **27**, 99–105.

Saxena, P.R. (1986). Pharmacology of cranial arteriovenous anastomoses. In: *Neural regulation of brain circulation*, (ed. C. Owman and J.E. Hardebo), Vol. 8, pp. 541–58, Elsevier Science Publishers, Amsterdam.

Saxena, P.R. and Verdouw, P.D. (1985). 5-Carboxamidotryptamine, a compound with high affinity for 5-hydroxytryptamine$_1$ binding sites, dilates arterioles and constricts arteriovenous anastomoses. *British Journal of Pharmacology*, **84**, 533–44.

Saxena, P.R., Mylecharane, E.J., and Heiligers, J. (1985). Analysis of the heart rate effects of 5-hydroxytryptamine in the cat; mediation of tachycardia by 5-HT$_1$-like receptors. *Naunyn-Schmiedeberg's Archives of Pharmacology*, **330**, 121–9.

Sicuteri, F., Testi, A., and Anselmi, B. (1961). Biochemical investigations in headache: increase in the hydroxyindoleacetic acid excretion during migraine attacks. *International Archives of Allergy*, **19**, 55–8.

Sicuteri, F., Anselmi, B., and Fanciullaci, M. (1973). The serotonin (5-HT) theory of migraine. *Advances in Neurology*, **4**, 383–94.

Sjaastad, O. (1975). The significance of blood serotonin levels in migraine. A critical review. *Acta Neurologica Scandinavica*, **51**, 200–10.

Smith, A.P. (1974). A comparison of the effects of prostaglandin E_2 and salbutamol by intravenous infusion on the airways obstruction of patients with asthma. *British Journal of Clinical Pharmacology*, **1**, 399–404.

Spierings, E.L.H. and Saxena, P.R. (1980). Anti-migraine drugs and cranial arteriovenous shunting in the cat. *Neurology*, **30**, 696–701.

Sumner, M.J., Humphrey, P.P.A., and Feniuk, W. (1987). Characterisation of the 5-HT$_1$-like receptor mediating relaxation of porcine vena cava. *British Journal of Pharmacology*, **92**, 574P.

Syvalahti, E., Kangasniemi, P., and Ross, B. (1979). Migraine headache and blood serotonin levels after administration of zimelidine, a selective inhibitor of serotonin uptake. *Current Therapeutic Research Clinical and Experimental*, **25**, 299–310.

Trevethick, M.A., Feniuk, W., and Humphrey, P.P.A. (1984). 5-Hydroxytryptamine-induced relaxation of neonatal porcine vena cava in vitro. *Life Sciences Part I Physiology and Pharmacology*, **35**, 477–86.

Trevethick, M.A., Feniuk, W., and Humphrey, P.P.A. (1986). 5-Carboxamidotryptamine: a potent agonist mediating relaxation and elevation of cyclic AMP in the isolated neonatal porcine vena cava. *Life Sciences Part I Physiology and Pharmacology*, **38**, 521–8.

Watts, A.D., Feniuk, W., and Humphrey, P.P.A. (1981). A pre-junctional action of 5-hydroxytryptamine and methysergide on noradrenergic nerves in dog isolated saphenous vein. *Journal of Pharmacy and Pharmacology*, **33**, 515–20.

Wolff, H.S. (1963). *Headache and other head pain* (2nd edn). Oxford University Press, London.

Discussion

PEATFIELD: Has the '5-HT$_1$-like' receptor (or 'dog saphenous vein receptor', if you will) been found in the human coronary arteries?

HUMPHREY: In all the experiments we have done in cats and dogs we have seen no effect of GR43175 on the coronary vasculature either *in vitro* or *in vivo*. In human coronary arteries, we and others have seen a small contraction in response to GR43175 in the few isolated vessels that we have looked at so far. So a few of these 5-HT$_1$-like receptors seem to be present in large human epicardial arteries. But, to put it in context, the thromboxane A_2 mimetic, u-46619, was a much more potent and effective spasmogen than 5-HT, which itself was more potent and effective than GR43175 (Connor *et al.* 1989). Indeed, we have shown that 5-HT acts predominantly through 5-HT$_2$ receptors, as judged by the effectiveness of ketanserin as an antagonist. I do not think that 5-HT is a major pathological mediator of spasm in these vessels because it is relatively so weak. Dr Edvinsson is now examining the effects of GR43175 on other human vessels, the meningeal and pial arteries, and the results may help to illuminate the precise locus of the pathology of migraine.

SANDLER: Does methiothepin provoke a migraine attack?

HUMPHREY: I do not know. It is a very 'dirty' drug, and I do not think it can be given to humans.

LANCE: We have used intravenous GR43175 in the model I described earlier. We recorded single cell discharges in response to stimulation of the superior sagittal sinus, middle meningeal artery and superficial temporal artery in the cat. Intravenous GR43175 had no consistent effect on the central discharge of these pain pathways, which supports Dr Humphrey's view that the action of GR43175 is peripheral.

FERREIRA: Is there any vasoconstrictor that mimics your 5-HT agonist — for example, angiotensin, endothelin, noradrenaline? Do they have some similarity in their pharmacological profile?

HUMPHREY: No. If you inject most known vasoconstrictors into an animal or human you get pressor responses and vasoconstriction in most vascular beds within the body. What struck us about methysergide was its very localized action at least in the dog; and, of course, GR43175 has a very localized action. Nevertheless, any vasoconstrictor (for example, 5-HT) seems to be able to alleviate a migraine headache. Did you ever use noradrenaline, Professor Lance?

LANCE: We ourselves have not infused noradrenaline but Harold G. Wolff (1963) did some classical experiments in which infusion of noradrenaline did alleviate a migraine headache.

SAXENA: Isometheptene, another sympathomimetic drug, has also been used (see Spierings and Saxena 1980).

SCHWARTZ: I would like to ask you a pharmacological question. Where would you place your 5-HT$_1$-like receptor in the classification that is used by people doing binding studies? Is it the receptor that has recently been cloned? Many years ago we published a paper showing that 5-HT has a high glycogenolytic activity in brain slices. It was a receptor-mediated process, and the response was similar to the one you found. The only compounds that were active, apart from methiothepin, were imipramine and imipramine-like drugs at rather high concentrations (Quach *et al.* 1982).

HUMPHREY: I can appreciate your question because the 5-HT receptor area is very confusing. As one of the members of the committee who wrote the Bradley paper on 5-HT receptor classification (Bradley *et al.* 1986), along with John Fozard and Pramod Saxena, I was very keen to discuss this with the committee simply because we had found the 'dog saphenous vein receptor' and it clearly did not fit in with the existing binding data. At this stage we use the appellation *5-HT$_1$-like*, which covers receptors that can be stimulated by 5-CT (5-carboxamidotryptamine) and blocked by methiothepin. The dog saphenous vein receptor does not appear to be similar to the 5-HT$_{1A}$, the 5-HT$_{1B}$, the 5-HT$_{1C}$, or the 5-HT$_{1D}$ receptors. We are doing binding studies with GR43175, and have found that the 5-HT$_{1D}$ site is not a homogeneous site. There appear to be two binding components to it and, for one of these, GR43175 is very selective. We may therefore finally end up with a binding site in the brain that we can equate with the receptor in dog saphenous vein, but we have yet to name it.

MOSKOWITZ: I was pleased that although vasoconstriction might prove to be the mechanism of action for GR43175, you did not infer that vasodilation is the cause of the pain. Vasoconstriction will change the geometry of the perivascular sensory fibres, and by so doing may change the electrical threshold for depolarization of these pain fibres. We might also consider why headaches are experienced in the head. If headaches are triggered by humoral or blood-mediated phenomena, why does the pain reside in the head and not in the arm or the kidney? Perhaps the uniqueness lies in the trigeminal nerve. But you have given another potential answer to this question; you have shown that cerebral vessels have specific vascular receptors, and this discovery is extremely exciting.

PEATFIELD: Are the cat arteriovenous shunts found in the head only?

HUMPHREY: Predominantly. We know, however, that there is also a small degree of shunting in some animals in the paws, for example.

PEATFIELD: Is that the explanation? Is the pain felt in the head because there are more shunts in our heads than elsewhere in our bodies?

HUMPHREY: One of the criticisms of the shunt hypothesis is that those domestic animals where functionally significant shunting has been demonstrated have a different craniovascular anatomy from humans. There appears to be no marked shunting in primates (Saxena 1987), although in cadavers there is evidence that some sort of carotid shunting takes place. Whether that is relevant to an ambulatory person's migraine is another matter! Certainly there is some anatomical evidence that shunting occurs in the meningeal vascular territory in humans. Perhaps one could bring all these hypotheses together in one unifying hypothesis.

VANE: Another organ in which it is very easy to demonstrate shunts is the kidney. Have you looked at the kidney?

HUMPHREY: Most of the shunting in anaesthetized dogs and cats is in the carotid circulation. There is some shunting elsewhere, but it is less than 5 per cent of the total.

VANE: Does your compound have any side-effects, such as changing urine flow?

HUMPHREY: In the studies we have done so far, it seems to be remarkably free from any major side-effects; minor effects such as scalp tingling and a transient feeling of faintness have been described. Interestingly, it not only aborts the headache, but the nausea, vomiting and other autonomic symptoms also seem to disappear. Again, we must return to the concept of a central inflammation such as that described by Moskowitz. The afferent stimuli may not only be producing the pain but also the other autonomic effects.

SAXENA: With the use of radioactive microspheres of four different diameters we were unable to find any large arteriovenous anastomoses in the kidneys. These shunt vessels were localized primarily in the skin, ears, and tongue. In the skin there is a heterogeneity, with some regions showing less and others showing more shunting. The greatest shunting was in the skin of the head (Saxena and Verdouw 1985).

VANE: If you look at the renal veins in an anaesthetized dog, you can see arterial blood coming into them in streams.

SAXENA: That is possible. Histologically or radiologically, the arteriovenous shunts can be located in many different tissues (for references, see Saxena 1987). On the other hand, the microsphere technique (where one usually uses spheres of 15 μm diameter) reveals arteriovenous shunts that are anatomically larger than 15 μm. Apparently, only small shunts are present in the kidneys.

LANCE: We must keep in mind the correlation between the basic science and the clinical picture. Migraine headache is not necessarily confined to the head. Many patients commonly complain of pain in the neck, shoulder, arm, and even down the entire half of the body. So whatever the influence that operates in the periphery (in the vasculature) to set up this neurovascular reflex responsible for pain, it can presumably also activate spinothalamic as well as trigeminothalamic pathways. So migraine is not simply a pain in the head.

FOZARD: Although you are keeping an open mind about the mode of action of GR43175, your bias is towards a vascular site of action. Yet in the dog saphenous vein, GR43175 is an effective inhibitor of transmitter release from the sympathetic *nerves*. The only information we have about the neuronal effects of this compound is from that particular tissue.

HUMPHREY: I do have an open mind, but we simply have great difficulty in finding the GR43175-sensitive receptor in other preparations. We cannot find it on the nerve terminals in lots of other places that we have looked. We have found it, however, in the femoral bed of the anaesthetized dog, where it must explain the vasodilatation that we have observed with methysergide and GR43175 (Feniuk *et al*. 1981, 1989). These agonists appear to turn off sympathetic drive in that vascular bed by an action on nerve terminals. We have systematically examined the role of 5HT$_1$-like receptors in the control of noradrenaline release, and have now turned our attention to their possible control of neurokinin release from nerves.

SCHWARTZ: What is the activity of your compound on 5-HT release in the brain — that is, on the autoreceptor?

HUMPHREY: We have not done this, but D.N. Middlemiss has some recent data on this. He believes the guinea-pig autoreceptor on serotoninergic brain neurones is like the receptor in dog saphenous vein (Middlemiss *et al*. 1988).

COPPEN: When you did preliminary clinical trials to test GR43175 as an acute treatment for severe migraine (Doenicke *et al*. 1988), was this a treatment of episodes?

HUMPHREY: No, that work was simply done to treat people who had a single headache that was established for between half an hour and up to 12 hours. The initial studies were uncontrolled.

COPPEN: Perhaps a useful strategy for treating headache is to give some treatment over the long term. Would this compound be something that you would want to give long term?

HUMPHREY: What has struck me from the clinical data is that the drug seems to work even when the headache is well established. Ergotamine, on the other hand, cannot readily effect pain reversal once the headache is established. However, when we have shown success with a long-established headache of, say, 12 hours, one could argue that the pain would have gone away anyway. We shall have to determine the true efficacy of the drug in large-scale clinical trials which are properly placebo-controlled.

COPPEN: How long does it take to act?

HUMPHREY: When given subcutaneously; it will normally be effective within about 20–30 minutes.

References

Bradley, P.B. *et al*. (1986). Proposals for the classification and nomenclature of functional receptors for 5-hydroxytryptamine. *Neuropharmacology*, **25**, 563–76.

Connor, H.E., Feniuk, W., and Humphrey, P.P.A. (1989). 5-HT contracts human coronary arteries predominantly via 5-HT$_2$ receptor activation. *European Journal of Pharmacology*, **161**, 91–4.

Doenicke, A., Brand, J., and Perrin, V.L. (1988). Possible benefit of GR43175, a novel 5-HT$_1$-like receptor agonist, for the acute treatment of severe migraine. *Lancet*, **i**, 1309–11.

Feniuk, W., Humphrey, P.P.A., and Watts, A.D. (1981). Modification of the vasomotor actions of methysergide in the femoral arterial bed of the anaesthetized dog by changes in sympathetic nerve activity. *Journal of Autonomic Pharmacology*, **1**, 127–32.

Feniuk, W., Humphrey, P.P.A., and Perren, M.J. (1989). The selective carotid arterial vasoconstrictor action of GR43175 in anaesthetized dogs. *British Journal of Pharmacology*, **96**, 83–90.

Middlemiss, D.N., Bremer, M.E., and Smith, S.M. (1988). A pharmacological analysis of the 5-HT receptor mediating inhibition of 5-HT release in the guinea-pig frontal cortex. *European Journal of Pharmacology*, **157**, 101–7.

Quach, T.T., Rose, C., Duchemin, A.M., and Schwartz, J.C. (1982). Glycogenolysis induced by serotonin in brain: identification of a new class of receptor. *Nature*, **298**, 373–5.

Saxena, P.R. (1987). The arteriovenous anastomoses and veins in migraine research. In *Migraine: therapeutic, conceptual and research aspects*, (ed. J.N. Blau), pp. 581–96. Chapman and Hall, London.

Saxena, P.R. and Verdouw, P.D. (1985). Tissue blood flow and arteriovenous shunting in pigs measured with microspheres of four different sizes. *Pfluegers Archiv European Journal of Physiology*, **403**, 128–35.

Spierings, E.L.H. and Saxena, P.R. (1980). Effect of isometheptene on the distribution and shunting of 15 μm microspheres throughout the cephalic circulation of the cat. *Headache*, **20**, 103–6.

Wolff, H.G. (1963). *Headache and other pain*, (2nd edn). Oxford University Press, New York.

13. Behavioural effects of m-chlorophenylpiperazine (m-CPP), a reported migraine precipitant

G. Curzon, G.A. Kennett, K. Shah, and P. Whitton

Introduction

Previous contributors to this volume have given many indications that 5-hydroxytryptamine (5-HT; serotonin) is involved in migraine. In particular, John Fozard has pointed out that many 5-HT antagonists with prophylactic activity bind strongly to 5-HT_2 and 5-HT_{1C} sites. We have recently been investigating three behavioural effects of the 5-HT agonist 1-(3-chlorophenylpiperazine) (m-CPP) and of the related compound 1-[(3-trifluoromethy)phenyl] piperazine (TFMPP). These are hypolocomotion, hypophagia, and anxiety. When we began this work, m-CPP and TFMPP were considered as putative 5-HT_{1B} agonists (Sills et al. 1984; Asarch et al. 1985; Hamon et al. 1986). However, the behavioural effects now appear more to suggest major agonist actions at 5-HT_{1C} sites (Kennett and Curzon 1988a,b; Kennett et al. 1989) and this agrees with recent binding data (Hoyer 1988) and with the stimulating effect of m-CPP on phosphoinositide hydrolysis in the 5-HT_{1C}-rich choroid plexus (Conn and Sanders-Bush 1987).

The anxiogenic effect may be relevant to migraine, as anxiety or stress are candidates for precipitating attacks of migraine, and it is therefore of great interest that Brewerton et al. (1988) recently reported that m-CPP precipitated headache in both control and migrainous subjects with a significantly greater incidence in the latter group. Seven out of eight of them reported that the headaches could not be distinguished from their naturally occurring symptoms, except possibly for the absence of prodromal signs.

This work and our own findings may suggest new avenues for migraine research. At the least, they raise a number of questions. This paper summarizes the evidence that the anxiogenic effect of m-CPP is mediated by 5-HT_{1C} receptors, that it is not merely a consequence of the hypolocomotor effect of m-CPP, and that it may also have implications for the mechanism and treatment of migraine.

Materials and methods

Animals

Male Sprague Dawley rats (200–250 g, Charles River, UK) were individually housed under a 12 h light/dark cycle (lights on 06.00 h) at 20 ± 2°C, with free access to food and water for at least five days before experimentation. In all three tests of anxiety, rats were injected in their holding rooms before being tested in a separate, quiet room. The boxes and open fields were carefully wiped with a damp cloth between anxiety tests.

Social interaction testing

This was conducted in a box with opaque walls on three sides and a glass front and top (height 30 cm; depth 27 cm; length 60 cm) under red light. On each of the two days immediately prior to experimentation, rats were individually habituated to the box for 10 min. On the third day, rats were injected subcutaneously in weight-matched pairs between 1300 and 1330 h, with a 5-HT receptor antagonist or vehicle and returned to their home cages. Twenty mins later they were injected intraperitoneally with *m*-CPP or 0.9 per cent NaCl, and again returned to their home cage. After a further 20 min, they were placed together with their weight-matched pair-mate in the social interaction box, and the resultant behaviour over the next 15 min was videotaped (camera and videorecorder, JVC).

m-CPP-induced hypophagia

Food was withdrawn between 1600 and 1800 h. On the following day, between 1300 and 1400 h, *m*-CPP was injected and, 20 min later, a weighed quantity of food was restored (200 g). Food intake was determined by weighing the food remaining after two hours.

Videotape analysis

Total interaction times and numbers of rectangles crossed in the interaction test were measured by using stopwatches and hand-held counters, respectively. Durations of individual components of behaviour during the test (grooming, self-grooming, mounting, sniffing, following, and boxing and biting) were analysed on a Sharp MZ80B microcomputer, with a modification of the 'BASIC' program described by Hendrie and Bennett (1983).

Drugs

The drugs — 1-(3-chlorophenyl) piperazine dihydrochloride (*m*-CPP), 1-naphthyl-piperazine (both Research Biochemicals Inc., Wayland, MA, USA), ICS 205 930 (Sandoz Ltd., Switzerland), and chlordiazepoxide hydrochloride (Roche Products Ltd., England) — were dissolved in 0.9 per cent saline and injected intraperitoneally (*m*-CPP and chlordiazepoxide) or subcutaneously (ICS 205 930) at the nape of the neck. (−)Propranolol hydroch-

TABLE 13.1. *Effects of m-CPP on locomotion and social interaction and on food intake*

m-CPP (mg kg^{-1})	Social interaction time (s)	Locomotion (rectangles crossed)	Food intake[†] (g 2h^{-1})
0	272 ± 20	102 ± 5	6.1 ± 0.5
0.2	176 ± 22*	95 ± 5	
0.5	116 ± 19**	105 ± 12	
1.0	76 ± 10**	67 ± 10*	5.4 ± 0.9
5.0			1.8 ± 0.4**

Means ± s.e.m; n= 5–12;
Differences from controls *p < 0.05; **p < 0.01.
[†]Results from Kennett and Curzon (1988*b*).

loride (ICI, Macclesfield, UK) was also dissolved in 0.9 per cent saline and injected subcutaneously after being brought to pH 6.5. Metergoline (Farmitalia), (+)cyanopindolol (Sandoz Ltd, Basel), ketanserin tartrate and ritanserin (Janssen, Beerse, Belgium), mianserin hydrochloride (Organon Laboratories Ltd, Newhouse, England), and cyproheptadine (Merck, Sharp and Dohme, Harlow, UK) were dissolved in 100–200 µl of 10 per cent acetic acid, made up to almost the required volume with 0.9 per cent saline, and brought to pH 6.5 before subcutaneous injection. All drugs were administered in volumes of 1 ml kg^{-1}.

Results and discussion

Effects of m-CPP on social interaction, locomotion, and food intake are shown in Table 13.1. It is clear that the decrease of social interaction is not simply due to decreased locomotion as it was markedly affected at doses below those that affected locomotion. Hypophagia occurred at only very high dosage in food-deprived rats but m-CPP was more hypophagic in freely feeding animals (Kennett and Curzon 1988*a*). m-CPP was comparably potent, not only in the social interaction test but also in another anxiety model, the light/dark box test (Kennett *et al.* 1989) and it is also anxiogenic at similar dosages in humans (Mueller *et al.* 1985; Charney *et al.* 1987).

Table 13.2 summarizes our results on the effects of 5-HT antagonists on the responses studied. Table 13.3 gives binding data of a number of drugs for 5-HT sites. More detailed information is provided by Hoyer (1988). m-CPP-induced hypoactivity was not blocked by drugs with a selectivity against 5-HT$_{1A}$ and 5-HT$_{1B}$ receptors — (−)pindolol, (−)propranolol, and (±)cyanopindolol — but was blocked by the non-selective 5-HT antagonist metergoline and by three drugs with high activity against 5-HT$_{1C}$ and 5-HT$_2$

TABLE 13.2. *Behavioural effects of mCPP: blockade by antagonists*

Antagonist	Dose (mg kg⁻¹)	Hypoactivity (m-CPP 5mg kg⁻¹)	'Anxiety'[†] (m-CPP 0.5 mg kg⁻¹)	Hypophagia (m-CPP 5mg kg⁻¹)
metergoline	5	+	+[‡]	+
(−) pindolol	2	−		−
(−) propranolol	16	−	−	+
(±) cyanopindolol	8	−	−	+
mianserin	2	+	+	+
cyproheptadine	2	+	+	−[§]
l-naphthyl-piperazine	2	+	+	+
ketanserin	0.2	−	−	−
ritanserin	0.6	−	−	−
chlordiazepoxide	5*		+	
ICS 205–930	0.05		+	

+ = blocked, − = not blocked. *mg day⁻¹ × 5.
[†]Decreased social interaction time, [‡]metergoline 2.5 mg kg⁻¹, [§] 10 mg kg⁻¹ cyproheptadine
Results given in full detail in Kennett and Curzon 1988a,b; Kennett et al. 1989.

TABLE 13.3. *Affinities for 5-HT receptors*

Drug	Receptor type (pK$_D$ values, −log mol l^{-1})					
	1A	1B	1C	1D	2	3
m-CPP	6.5	6.6	7.7		6.7	(7.3)
methysergide	7.6	5.8	8.6		8.6	
cyproheptadine	6.5	5.3	7.9		8.5	(<5)
pizotifen	6.2	5.5	8.1	5.6	7.8	
(−)propranolol	6.8	7.3	6.8	5.5	5.7	5.7
mianserin	6.0	5.2	8.0	6.4	8.1	
ketanserin	5.9	5.7	7.0	6.0	8.9	(<5)
ritanserin	5.4	4.0	8.7		9.3	
l-naphthylpiperazine	7.2	6.6	8.2		7.2	
atenolol	3.3	3.8	4.0		4.0	

Data from Hoyer (1988) except for 5-HT$_3$ affinities (Kilpatrick *et al.* 1988)

sites, mianserin, cyproheptadine and 1-naphthyl-piperazine. Ketanserin and ritanserin, which are selective against 5-HT$_2$ sites but also have quite a high affinity for 5-HT$_{1C}$ sites, were inactive at concentrations sufficient to block a 5-HT$_2$ receptor-dependent behaviour, 5-hydroxytryptophan-induced head-twitches. The ID$_{50}$ values for inhibition of the latter were 0.036 mg kg^{-1} (ketanserin) and 0.19 mg kg^{-1} (ritanserin); (Kennett and Curzon 1989).

The pharmacological profile for blockade of the anxiety response to *m*-CPP (decreased social interaction time) was identical with that described above, except that two of the drugs — (−)pindolol and l-naphthyl-piperazine — were not tested. These results suggest that activation of 5-HT$_{1C}$ receptors by *m*-CPP causes both the hypolocomotor and the anxiogenic responses. The latter effect is not merely a consequence of the former. This is indicated by their different dose dependencies (Table 13.1) and also by anxiolytic treatment (with chronic chlordiazepoxide), which prevents only the anxiogenic response. This response was also prevented by the 5-HT$_3$ antagonist ICS 205–930. While *m*-CPP itself has an appreciable affinity for 5-HT$_3$ sites (Kilpatrick *et al.* 1988), the blockade of its hypolocomotor and anxiogenic effects by cyproheptadine suggests that these effects are not explicable by this 5-HT$_3$ affinity, because cyproheptadine has little 5-HT$_3$ binding affinity but binds strongly to 5-HT$_{1C}$ sites.

Table 2 also shows the effects of 5-HT antagonists on *m*-CPP-induced hypophagia. Apart from the lack of effect of (−)pindolol and cyproheptadine, these findings are consistent with an involvement of both 5-HT$_{1B}$ and 5-HT$_1$ receptors, as discussed in detail elsewhere (Kennett and Curzon 1988*b*). A role for agonist action at 5-HT$_{1C}$ rather than at 5-HT$_2$ sites is

178   G. Curzon et al.

strongly indicated (G.A. Kennett and G. Curzon, unpublished results) by a comparison of the ID_{50} values of antagonists against the hypophagia, and against the 5-HT$_2$ receptor-dependent 5-hydroxytryptophan-induced head-twitch, with the corresponding affinities (Hoyer 1988) for 5-HT$_{1C}$ and 5-HT$_2$ sites.

These findings raise numerous questions. Is m-CPP headache a useful research tool? Is the anxiety-like effect of m-CPP in rats a useful test-bed for migraine prophylactics? Do drugs that block its actions at 5-HT$_{1C}$ sites tend to prevent migraine attacks? Table 13.3 gives affinities for 5-HT binding sites of some prophylactic and other drugs. While prophylaxis is not necessarily associated with a high affinity for 5-HT$_{1C}$ (and 5-HT$_2$) sites (that is, atenolol), the high affinity of some prophylactic drugs (e.g. methysergide, cyproheptadine, pizotifen and possibly ($-$)propranolol; Peatfield et al. 1986) raises questions about compounds such as mianserin and ritanserin. The lack of convincing evidence for prophylaxis by ketanserin points to 5-HT$_{1C}$ rather than to 5-HT$_2$ antagonism as being beneficial. Finally, although such effects do not necessarily imply 5-HT$_{1C}$ site abnormalities in migraine-prone subjects, they do raise this possibility.

References

Asarch, K.E., Ransom, R.W., and Shih, J.S. (1985). 5-HT$_{1A}$ and 5-HT$_{1B}$ selectivity of two phenylpiperazine derivatives: evidence for 5-HT$_{1B}$ heterogeneity. *Life Sciences*, **36**, 1265–73.

Brewerton, T.D., Murphy, D.L., Mueller, E.A., and Jimerson, D.C. (1988). Induction of migraine-like headaches by the serotonin agonist m-chlorophenyl-piperazine. *Clinical Pharmacology and Therapeutics*, **43**, 605–9.

Charney, D.S., Woods, S.W., Goodman, W.K., and Heninger, G.R. (1987). Serotonin function in anxiety. II: Effects of the serotonin agonist mCPP in panic disorder patients and healthy subjects. *Psychopharmacology* **92**, 14–24.

Conn, P.J. and Sanders-Bush, E. (1987). Relative efficacies of piperazines at the phosphoinositide hydrolysis-linked serotoninergic (5-HT$_2$ and 5-HT$_{1C}$) receptors. *Journal of Pharmacology and Experimental Therapeutics*, **242**, 552–7.

Hamon, M., Cossery, J-M., Spampinato, U., and Gozlan, H. (1986). Are there selective ligands for 5-HT$_{1A}$ receptor binding sites in brain? *Trends in Pharmacological Sciences*, **7**, 336–7.

Hendrie, C.A. and Bennett, S. (1983). A microcomputer technique for the detailed analysis of animal behavior. *Physiology and Behavior*, **30**, 233–5.

Hoyer, D. (1988). Functional correlates of serotonin 5-HT$_1$ recognition sites. *Journal of Receptor Research*, **8**, 59–81.

Kennett, G.A. and Curzon, G. (1988a). Evidence that mCPP may have behavioural effects mediated by central 5-HT$_{1C}$ receptors. *British Journal of Pharmacology*, **94**, 137–47.

Kennett, G.A. and Curzon, G. (1988b). Evidence that hypophagia induced by mCPP and TFMPP requires 5-HT$_{1C}$ and 5-HT$_{1B}$ receptors; hypophagia induced by RU 24969 only requires 5-HT$_{1B}$ receptors. *Psychopharmacology*, **96**, 93–100.

Kennett, G.A., Whitton, P., Shah, K., and Curzon, G. (1989). Anxiogenic-like effects of mCPP and TFMPP in animal models are opposed by 5-HT$_{1C}$ receptor antagonists. *European Journal of Pharmacology*, **164**, 445–54.

Kilpatrick, G.J., Jones, B.J., and Tyers, M.B. (1988). Identification and distribution of 5-HT$_3$ receptors in rat brain using radioligand binding. *Nature*, **330**, 746–8.

Mueller, E.A., Murphy, D.L., and Sunderland, T. (1985). Neuroendocrine effects of m-chlorophenylpiperazine, a serotonin agonist, in humans *Journal of Clinical Endocrinology and Metabolism*, **61**, 1179–84.

Peatfield, R.C., Fozard, J.R., and Rose, F.C. (1986). Drug treatment of migraine. In *Handbook of clinical neurology*, (ed. P.J. Vinken, G.W. Bruyn, and H.L. Klawans), Vol. 4, pp. 173–216. Elsevier, Amsterdam.

Sills, M.A., Wolfe, B.B., and Frazer, A. (1984). Determination of selective and non-selective compounds for the 5-HT$_{1A}$ and 5-HT$_{1B}$ receptor subtypes in rat frontal cortex. *Journal of Pharmacology and Experimental Therapeutics*, **231**, 480–7.

Discussion

SANDLER: These triazolo compounds, such as alprazolam, are well known for interacting (some as inverse agonists) with the benzodiazepine receptor. What proportion of trazodone is metabolized to *m*-chlorophenylpiperazine (*m*-CPP)?

CURZON: Plasma levels of *m*-CPP in patients on trazodone are about 40% of those of the parent drug (Suckow 1983).

SANDLER: Is it correct that headache may be a side-effect of trazodone?

CURZON: Yes, and the work of Brewerton *et al.* (1988) strongly points to a migrainogenic effect of *m*-CPP.

SANDLER: Why are you sure that *m*-CPP is a specific drug? Why do you think that its anxiogenic action may be because of the 5-HT$_{1C}$ receptor?

CURZON: Our evidence (Kennett *et al.* 1989) about the effects of *m*-CPP on rat models of anxiety, and their blockade by other drugs, strongly points to 5-HT$_{1C}$ sites. However, the degree to which these sites and 5-HT$_3$ or benzodiazepine receptors mediate non-drug-induced anxiety is quite unknown.

SANDLER: Do you know, Dr Humphrey, whether *m*-CPP acts on the dog's saphenous vein receptor?

HUMPHREY: It would seem that the drug can stimulate or block most 5-HT (5-hydroxytryptamine; serotonin) receptors. Nevertheless, I accept that Professor Curzon in his rat model has evidence, from his tests with all the antagonists, that *m*-CPP is acting through a 5-HT$_{1C}$ mechanism. But because *m*-CPP *is* a non-specific or 'dirty' drug, one cannot extrapolate from the rat experiments to headache in humans. Who knows why it causes a headache in humans?

CURZON: We do not know whether 5-HT$_{1C}$ sites are involved in spontaneous migraine. *m*-CPP binds to many 5-HT receptor subtypes and also to other sites. In fact, when we first obtained behavioural data to suggest that it acted at 5-HT$_{1C}$ sites, I felt rather cautious because at that time it was being referred to as a 5-HT$_{1B}$ drug. However, the most recent binding data (Hoyer 1988) indicate that *m*-CPP binds strongly to the 5-HT$_{1C}$ receptor. We also found that (at appropriate concentrations) antagonists to 5-HT$_{1A}$, 5-HT$_{1B}$, and 5-HT$_2$ receptor subtypes did not block the *m*-CPP effects, but 5-HT$_{1C}$ antagonists did. The extent to which the 5-HT$_{1C}$-dependent effect of *m*-CPP in the rat is a model of migraine in the human will need much more investigation. Nevertheless, as *m*-CPP is reported to cause migraine attacks and anxiety in the human and anxiety-like behaviour in the rat, the latter effect if worth consideration as a possible model.

ZIEGLER: Would you please comment on ipsapirone? This seems to be the drug that is the antagonist to m-CPP, especially with respect to the anxiogenic responses.

CURZON: Ipsapirone, buspirone, gepirone, and 8-OH-DPAT (8-hydroxy-2-(di-n-propylamino)tetralin — are all 5-HT$_{1A}$ agonists. At lower doses they are selective for 5-HT$_{1A}$ presynaptic sites at the cell body and thus decrease 5-HT release from terminals to postsynaptic sites. We have shown this by injecting 8-OH-DPAT into the raphé, and by detecting a reduction in 5-HT levels at a dialysis probe implanted into a terminal region. If activation of postsynaptic 5-HT$_{1C}$ or other 5-HT sites is anxiogenic, it seems reasonable that drugs that decrease 5-HT release to such sites will be anxiolytic.

ZIEGLER: Would you conclude that it would be worthwhile to try ipsapirone as a migraine prophylactic drug?

CURZON: This raises a rather general question: do antidepressant drugs and anxiolytic drugs decrease the incidence or severity of migraine attacks?

WELCH: Trazodone has been used in the prophylaxis of migraine but anecdotal evidence suggests that this was not very successful.

DE BELLEROCHE: Do the human results on induction of migraine occur at low enough drug concentrations to suggest that the drug would be selective for the 5-HT$_{1C}$ sites?

CURZON: Yes. The doses of m-CPP used in humans to produce anxiety and headache are similar to the doses that we find are effective in the rat anxiety model.

DE BELLEROCHE: The 5-HT$_{1C}$ receptor sites are restricted, as I understand, to the choroid plexus in the brain, and it is difficult to understand the mechanism that might be involved in inducing anxiety.

FOZARD: Autoradiography reveals that 5-HT$_{1C}$ sites are indeed relatively restricted in their distribution. Recently, the mRNA for the 5-HT$_{1C}$ sites has been mapped (Julius et al. 1988), and has been shown to have a far broader distribution than the sites themselves. We have to keep an open mind about where the 5-HT$_{1C}$ sites might be and how they might appear in key areas to play a role in anxiety.

CURZON: The way people are looking at 5-HT$_{1C}$ sites at the moment reminds me of how we tended to look at dopamine 20 years ago. The high concentration of dopamine in the basal ganglia led people to believe that that was the only place where it mattered. Then dopamine was found to occur in the cortex, and elsewhere, at levels that were much lower than in the basal ganglia but quite comparable with values for other transmitters such as 5-HT or noradrenaline. 5-HT$_{1C}$ sites have a tremendous concentration in the choroid plexus, but they also exist in many other places and could have functions there.

References

Brewerton, T.D., Murphy, D.L., Mueller, E.A., and Jimerson, D.C. (1988). Induction of migraine-like headaches by the serotonin agonist m-chlorophenyl-piperazine. *Clinical Pharmacology and Therapeutics*, **43**, 605–9.

Hoyer, D. (1988). Functional correlates of serotonin 5-HT$_1$ recognition sites. *Journal of Receptor Research*, **8**, 59–81.

Julius, O., McDermott, A.B., Axel, R., and Jessell, T.M. (1988). Molecular characterization of a functional cDNA encoding the serotonin 1C receptor. *Science*, **241**, 558–64.

Kennett, G.A., Whitton, P., Shah, K., and Curzon, G. (1989). Anxiogenic-like effects of mCPP and TFMPP in animal models are opposed by 5-HT$_{1C}$ receptor antagonists. *European Journal of Pharmacology*, **164**, 445–54.

Suckow, R.F. (1983). A simultaneous determination of trazodone and its metabolite 1-*m*-chlorophenylpiperazine in plasma by liquid chromatography with electrochemical detection. *Journal of Liquid Chromatography*, **6**, 2195–208.

14. 5-HT receptors and migraine

Pramod R. Saxena

Introduction

Migraine is a vascular headache but its pathophysiology is complex and multifactorial. Of the many pathophysiological factors that are implicated in migraine, changes in the metabolism of 5-hydroxytryptamine (5-HT) are the best documented. During the headache phase of migraine urinary excretion of 5-hydroxyindoleacetic acid increases, whereas the blood 5-HT concentration decreases. Furthermore, in migraine patients reserpine precipitates a headache that can be alleviated by 5-HT (Tandon *et al.* 1969; Lance 1982).

In the light of recent developments in the characterization and classification of the receptors for 5-HT, the purpose of this paper is to discuss the relationship between the neural and cephalovascular 5-HT receptors and the antimigraine action of drugs.

5-HT receptor classification

Three main kinds of 5-HT receptors (5-HT$_1$-like, 5-HT$_2$, and 5-HT$_3$ receptors) mediate functional responses to 5-HT (Table 14.1; Bradley *et al.* 1986; Humphrey and Feniuk 1988). Only 5-HT$_2$ and 5-HT$_3$ receptors have so far been well characterized, by the use of selective antagonists. No such compound is yet available for 5-HT$_1$-like receptors. These receptors, having a nanomolar affinity for 5-HT, are heterogeneous in nature but the exact association with the 5-HT$_1$ binding-site subtypes is unclear.

Neural 5-HT Receptors

5-HT receptors are present on peripheral and central neurones; the main functional responses are listed in Table 14.1. It is postulated that 5-HT$_3$ receptors serve as 'transducers' for painful stimuli that originate from blood vessels (for example, as a result of an overactivity of raphé neurones), and the resulting peripheral nociceptive input is then transmitted, via afferent fibres, to the dorsal horn cells (Richardson *et al.* 1986; Raskin 1988; Fozard, this volume). The nociceptive afferents synapse with the spinothalamic fibres in the periaqueductal gray region of the spinal cord. The transmission in the nociceptive afferents can be inhibited by serotoninergic fibres that

TABLE 14.1. *Classification of, and some functional responses mediated by, 5-HT receptors*

Receptor or its subtype	Agonists	Antagonists	Binding site	Functional responses
5-HT$_1$-like*	5-HT; 5-CT	Methiothepin[†] Methysergide[†]	5-HT$_1$	Behavioural changes; centrally evoked hypotensive response.
5-HT$_{1A}$	5-HT; 5-CT; 8-OH-DPAT; RU 24969	Methiothepin Cyanopindolol, Methysergide	5-HT$_{1A}$	Autoreceptor in the rat brain.
5-HT$_{1B}$	5-HT; 5-CT; RU 24969	Methiothepin, Cyanopindolol	5-HT$_{1B}$	
Unnamed[‡]	5-HT; 5-CT; AH25086; GR43175	Methiothepin, Methysergide[§]	Not yet found[¶]	Contraction of cranial arteries (basilar, pial) and arteriovenous anastomoses in the carotid region; inhibition of noradrenaline release.
Unnamed[‡]	5-HT; 5-CT	Methiothepin, Methysergide	Not yet found[¶]	Vascular smooth muscle relaxation; hypotension.
5-HT$_2$	5-HT; α-CH$_3$-5-HT	Ketanserin, Cyproheptadine, Methysergide, Methiothepin	5-HT$_2$	Contraction of various vascular, gastrointestinal, and bronchial smooth muscles; platelet aggregation; head twitch and convulsion.
5-HT$_3$	5-HT; 2-CH$_3$-5-HT	MDL 72222, ICS 205–930, BRL 43694, GR38032	5-HT$_3$	Membrane depolarization; dermal pain; and flare response.

*Heterogeneous receptors;

[†]Non-selective antagonist (also blocks 5-HT$_2$ receptors);

[‡]Receptor type is not yet named;

[§]Partial agonist;

[¶]Does not correlate with either 5-HT$_{1C}$ or 5-HT$_{1D}$ binding sites. The table is based on Bradley *et al.* (1986), Humphrey and Feniuk (1988), and Saxena *et al.* (1989).

descend from the nucleus raphé magnus. Since this inhibitory response is not blocked by 5-HT$_2$ receptor antagonists, Richardson *et al.* (1986) suggest that this receptor could be 5-HT$_1$-like in nature.

Cephalovascular 5-HT receptors

Isolated cerebral and extracerebral cephalic vessels usually contract in response to 5-HT. The 5-HT-induced contraction of large 'conducting' cephalic vessels is, as in other large peripheral vessels, often mediated via 5-HT$_2$ receptors. However, in several instances — for example in human, dog, and guinea-pig basilar arteries — 5-HT$_1$-like receptors are involved in addition to, or in place of, 5-HT$_2$ receptors (Table 14.1; see Saxena *et al.* 1989). *In vivo*, 5-HT can cause either a constriction or a dilatation of cephalic vessels. Early studies from our laboratory showed that administration of 5-HT into the canine common carotid artery elicited vasoconstriction that was not, or was only slightly, affected by mianserin, cyproheptadine, or methysergide (see Saxena 1972), all of which powerfully antagonize responses mediated by 5-HT$_2$ receptors. We therefore concluded that the 5-HT receptors in the carotid circulation belong to a new type. Subsequently, it was shown that methysergide selectively constricted carotid vessels, probably by acting as an agonist at these 'atypical' 5-HT receptors (Saxena 1974).

Recently, we studied the nature of 5-HT receptors in the porcine carotid circulation, by using a combination of electromagnetic flowmetry and radioactive microspheres. 5-HT and 5-carboxamidotryptamine (5-CT), an agonist at 5-HT$_1$-like receptors, redistributed the carotid arterial blood flow (which was either unchanged or decreased) in favour of extracerebral cephalic tissue, at the expense of the fraction shunted via cephalic arteriovenous anastomoses (Saxena and Verdouw 1982, 1985). The increase in blood flow to the extracerebral structures was most marked in the cranial skin and ears, the colour of which changed to bright red. In animals treated with 5-HT$_2$ antagonists (for example, ketanserin), total carotid blood flow increased after 5-HT administration, and the vasodilator effect on the extracerebral arterioles was enhanced without much change in the arteriovenous anastomotic constriction. In contrast, methiothepin, a mixed 5-HT$_1$-like and 5-HT$_2$ receptor antagonist, antagonized the effects of 5-HT on both arterioles and arteriovenous anastomoses (Table 14.2; Saxena *et al.* 1986). Therefore, we concluded that the porcine carotid vascular bed has three different 5-HT receptor populations: constrictor 5-HT$_2$ receptors on the main carotid artery, dilator 5-HT$_1$-like receptors on carotid arterioles, and constrictor 5-HT$_1$-like receptors on cephalic arteriovenous anastomoses. Table 14.2 also shows that some agonists (methysergide, BEA 1654, 8-OH-DPAT, and GR43175) constrict arteriovenous anastomoses without eliciting much arteriolar vasodilatation. This result suggests that the 5-HT$_1$-like receptors on arteriovenous anastomoses and arterioles are heterogeneous. The constric-

TABLE 14.2. 5-HT receptors and drug effects on arterioles and on arteriovenous anastomoses (AVAs) in the porcine carotid artery bed

Drug	Arterioles	AVAs	Antagonism by:	Resistance to:	Receptor type
5-HT	– – – –	+ + + +	Methiothepin	Cyproheptadine, Ketanserin, WAL 1307, MDL 72222	5-HT$_1$-like
5-CT	– – – –	+ + + +		Cyproheptadine	5-HT$_1$-like
Methysergide	–	+ + +			5-HT$_1$-like
BEA 1654	– –	+ + +		Ketanserin	5-HT$_1$-like
GR43175*	0	+ + + +			5-HT$_1$-like
AH25086*	0	+ + + +			5-HT$_1$-like
8-OH-DPAT	–	+ + + +	Methiothepin	Ketanserin	5-HT$_1$-like
Ipsapirone	0	0			
Ergotamine	0	+ + + +		Methiothepin	Not known

8-OH-DPAT, 8-hydroxy-2-(di-*n*-propylamino) tetralin.

–, dilatation; +, contraction; 0, no effect. The number of '–' and '+' signs indicates the magnitude of the effect.

*Data from the cat.

The table is based on Saxena *et al.* (1989).

tion of arteriovenous anastomoses by 8-OH-DPAT tempts one to classify the 5-HT$_1$-like receptors on arteriovenous anastomoses as belonging to the 5-HT$_{1A}$ subtype, but ipsapirone, which also exhibits a high affinity for 5-HT$_{1A}$ recognition sites, proved to be inactive (Bom *et al.* 1989). Lastly, it may be noted that the effect of ergotamine on arteriovenous anastomoses, being unaffected by methiothepin, is mediated by neither 5-HT$_1$-like nor 5-HT$_2$ receptors (Bom *et al.* 1988).

The cephalovascular pharmacological properties of 5-HT — constriction of large extracerebral arteries (mediated by 5-HT$_1$-like and/or 5-HT$_2$ receptors) and arteriovenous anastomoses (5-HT$_1$-like receptors), and dilatation of arterioles (5-HT$_1$-like receptors) — suggest a role for 5-HT in the distribution of arterial blood flow. There is evidence for the presence of 5-HT neurones, and co-localization of 5-HT in the sympathetic neurones at some cranial neurovascular terminals, and the plasma 5-HT concentrations can reach values as high as 10–300 nM (see Fozard, this volume; Saxena *et al.* 1989). Thus, following a decrease in endogenous 5-HT activity during migraine (Lance 1982), large arteries and arteriovenous anastomoses may excessively dilate to initiate a nociceptive sensation and cause increased arteriovenous anastomotic shunting (see my next chapter in this volume), tissue ischaemia, and oedema.

5-HT receptor profile of antimigraine drugs

The 5-HT receptor profile of a number of new and established antimigraine drugs is presented in Table 14.3. With respect to 5-HT$_1$-like receptors it is obvious that the selective agonists at the distinct subtype that mediates contractions of extracerebral cephalic arteries and arteriovenous anastomoses (AH25086 and GR43175) are effective in the treatment of acute migraine attacks (Brand *et al.* 1987; Humphrey *et al.* 1988, and in this volume; Doenicke *et al.* 1988). These drugs do not penetrate into the central nervous system and, therefore, it seems likely that the site of their antimigraine action is in the extracerebral cephalic vasculature. The same appears to be true for ergotamine, though the drug fails to stimulate 5-HT$_1$-like receptors (Bom *et al.* 1988). In addition, ergotamine (oral bioavailability 5 per cent) does not readily penetrate into the central nervous system (Perrin 1985). It is, therefore, doubtful that its antimigraine action is due to stimulation of putative spinal 5-HT$_1$-like receptors that interfere with pain transmission via primary nociceptive afferents (Richardson *et al.* 1986; Raskin 1988).

Some antimigraine drugs are potent 5-HT$_2$ receptor antagonists, but several other antagonists at 5-HT$_2$ and/or 5-HT$_1$-like receptors (ketanserin, ritanserin, cyproheptadine, mianserin, methiothepin, and metergoline) are not very effective in migraine therapy. Therefore, it appears that additional properties — a constriction of extracerebral cephalic vessels with methysergide, ergotamine, and dihydroergotamine, and an antidepressant

TABLE 14.3. *Profile of potential and proven antimigraine drugs in relation to 5-HT$_1$-like receptors*

Antimigraine drug	5-HT$_1$-like receptor	5-HT$_2$ receptor	5-HT$_3$ receptor	Penetration into the CNS
AH25086	Agonist*	Inactive	Inactive	Poor or none
GR43175	Agonist*	Inactive	Inactive	Poor or none
Methysergide	Partial agonist*†	Antagonist‡	Inactive	Possibly yes
Ergotamine	Inactive	Antagonist	Inactive	Poor or none
Dihydroergotamine		Antagonist	Inactive	
Pizotifen	Inactive	Antagonist	Inactive	Possibly yes
Propranolol	Weak antagonist§	Inactive	Inactive	
MDL 72222	Inactive	Inactive	Antagonist¶	Rapid

CNS, central nervous system.
*Action is selective on 5-HT$_1$-like receptors that mediate the contraction of cephalic arteries and arteriovenous anastomoses;
† Antagonists of 5-HT$_1$-like receptors (methiothepin, metergoline) have no antimigraine activity;
‡ Many other 5-HT$_2$ antagonists (ketanserin, retanserin, cyproheptadine) have not proved very effective in migraine therapy;
§ Other antimigraine β-adrenoceptor antagonists (atenolol, timolol) have no affinity for 5-HT$_1$-like receptors;
¶ ICS 205–930, and probably some other antagonists at 5-HT$_3$ receptors, are not very effective in migraine.

action with pizotifen — are more important than the 5-HT$_2$ receptor antagonism for a therapeutic action in migraine.

The idea that 5-HT$_3$ receptors play a crucial role in pain transduction in migraine by depolarizing primary nociceptive afferents on cephalic vessels has been advocated by Fozard (this volume). This suggestion seemed to be initially supported by the effectiveness of a 5-HT$_3$ receptor antagonist, MDL 72222, in aborting acute migraine attacks (Loisy et al. 1985). However, another 5-HT$_3$ receptor antagonist, ICS 205–930, has proved to be ineffective in the treatment of acute migraine attacks (X. Lataste, unpublished paper from International Congress on Cardiovascular Pharmacology of 5-HT, Amsterdam, October 1988). Moreover, several newer 5-HT$_3$ receptor antagonists have been undergoing clinical trial for some time (Fozard 1987), but none of them has so far been reported to be of value in migraine.

Concluding remarks

A number of new and established antimigraine drugs interact with 5-HT receptors. Selective agonists at the 5-HT$_1$-like receptor subtype that mediates contractions of cephalic vessels are effective in the treatment of acute migraine attacks. Some antimigraine drugs antagonize 5-HT$_2$ receptors (methysergide, ergotamine, dihydroergotamine, and pizotifen), or 5-HT$_1$-like receptors (methysergide and propranolol). But many antagonists at 5-HT$_2$ and/or 5-HT$_1$-like receptors (ketanserin, ritanserin, cyproheptadine, mianserin, methiothepin, and metergoline) have not found much use in migraine therapy. Possibly, additional properties of such antimigraine drugs, for example, the vasoconstriction in the extracerebral cephalic circulation with methysergide, ergotamine and dihydroergotamine, and the antidepressant action with pizotifen, may be involved in their therapeutic action. Though MDL 72222, a 5-HT$_3$ receptor antagonist, is reported to be effective against acute migraine attacks, other such drugs are not. Therefore within the bounds of serotoninergic mechanisms, the antimigraine action seems to depend mainly on agonism at the 5-HT$_1$-like receptor subtype that mediates craniovascular contraction, and the antagonism at 5-HT$_2$ or 5-HT$_3$ receptors does not seem to be essential for antimigraine action.

For a discussion of this chapter see that at the end of Chapter 15.

References

Bom, A.H., Heiligers, J., Saxena, P.R., and Verdouw, P.D. (1988). Changes in carotid blood flow and its distribution by 5-hydroxytryptamine and ergotamine. *Pharmaceutisch Weekblad (Scientific edition)*, **10**, 226.
Bom, A.H., Verdouw, P.D., and Saxena, P.R. (1989). Carotid haemodynamics in

pigs during infusions of 8-OH-DPAT: reduction in arteriovenous shunting is mediated by 5-hydroxytryptamine$_1$-like receptors. *British Journal of Pharmacology*, **96**, 125–32.

Bradley, P.B., Engel, G., Feniuk, W., Fozard, J.R., Humphrey, P.P.A., Middlemiss, D.N., Mylecharane, E.J., Richardson, B.P., and Saxena, P.R. (1986). Proposals for the classification and nomenclature of functional 5-hydroxytryptamine receptors. *Neuropharmacology*, **25**, 563–76.

Brand, J., Hadoke, M., and Perrin, V.L. (1987). Placebo-controlled study of a selective 5-HT$_1$-like agonist, AH25086B, in relief of acute migraine. *Cephalalgia*, **7** (Suppl. 6), 402.

Doenicke, A., Brand, J., and Perrin, V.L. (1988). Possible benefit of GR43175, a novel 5-HT$_1$-like receptor agonist, for the treatment of severe migraine. *Lancet*, **i**, 1309–11.

Fozard, J.R. (1987). 5-HT: the enigma variations. *Trends in Pharmacological Sciences*, **8**, 501–6.

Humphrey, P.P.A. and Feniuk, W. (1988). Pharmacological characterization of functional neuronal receptors for 5-hydroxytryptamine. In *Neuronal messengers in vascular function*, (ed. A. Nobin, C. Owman, and B. Arneklo-Nobin), pp. 3–19, Elsevier, Amsterdam.

Humphrey, P.P.A., Feniuk, W., Perren, M.J., Connor, H.E., Oxford, A.W., Coates, I.H. and Butina, D. (1988). GR43175, a selective agonist for the 5-HT$_1$-like receptor in the dog saphenous vein. *British Journal of Pharmacology*, **94**, 1123–32.

Lance, J.W. (1982). *Mechanism and management of headache.* Butterworth, London.

Loisy, C., Beorchia, S., Centzone, V., Fozard, J.R., Schechter, P.J., and Tell, G.P. (1985). Effects on migraine headache of MDL 72222, an antagonist at neuronal 5-HT receptors. Double-blind, placebo-controlled study. *Cephalalgia*, **5**, 79–82.

Perrin, V.L. (1985). Clinical pharmacokinetics of ergotamine in migraine and cluster headache. *Clinical Pharmacokinetics*, **10**, 334–52.

Raskin, N.H. (1988). *Headache*, (2nd edn) Churchill Livingstone, New York.

Richardson, B.P. *et al.* (1986). Defective serotonergic transmission: a possible cause of migraine and a basis for the efficacy of ergot compounds in the treatment of attacks. In *Recent trends in the management of migraine* (ed. J.W. Lance), pp. 9–21, Editio Cantor, Aulendorf.

Saxena, P.R. (1972). The effects of antimigraine drugs on the vascular responses evoked by 5-hydroxytryptamine and related biogenic substances on the external carotid bed of dogs: possible pharmacological implications to their antimigraine action. *Headache*, **12**, 44–54.

Saxena, P.R. (1974). Selective vasoconstriction in carotid vascular bed by methysergide: possible relevance to its antimigraine effect. *European Journal of Pharmacology*, **27**, 99–105.

Saxena, P.R. and Verdouw, P.D. (1982). Redistribution by 5-hydroxytryptamine of carotid arterial blood at the expense of arteriovenous blood flow. *Journal of Physiology (London)*, **332**, 501–20.

Saxena, P.R. and Verdouw, P.D. (1985). 5-Carboxamide tryptamine, a compound with high affinity for 5-hydroxytryptamine$_1$ binding sites, dilates arterioles and constricts arteriovenous anastomoses. *British Journal of Pharmacology*, **84**, 533–44.

Saxena, P.R., Duncker, D.J., Bom, A.H., Heiligers, J., and Verdouw, P.D. (1986).

Effects of MDL 72222 and methiothepin on carotid vascular responses to 5-hydroxytryptamine in the pig: evidence for the presence of '5-hydroxytryptamine$_1$-like' receptors. *Naunyn Schmiedeberg's Archives of Pharmacology*, **333**, 198–204.

Saxena, P.R., Bom, A.H., and Verdouw, P.D. (1989). Characterization of 5-hydroxytryptamine receptors in the cranial vasculature. *Cephalalgia*, **9**, (Suppl. 9), 15–22.

Tandon, R.N., Sur, B.K., and Nath, K. (1969). Effect of reserpine injections in migrainous and normal control subjects, with estimations of urinary 5-hydroxyindole acetic acid. *Neurology*, **19**, 1073–9.

15. Is there still a case for the shunt hypothesis in migraine?

Pramod R. Saxena

Introduction

There can be no doubt that migraine is associated with changes in the cephalic (cerebral and non-cerebral) circulation; the doubts, however, concern the cause and nature of such changes. In a majority of migraine patients with 'aura', the cerebral blood flow decreases, but in 'classical' migraine patients both decreases and increases have been reported (Meyer *et al.* 1987; Lauritzen and Olesen 1987). In the non-cerebral cephalic circulation, vasodilatation and increased pulsations are observed principally on the side of the migraine headache (Drummond and Lance 1983; Meyer *et al.* 1987), but the idea of simple vasodilatation is paradoxical to the facial pallor and laxity of tissues usually noticed during the headache. To resolve this paradox, Heyck (1969) suggested that vasodilatation involves cephalic arteriovenous anastomoses.

Arteriovenous anastomoses and the shunt hypothesis

Arteriovenous anastomoses are precapillary communications between arteries and veins (Fig. 15.1) and are present in the skin of various regions including the cheeks, lips, forehead, nose and ears, nasal mucosa, and eyes (Sherman 1963; Saxena and Verdouw 1985) as well as in the human dura mater (Rowbotham and Little 1965). Arteriovenous anastomoses are innervated by vasoconstrictor adrenergic and vasodilator cholinergic, dopaminergic, and purinergic neurones (Bell and Lang 1979; Hillman *et al.* 1982; Molyneux and Harmon 1982). Besides, they may also be under hormonal constrictor (serotoninergic) and vasodilator (β-adrenergic) influences, because 5-hydroxytryptamine (5-HT), via 5-HT_1-like receptors, and β-adrenoceptor antagonists constrict the arteriovenous anastomoses (see Cohen and Coffman 1981; Saxena 1987, this volume).

The lumen of the arteriovenous anastomoses is much wider than that of the capillaries (whose diameter is about 5 μm) and, in many cases, may be more than 100 μm in diameter (Sherman 1963; Saxena and Verdouw 1985). Since blood flow in a vessel is proportional to the fourth power of the vessel

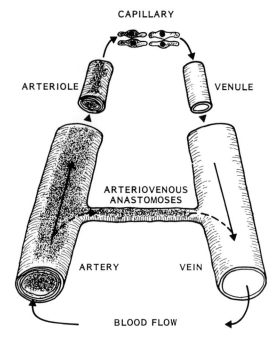

FIG. 15.1. A diagrammatic representation of arteriovenous anastomoses. The arteriovenous anastomoses are present in the skin of various regions, in the nasal mucosa, the eyes and the dura mater.

diameter, the arteriovenous anastomoses form 'low-resistance' bridges, which can quickly shunt a large amount of blood from the arteries to the veins, bypassing the tissue capillaries. Thus, opening of cephalic arteriovenous anastomoses, which results in increased cephalic arteriovenous shunting — as postulated in migraine — can explain the low diastolic arterial pressure, arterial pulsations, tissue ischaemia, and oedema observed (Heyck 1969; Saxena 1978, 1987). The dilated and pulsating cephalic vessels, as well as the tissue ischaemia and oedema, may then increase the activity of primary nociceptive afferents, to cause the headache.

Points in favour of the shunt hypothesis

The following points favour the involvement of the opening of arteriovenous anastomoses in the pathophysiology of migraine.

1. It has been reported that blood flow in the external carotid artery increases (see Meyer *et al.* 1987), and that the difference between the oxygen content of arterial and jugular venous blood (the AV O_2 content difference) decreases on the side of the migraine headache (Heyck 1969).

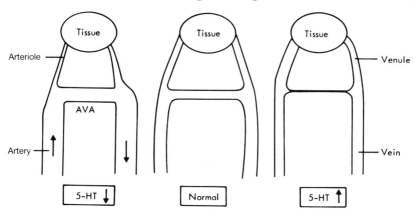

FIG. 15.2. Schematic representation of the presumed role of 5-hydroxytryptamine (5-HT) in the distribution of arterial blood into nutrient (tissue) and non-nutrient (arteriovenous anastomotic; AVA) parts. The arrows in the arteries and vein indicate the direction of blood flow, whereas those next to '5-HT' denote a decrease (↓) or an increase (↑) in the concentration of 5-HT in the blood.

2. The AV O_2 content difference is normalized after spontaneous and drug-induced alleviation of headache (Heyck 1969).

3. The skin temperature decreases on the side of the headache in a substantial proportion of migraineurs (Drummond and Lance 1983).

4. Migraine seems to be a 'low 5-HT syndrome' (Lance 1982) and the pharmacological properties of 5-HT (constriction of large arteries and arteriovenous anastomoses, and dilatation of arterioles) suggests that its deficiency can result in increased shunting of arterial blood (Fig. 15.2; Saxena 1987, this volume).

5. A number of proven and effective antimigraine drugs affect arteriovenous shunting. Thus, ergotamine increases AV O_2 content difference and selectively decreases the external carotid blood flow, both in animals (Saxena 1972) and humans (Fig. 15.3; Puzich *et al.* 1983), mainly by acting on cephalic arteriovenous anastomoses (Johnston and Saxena 1978; Spierings and Saxena 1980*a*). Dihydroergotamine (Spierings and Saxena 1980*a*), methysergide (Saxena and Verdouw 1984), isometheptene (Spierings and Saxena 1980*b*), and clonidine (Verdouw *et al.* 1984) also decrease both the total carotid and the arteriovenous anastomotic blood flow in animals, while propranolol reduces the arteriovenous shunting in human digital circulation (Cohen and Coffman 1981).

6. Selective agonists at the 5-HT_1-like receptor subtype, which mediate contractions of cephalic arteries and arteriovenous anastomoses (AH25086, GR43175), and which do not penetrate into the central nervous system, are effective in the treatment of acute migraine attacks (see Saxena, this volume; Humphrey *et al.*, this volume).

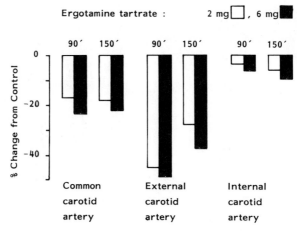

FIG. 15.3. The effect of oral administration of ergotamine on the velocity of blood flow in the carotid vessels of migraine patients outside the headache period. Note that ergotamine mainly affects the external carotid circulation. (This figure is redrawn from Puzich *et al.* 1983).

Points against the shunt hypothesis

Some points that may be considered as being against the shunt hypothesis concern the measurement of extracranial blood flow in migraine patients.

1. The clearance of intradermal ^{24}Na, which is used as an index of cutaneous blood flow, increases during a migraine attack, more prominently on the side of the headache (Elkind *et al.* 1964).

2. Sakai and Meyer (1978) used a ^{133}Xe inhalation method and found that the contribution of extracerebral tissues to cephalic blood flow increases during migraine.

Although the disappearance of indicators (such as ^{24}Na and ^{133}Xe) is regarded as an index of tissue (nutrient) blood flow, it cannot be ruled out that the indicator concentration may also be influenced by changes in arteriovenous anastomotic blood flow. No study seems yet to have addressed this question.

Concluding remarks

The view that migraine headaches result from a sudden opening of cephalic arteriovenous anastomoses, probably in the dura mater and skin, is supported by a number of findings: the pallor and coldness of the skin, and the narrowing of the difference between the oxygen content of arterial and jugular venous blood on the side of the migraine headache; and the constriction of large arteries and arteriovenous anastomoses by a number of proven and effective antimigraine drugs (ergotamine, dihydroergotamine, and methysergide). Similar pharmacological effects are observed with 5-HT; its blood concentration is reported to decrease in migraine, and it can alleviate migraine pain. Further indications in favour of the shunt hypothesis are provided by two new compounds (AH25086, GR43175), which are highly selective agonists at the 5-HT$_1$-like receptor subtype that mediates contractions of cephalic arteries and arteriovenous anastomoses. These 5-HT$_1$-like receptor agonists do not penetrate into the central nervous system but are very effective in the treatment of acute migraine attacks. Thus, there is a reasonable body of evidence to answer in the affirmative the title question of my paper: 'Is there still a case for the shunt hypothesis in migraine?', at least for some migraine patients. The involvement of cephalic arteriovenous anastomoses, both inside the cranium (in the dura mater) and outside the cranium (in the skin), may not necessarily be a *primary* event and, instead, may represent the *final* outcome of the neurovascular changes that occur in migraine.

Lastly, I would like to make the following suggestions for further investigations into the role of arteriovenous anastomoses in migraine.

1. It would be useful to measure the arteriovenous oxygen differences in migraine in a large series of patients, not only before and after the migraine attack but also before and after drug treatment.

2. Special attention should be paid to the measurement of extracerebral blood flow in migraine, before and after the administration of drugs effective in aborting migraine attacks.

3. Attempts could be made to investigate the effects of antimigraine drugs on the shunting of human albumin microspheres in the human forearm.

4. More fundamental studies should be undertaken to help reveal the location, type of physiological regulation, and type of pharmacological control of arteriovenous anastomoses.

Acknowledgements

I would like to thank Dr Barry Cox (Pharmaceutical Division, I.C.I., U.K.) for Figure 1, which is redrawn from a slide provided by him. I also thank Dr Puzich and co-workers and *Deutsche Medizinisches Wochenschrift* for the data shown in Figure 15.2.

References

Bell, C. and Lang, W.J. (1979). Evidence for dopaminergic vasodilator innervation of the canine paw pad. *British Journal of Pharmacology*, **67**, 337–43.
Cohen, R.A. and Coffman, J.D. (1981). Beta-adrenergic vasodilator mechanism in the finger. *Circulation Research*, **49**, 1196–202.

Drummond, P.D. and Lance, J.W. (1983). Extracranial vascular changes and the source of pain in migraine headaches. *Annals of Neurology*, **13**, 32–7.

Elkind, A.H., Friedman, A.P., and Grossman, J. (1964). Cutaneous blood flow in vascular headaches of the migraine type. *Neurology*, **14**, 24–30.

Johnston, B.M. and Saxena, P.R. (1978). The effect of ergotamine on tissue blood flow and the arteriovenous shunting of radioactive microspheres in the head. *British Journal of Pharmacology*, **63**, 541–9.

Heyck, H. (1969). Pathogenesis of migraine. *Research and Clinical Studies in Headache*, **2**, 1–28.

Hillman, P.E., Scott, N.R., and Van Tienhoven, A. (1982). Vasomotion in chicken foot: dual innervation of arteriovenous anastomoses. *American Journal of Physiology*, **242**, R582–R590.

Lance, J.W. (1982). *Mechanism and management of headache*. Butterworth, London.

Lauritzen, M. and Olesen, J. (1987). Leão's spreading depression. In *Migraine: therapeutic conceptual and research aspects* (ed. J.N. Blau), pp. 387–402. Elsevier, Amsterdam.

Meyer, J.S., Hata, T., and Imai, A. (1987). Evidence supporting a vascular pathogenesis of migraine and cluster headache. In *Migraine: therapeutic, conceptual and research aspects* (ed. J.N. Blau), pp. 265–302. Elsevier, Amsterdam.

Molyneux, G.S. and Harmon, B. (1982). Innervation of the arteriovenous anastomoses in the web of the foot of the domestic duck, *Anas platyrhynchos*; structural evidence for the presence of non-adrenergic non-cholinergic nerve. *American Journal of Anatomy*, **135**, 119–28.

Puzich, R., Girke, W., Heidrich, H., and Rischke, M. (1983). Dopplersonographische Untersuchungen der extrakraniellen Hirngefäse bei Migräne-Patienten nach Gabe von Ergotamintartrat. *Deutsche Medizinisches Wochenschrift*, **108**, 457–61.

Rowbotham, G.F. and Little, E. (1965). New concepts on the aetiology and vascularization of meningiomata; the mechanisms of migraine; the chemical process of the cerebrospinal fluid; and the formations of the collections of blood or fluid in the subdural space. *British Journal of Surgery*, **52**, 21–4.

Sakai, F. and Meyer, J.S. (1978). Regional cerebral hemodynamics during migraine and cluster headaches measured by the ^{133}Xe inhalation method. *Headache*, **18**, 122–32.

Saxena, P.R. (1972). The effects of antimigraine drugs on the vascular responses evoked by 5-hydroxytryptamine and related biogenic substances on the external carotid bed of dogs: Possible pharmacological implications to their antimigraine action. *Headache*, **12**, 44–54.

Saxena, P.R. (1978). Arteriovenous shunting and migraine. *Research and Clinical Studies in Headache*, **6**, 89–102.

Saxena, P.R. (1987). The arteriovenous anastomoses and veins in migraine research. In *Migraine — therapeutic, conceptual and research aspects*, (ed. J.N. Blau), pp. 581–96. Elsevier, Amsterdam.

Saxena, P.R. and Verdouw, P.D. (1984). Effects of methysergide and 5-hydroxytryptamine on carotid blood flow distribution in pigs: further evidence for the presence of atypical 5-HT receptors. *British Journal of Pharmacology*, **82**, 817–26.

Saxena, P.R. and Verdouw, P.D. (1985). Tissue blood flow and arteriovenous shunting in pigs measured with microspheres of four different sizes. *Pfluegers Archiv European Journal of Physiology*, **403**, 128–35.

Spierings, E.L.H. and Saxena, P.R. (1980*a*). Antimigraine drugs and cranial arter-iovenous shunting in the cat. *Neurology*, **30**, 696–701.

Spierings, E.L.H. and Saxena, P.R. (1980*b*). Effect of isometheptene on the dis-tribution and shunting of 15 μm microspheres throughout the cephalic circulation of the cat. *Headache*, **20**, 103–6.

Sherman, J.L. (1963). Normal arteriovenous anastomoses. *Medicine*, **92**, 247–67.

Verdouw, P.D., Duncker, D.J., and Saxena, P.R. (1984). Poor vasoconstrictor response to adrenergic stimulation in the arteriovenous anastomoses present in the carotid vascular bed of young Yorkshire pigs. *Archives Internationales de Pharma-codynamie et de Thérapie*, **272**, 56–70.

Discussion following the preceding two chapters

CURZON: One of your points in favour of the shunt hypothesis was that migraine is a low 5-HT (serotonin) syndrome. This is confusing because extracerebral 5-HT and brain 5-HT are two completely separate pools. Although migraine may be related to a low vascular (extracerebral) 5-HT level, that tells us nothing about what is happening in central neurones.

SAXENA: Your point is taken. I was talking of vascular 5-HT. Nevertheless some vessels are probably innervated from the raphé nucleus (Reinhard *et al.* 1979). These fibres may also be less active.

OLESEN: You have done very important pharmacological work in characterizing receptors and so on. But I think it is hasty to proceed, from there, to talk about the shunt hypothesis in migraine. These animal experiments with microspheres are far removed from the clinical syndrome of migraine. Kai Jensen and I have studied blood flow in muscle, subcutaneous tissue, and extracranially, during migraine attacks and we found that the blood flow was normal (Jensen and Olesen 1985; Jensen 1987). As you mentioned, there are no functioning shunts in the brain in humans, which is also true during a migraine attack. We can see this clearly from our clearance curves. So these points are against the concept. You say that the shunts are in the extracranial territory, where the migraine pain originates. However, in the extracranial or extracerebral territory, arteriovenous anastomoses will mostly be found in the nose and ears, which are not the sites of pain in migraine patients. One is left with the possibility that if shunts are operating they must be in the meningeal circulation. And we have yet to see evidence that the arteriovenous anastomoses in the meningeal circulation respond differently from those in the nose and ears.

SAXENA: You measured blood flows using the xenon clearance curve. With clear-ance of xenon you cannot distinguish between the arteriovenous anastomotic (non-nutrient) and arteriolar (tissue-nutrient) components of arterial blood flow. Hence, these observations are not necessarily against changes in shunt flow during migraine. Secondly, arteriovenous anastomoses are located not only in the head skin, nose and lips, but also within the cranium in meningeal vessels in humans (Rowbotham and Little 1965). We are planning to study the effects of antimigraine drugs on meningeal arteriovenous anastomoses. Lastly, in pharmacological experi-ments a number of established and new antimigraine drugs, including ergotamine and GR43175, have a very selective vasconstrictor action on the cephalic arterio-venous anastomoses in microgram doses. This ought to be telling us something.

I am simply appealing to you, as clinicians, to examine this possibility further and not to dismiss it out of hand. If there is shunting of blood during migraine (probably secondarily to changes in the central nervous system), let us not think only in terms of tissue ischaemia, but let us also consider that vasodilatation *per se* may be involved. Vasodilatation might increase the activity of nociceptive afferent fibres and cause migraine headache. In humans there is no way to locate arteriovenous anastomoses in the head circulation other than by histological methods, and that has now been done. (It would, of course, be ethically acceptable to study peripheral shunting in humans).

OLESEN: What about the lack of migraine pain in the nose and ears, and the fact that shunting is not painful in any other part of the body such as the fingers or the feet?

SAXENA: One should distinguish between shunting phenomena, as such, and the pain. As I said, there may be arteriovenous anastomotic dilatation which could increase afferent nerve traffic to the brain, from where the pain can be referred to another site. Moreover, dilatation of the arteriovenous anastomoses in the cephalic circulation may be selective during migraine attacks.

BLAU: The nose can be involved in migraine. A proportion of patients have a congested nose, while others have the opposite: they have dry noses, and at the end of an attack their noses begin to run (Blau 1988). I suspect this observation is an epiphenomenon of what is going on inside the head.

PEATFIELD: Have you any thoughts on the mode of action of nimodipine in migraine from your pharmacological experiments?

SAXENA: In our experiments nimodipine and nifedipine increase tissue blood mainly to the muscles (not to skin as with 5-HT) and only 'passively' cause a small decrease in arteriovenous anastomotic blood flow (Duncker *et al.* 1987). These drugs are not very effective in the treatment of migraine.

VANE: As I understand the microsphere technique, you are measuring the proportion of the cardiac output that goes to a particular organ or tissue?

SAXENA: Yes; or the proportion of arterial blood flow, if the microspheres are injected into an artery.

VANE: You said that the skin, which gets about 10 per cent of the total cardiac output, has an enormous amount of shunting in it. Why do you therefore not see these microspheres coming through into the lungs, when you have such big shunts?

SAXENA: Indeed I do. The microspheres escape through the arteriovenous anastomoses and appear in the venous blood. If one withdraws a venous blood sample during injection of microspheres into the left ventricle or into an artery, one can demonstrate their presence in the sampled venous blood. Ultimately, the microspheres in the venous blood reach the lungs, via the right side of the heart and the pulmonary artery, and they remain trapped there.

VANE: My second concern is that when you talk about carotid vasoconstriction you seem to use this synonymously with shunt mechanisms. Is that so? When there is vasoconstriction of the carotid vascular bed, does this mean there is a closing down of shunts?

SAXENA: It depends on the drug. For example, with lower doses of ergotamine, the reduction in carotid blood flow (measured with an electromagnetic blood flow meter) is largely due to a constriction of arteriovenous anastomoses. With larger doses, ergotamine also reduces arteriolar (tissue) blood flow (Johnston and Saxena 1978; Spierings and Saxena 1980). With 5-HT, there may or may not be any reduction in the total carotid blood flow because the arteriovenous anastomotic portion decreases and the arteriolar fraction increases (Saxena and Verdouw 1982). Dr Humphrey showed experiments with GR43175 which suggest a selectivity for the shunt vessels, but no effect on the arterial circuit. The same is true for methysergide, 8-OH-DPAT (8-hydroxy-2(di-*n*-propylamino)tetralin) and BEA-1654 (Saxena 1987). So, carotid vasoconstriction does not imply ischaemia of the brain. In animal models that we use, very little blood is supplied via the carotid arteries into the brain. More goes via the vertebral arteries. Carotid vasoconstriction mainly affects these shunts and the extracerebral circulation.

HUMPHREY: In some of our experiments we injected the spheres up the carotid artery, and saw vasoconstriction of the arteriovenous anastomoses, but blood flow to the brain increased. When the microspheres are injected into the heart, and GR43175 is given intravenously, we showed that the drug has no effect on the distribution of vertebral artery flow. So one is not compromising cerebral blood flow at all, either from the vertebral or the carotid side.

SAXENA: Even ergotamine does not decrease cerebral blood flow in the animal experiments that we did (Johnston and Saxena 1978).

VANE: This all seems to point towards its being, if headache is a vascular disease, a disease of the larger vessels rather than the smaller vessels.

SAXENA: Yes. That is what I am trying to convey.

References

Blau, J.N. (1988). A note on migraine and the nose. *Headache*, **28**, 495.

Duncker, D.J., Yland, M., van der Weij, L.P., Verdouw, P.D., and Saxena, P.R. (1987). Enhancement of vasoconstrictor and attenuation of vasodilator effects of 5-hydroxytryptamine by the calcium channel blockers, nimodipine and nifedipine in the pig. *European Journal of Pharmacology*, **136**, 11–21.

Jensen, K. and Olesen, J. (1985). Temporal muscle blood flow in common migraine. *Acta Neurologica Scandinavica*, **72**, 561–70.

Jensen, K. (1987). Subcutaneous blood flow in the temporal region of migraine patients. *Acta Neurologica Scandinavica*, **75**, 310–8.

Johnston, B.M. and Saxena, P.R. (1978). The effect of ergotamine on tissue blood flow and the arteriovenous shunting of radioactive microspheres in the head. *British Journal of Pharmacology*, **63**, 541–9.

Reinhard, J.F., Liebman, J.E., Schlosberg, A.T., and Moskowitz, M.A. (1979). Serotonin neurons project to small blood vessels in the brain. *Science*, **206**, 85–7.

Rowbotham, G.F. and Little, E. (1965). New concepts on the aetiology and vascularization of meningiomata; the mechanisms of migraine; the chemical process of the cerebrospinal fluid; and the formations of the collections of blood or fluid in the subdural space. *British Journal of Surgery*, **52**, 21–4.

Saxena, P.R. (1987). The arteriovenous anastomoses and veins in migraine research. In *Migraine: therapeutic, conceptual and research aspects*, (ed. J.N. Blau), pp. 581–96. Chapman and Hall, London.

Saxena, P.R. and Verdouw, P.D. (1982). Redistribution by 5-hydroxytryptamine of carotid arterial blood at the expense of arteriovenous blood flow. *Journal of Physiology (London)*, **332**, 501–20.

Spierings, E.L.H. and Saxena, P.R. (1980). Antimigraine drugs and cranial arteriovenous shunting in the cat. *Neurology*, **30**, 696–701.

16. General discussion I

5-HT uptake, platelets, and migraine

COPPEN: 5-HT (5-hydroxytryptamine; serotonin) has been studied in relation to migraine for about 20 years, but in relation to depression for about 30 years. The relationship between migraine and depression is fascinating. The prodromal symptoms of migraine (Blau, this volume) are very much like those of an affective disorder. Over the last 10 years 5-HT uptake by the platelets has been studied with interest. The platelet is readily accessible for study, and some of its transport systems may have something in common with those in the central nervous system. The variant that is most abnormal in depression is 5-HT V_{max}, the maximum 5-HT uptake by the platelet. At least 20 reports describe a significant decrease in 5-HT V_{max} during depression, and after recovery (Coppen *et al.* 1978, 1979). The feature is a trait abnormality. There is a seasonal variation in 5-HT V_{max} both in depressives and in normal controls, and there are seasonal changes in affective depressive disorders, too. It would be interesting to know if anyone had observed a seasonal variation in migraine. There is now very good evidence that lithium treatment restores the decreased 5-HT V_{max} to normal levels. The advent of treatment with lithium has had an astounding effect on psychiatry: it has reduced both the long-term morbidity and the long-term mortality of patients with both unipolar and bipolar illness (Coppen and Peet 1979). Migraine is more difficult to study than depression because the episodes are so much shorter (an attack of depression can last several months). In a group of 25 depressed patients who were vulnerable to migraine, we have found that their 5-HT V_{max} was a little low, but not significantly so. We subsequently reviewed those patients who had had an attack of migraine within five days of the measurement, and found that they had a decreased 5-HT V_{max}. This was quite different from the results on depression, where there is a decreased 5-HT V_{max} during and after a depressive episode.

WELCH: Are your results age-adjusted and sex-matched, to allow for variations related to age or gender?

COPPEN: Yes; we have taken those into account, and the difference is not related to age or sex. Because lithium has a profound effect on the morbidity of affective disorders, it would be interesting to know what effect it has on migraine.

PEATFIELD: We attempted a preliminary study of this. Although it was not a controlled, double-blind approach, we found that some patients' migraine became *worse* after lithium treatment (Peatfield and Clifford Rose 1981).

COPPEN: There is evidence that some untreated depressive patients have a higher incidence of migraine than the normal population. In our lithium clinic, we have 150 patients who have been on long-term treatment with lithium. We found that these patients scored fewer headache answers on the Waters' questionnaire than did the control population (Abou-Saleh and Coppen 1983). Individual patients with both affective disorders and migraine report that lithium leaves their migraine either unchanged (50 per cent) or with some improvement (50 per cent). After prescribing lithium to hundreds of patients I have never known anyone have to stop the treatment *because* of headaches.

PEATFIELD: It may be difficult to distinguish between misery and migraine. You are generally helping your patients' depression rather than positively helping the ones who have migraine. Your population of hospitalized depressive patients is also an atypical one, of course.

COPPEN: A real test of the benefits of lithium treatment for migraine would be to monitor patients over at least three months, because the 5-HT V_{max} changes take at least six weeks to happen.

Another compound of interest here is mianserin, on which we did some early clinical studies (Coppen *et al.* 1976). Mianserin, too, increase 5-HT V_{max}, and it was first developed as a possible antimigraine drug. Pauline Munro did a 16-week, double-blind controlled study, based on diaries kept by the patients who were treated with mianserin (Munro *et al.* 1985). She found that mianserin reduced the patients' own severity rating of their migraine attacks and also significantly reduced the mean number of migraines per four-week period. So this sort of antidepressant does seem to have an effect. There seems to be a short-term change in the 5-HT V_{max} of 'normal' migraine patients, but a much longer term change when the patients also have affective disorders.

PEATFIELD: I believe that Geaney *et al.* (1984) did some work on the imipramine binding sites in migraine.

GLOVER: Yes. They found a significant reduction in B_{max}, an index of the total number of imipramine binding sites.

WELCH: How do you interpret the low 5-HT V_{max} measurements that you recorded, Dr Coppen? Some patients, as you said, would have been measured five days before an attack while some were measured five days after an attack.

COPPEN: It may have some peripheral vascular significance if the platelets are not taking up the circulating 5-HT in plasma.

WELCH: So some of them might have already released 5-HT from the platelets whereas others might have been about to release platelet 5-HT?

GLOVER: There is a problem, technically, about macroaggregates: they might have been taking up less 5-HT because of what was going on in the platelet-release reaction.

MOSKOWITZ: What happens to platelets during spreading depression, when there is a profound decrease in blood flow disturbance in the microcirculation?

GARDNER-MEDWIN: We did a few experiments on this in rabbits anaesthetized with urethane and chloralose (Gardner-Medwin and Boullin 1985). We induced spreading depression with potassium chloride on the pial surface and measured platelet 5-HT content in systemic blood. We also assayed for any platelet releasing factor in the plasma. We did not find any significant differences caused by spreading depression, but this was very preliminary and would need a larger study to confirm it. The negative result in any case might not extrapolate to humans.

CURZON: Is anything known about abnormalities of the hypothalamo-pituitary-adrenal axis in migraine? For example, is the dexamethasone suppression test abnormal in migrainous patients who are not also depressives?

COPPEN: I do not know. Lithium produces a lot of neuroendocrine disturbances — for example, the prolactin response to intravenous tryptophan. This abnormality is normalized by lithium, which suggests that it has some impact on the central serotoninergic processes. But I do not know of any similar investigations in migraine.

ROSE: Rao and Pearce (1971) did a study on hypothalamic function (mainly insulin responsiveness) but published work since then has given variable results.

COPPEN: It is certainly less easy to study migraine than depression because it consists of sporadic attacks rather than a long-term altered state.

The blood–brain barrier and the pain of migraine

VANE: Is headache a vascular or an extravascular phenomenon? There is a lot of evidence suggesting that it originates within the circulation, including the fact that it can be pulsatile. But, more importantly, drugs like aspirin do not cross the blood–brain barrier. Lim *et al.* (1964), many years ago, showed in cross-perfusion experiments in dogs that the pain associated with injecting bradykinin into the spleen perfused by blood from a second dog could not be stopped by giving aspirin to the central nervous system of the first dog. However, it was blocked by injection of aspirin into the blood perfusing the spleen. One can extend that argument to say that the effects of aspirin on headache are probably through a peripheral action and not through an action within the brain. And I believe that Dr Humphrey's work with GR43175 shows little evidence that it crosses the blood–brain barrier.

HUMPHREY: That's right. In unpublished experiments we measured this in the mouse and found that less than 0.01 per cent of the drug entered the brain.

MOSKOWITZ: What about in the blood vessel itself? Does it get beyond the endothelium?

HUMPHREY: I would not expect it to get past the tight junctions in the endothelium of the cerebral vasculature.

VANE: Both propranolol and atenolol are used in migraine treatment to some extent. I do not know which is the more effective treatment, but I do know that propranolol gets into the brain more so than atenolol. Is one of them better than the other?

ROSE: There are arguments for both drugs; some would say that atenolol is better because of its different selectivity. It certainly works, which is the important point here.

VANE: Substances that do not easily get into the brain, such as aspirin, atenolol and GR43175 seem to work well in headache and also in migraine. To me, this evidence points to migraine being an intravascular phenomenon.

CURZON: Those arguments suggest that the *pain* is vascular; that does not mean that the *origin* is vascular.

MOSKOWITZ: As we discussed before, the only structures within the cranium that are pain-sensitive are blood vessels, so there is no question that the blood vessels are intermittently involved in the generation of that pain.

ROSE: What about the meninges?

MOSKOWITZ: Only the meninges immediately adjacent to the blood vessels are pain-sensitive. So there is no question about the importance of the vessels. This original work by Penfield and NcNaughton (1940), Ray and Wolff (1940) and McNaughton (1938) has held up to scrutiny. This relationship holds in the pia and the dura mater, obviously within the limits of their testing techniques.

FOZARD: How does aspirin lower temperature if it does not get into the brain?

VANE: It might block the release of interleukin 1 in the periphery. The high endothelial cells in the temperature-regulating centre probably release PGE_2 under the influence of interleukin 1.

ZIEGLER: Professor Vane stated that propranolol enters the brain while atenolol will be excluded. Since both drugs have been found to be of some value in the prophylactic treatment of migraine, this might suggest that migraine pain has a vascular origin. It has been shown, however, that atenolol is able to penetrate the blood–brain barrier (Cruickshank and Neil-Dwyer 1985), admittedly at a lower rate and to a smaller extent than propranolol. In migraine treatment, atenolol is given chronically, and it becomes effective only after two or three weeks. During such chronic treatment there may be enough time for effective concentrations of atenolol to accumulate within the brain. Nevertheless, I agree that the significance of the blood–brain barrier should be taken into account.

MOSKOWITZ: We should consider the possible differences between the integrity of the blood–brain barrier for large, pain-sensitive vessels at the base of the brain and that for the smaller pial vessels. If there is no difference, one must postulate another locus of drug action that does not require the integrity of a blood–brain barrier. This relates to our paper (Moskowitz and Buzzi, this volume) about the cavernous sinus and the juxtaposition of artery, nerve, and venous sinus. Since the cavernous sinus is a convergence point for sensory fibres that innervate cerebral vessels, and since it resides outside the barrier, it is a potential site for drug action. Another potential place for drugs to act is in the trigeminal ganglion itself, which receives blood primarily from the external carotid circulation. Hence, a drug that does not cross the blood–brain barrier may, nevertheless, have access to perivascular pain fibres that innervate the circle of Willis.

FOZARD: Dr van Brummelen and his colleagues (Blauw *et al.* 1988) have some surprising results from their infusions of 5-HT into the human forearm. Their dose–response curve showed that even in very low amounts (1 ng ml^{-1} min^{-1}) 5-HT could trigger an immediate increase in blood flow measured plethysmographically. There was also a secondary phase of vasodilatation. If they simultaneously infused a 5-HT$_3$ receptor antagonist (ICS 205-930) there was complete suppression not only of the first phase but also of the second phase. How might one interpret this? ICS 205-930 is a highly selective 5-HT$_3$ receptor antagonist, which implies that 5-HT at this dose must be activating the 5-HT$_3$ receptors to cause vasodilatation. One possible explanation is that 5-HT makes contact with the sensory nerve fibres, within the vessel wall; but, it must first penetrate beyond the endothelial layer, the basement membrane, and the media smooth muscle layer!

VANE: It might only have to make contact with the surface endothelial receptors.

FOZARD: As yet, 5-HT$_3$ receptors have not been found in any other tissues than neurones. Endothelial 5-HT receptors do, however, exist but they are '5-HT$_1$-*like*'. 5-HT may act to stimulate the terminals of sensory fibres and induce axon-reflex vasodilatation. If this is so, then perhaps ergotamine or GR43175 could also penetrate to a crucial part of the pain-sensing neuronal circuitry. I believe that the activation of perivascular sensory fibres is critical in generating the pain of migraine. If compounds such as GR43175 have the capacity to hyperpolarize such fibres (and this appears to happen in at least one neuronal system in the dog saphenous vein), then it is possible that a relatively weak, neurochemical depolarization of these sensory nerve endings would be suppressed.

SAXENA: We have published some similar results to this. With 5-HT, we saw an increase in tissue blood flow and a decrease in arteriovenous anastomotic blood flow. The increase in tissue blood flow by 5-HT was reduced by the 5-HT$_3$ receptor antagonist MDL 72222, but was completely blocked by methiothepin (Saxena *et al.* 1986). In humans, Blauw *et al.* (1988) have reported that the 5-HT-induced initial vasodilatory response is blocked by ICS 205-930. This effect of 5-HT in the human is probably due to an axon-like reflex originating from the dermal sensory afferents and not necessarily from the blood vessels.

VANE: What is missing is that we do not have an animal model of migraine. Until the new MDL or GR drugs are evaluated clinically for an effect on migraine, everything remains a hypothesis. Going back for a moment to platelets and 5-HT, the only way I can account for a unilateral headache in terms of platelets that release 5-HT is to suppose that the platelets are sticking unilaterally to the wall of a vessel and releasing their 5-HT into that area of the wall, if platelets have any sort of job to do in that particular situation.

SANDLER: The platelets may just represent epiphenomena, responding to the same noxious stimuli that act elsewhere.

VANE: I do not think there will be much 5-HT in the circulation, as John Fozard said in his paper (Fozard, this volume). But the delivery of 5-HT to the vascular wall via the platelets (if they stick) is testable by experiment. In patients with atherosclerosis one can inject indium-labelled platelets and scan to find the 'hot spots' where they stick to the atherosclerotic plaques. This technique could be tried in migraine patients, too.

WELCH: It has been tried in carotid atherosclerosis and, whereas it works extremely well in primates, the St Louis group found it to be such a variable technique in humans that they did not pursue it. It has not evolved as a clinical technique.

HUMPHREY: It is generally felt that $5-HT_3$ antagonists do not work acutely in migraine. This belief is mostly anecdotal, as much of the evidence has not been published. On the other hand, there is at least one study that says that MDL 72222 does work. Can its actions be differentiated in your tests, Professor Saxena, from the other $5-HT_3$ antagonists?

SAXENA: We have mainly used MDL 72222 in our experiments but Blauw *et al.* (1988) have used ICS 205-930 in humans and found comparable results. G.J. Blauw has done a couple of experiments with us in pigs and has found ICS 205-930 and MDL 72222 to be effective in attenuating the vasodilator response to 5-HT.

BLAU: I thought that every drug was nowadays recognized as having a certain propensity for crossing the blood–brain barrier. We know from experiments from 100 years ago with injection of vital dyes (which combine with a big molecule like albumin) that in certain areas of the brain — area postrema and some of the basal areas — there is blue staining. And they may just be the vital areas for migraine. A small amount of a drug crossing through to the brain may be the vital link in migraine. This is an important point that the pharmacologists among us might like to consider. As for the pulsatile quality of the migraine headache, Jes Olesen (1978) did a study in Copenhagen in which patients were asked during attacks whether their headache was throbbing: only 47 per cent said that it was throbbing at that time. I wonder in what proportion of the *total* migraine attack the headache was throbbing. The throbbing may not mean a great deal in terms of the pathogenesis of migraine. Finally, there is a universal cry for an animal model for migraine. But until a rat can talk there will not be an animal model for migraine. Even taking histories of migraine from patients, who can talk, can be quite difficult!

VANE: Until a drug is shown clinically to have been a success or failure, everything else we know about it contributes only hypothesis to its mode of action. Once a specific drug, such as a 5-HT antagonist or a 5-HT agonist, can be shown to have an effect clinically, then we are on much firmer ground.

BLAU: We need to dissect the pharmacological process in some way. Perhaps different groups of patients will respond to different drugs. If we look at the origin of migraine as being one pathway, we may be wrong. There may not only be different pathways, but different types of patient responses, or even different stages, suitable for treating in different ways.

VANE: In 1970 there were 15 different hypotheses as to how aspirin-like drugs worked. We were lucky enough to find that they inhibited prostaglandin formation (Vane 1971) and the other 14 hypotheses gradually went away. We had a biochemical intervention. This is what Pat Humphrey is working towards; it is what John Fozard is working towards — a specific compound that has a specific reaction with a specific receptor. And if those have an effect in the clinic — because there *is* no animal model — then many of the other hypotheses will fall by the wayside.

CURZON: I agree with Dr Blau that there can be no perfect animal models for affective states. Nevertheless, some models could have similarities with proposed or possible mechanisms for migraine. Models used in the pharmaceutical industry may have no connection with particular disorders but they nevertheless have a useful predictive ability for testing out drugs. Other models help us to consider particular diseases.

FERREIRA: If we find clinically that both 5-HT antagonists and 5-HT agonists help to relieve migraine, these results need not contradict each other. If both work, the antagonist is blocking somewhere in the circuit while the agonist is acting *at a vascular site*. 5-HT antagonists may block the pain mechanism at a different site from the one where 5-HT agonists act.

WELCH: Migraine, itself, is extremely difficult to define. Until we find a specific drug that acts against the specific condition, we are unlikely to understand fully the mechanism of a migraine attack.

References

Abou-Saleh, M.T. and Coppen, A. (1983). Subjective side-effects of amitriptyline and lithium in affective disorders. *British Journal of Psychiatry*, **142**, 391–7.

Blauw, G.J., Van Brummelen, P., and Van Zweiten, P.A. (1988). Serotonin induced vasodilatation in the human forearm is antagonized by the selective 5-HT$_3$ receptor antagonist ICS 205–930. *Life Sciences*, **43**, 1441–9.

Coppen, A. and Peet, M. (1979). The long term management of patients with affective disorders. In *Psychopharmacology of affective disorders*, (ed. E. Paykel and A. Coppen). pp. 248–56. Oxford University Press, Oxford.

Coppen, A., Gupta, R., Montgomery, S., Bailey, J., Burns, B., and de Ridder, J.J. (1976). Mianserin hydrochloride: a novel antidepressant. *British Journal of Psychiatry*, **129**, 342–5.

Coppen, A., Swade, C., and Wood, K. (1978). Platelet 5-hydroxytryptamine accumulation in depressive illness. *Clinica Chimica Acta*, **87**, 165–8.

Coppen, A., Carroll, D., and Wood, K. (1979). Platelet 5-HT accumulation and migraine. *Lancet*, **ii**, 914.

Gardner-Medwin, A.R. and Boullin, D.J. (1985). Platelet function during spreading depression: implications for migraine. In *Migraine: clinical and research advances*, (ed. F.C. Rose), pp. 126–9. Karger, Basel.

Geaney, D.P., Rutterford, M.G., Elliott, J.M., Schachter, M., Peet, K.M.S., and Grahame-Smith, D.G. (1984). Decreased platelet 3H-imipramine binding sites in classical migraine. *Journal of Neurology, Neurosurgery and Psychiatry*, **47**, 720–3.

Lim, R.K.S., Guzman, F., Rodgers, D.W., Goto, K., Braun, C., Dickerson, G.D., and Engle, R.J. (1964). Site of action of narcotic and nonnarcotic analgesics determined by blocking bradykinin-evoked visceral pain. *Archives Internationales de Pharmacodynamie et de Therapie*, **152**, 25–58.

McNaughton, F. (1938). The innervation of the intracranial blood vessels and dural sinuses. *Association for Research into Nervous and Mental Disease*, **18**, 178–200.

Munro, P., Swade, C., and Coppen, A. (1985). Mianserin in the prophylaxis of migraine: a double-blind study. *Acta Psychiatrica Scandinavica*, **72**, Suppl. 320, 98–103.

Olesen, J. (1978). Some clinical features of the acute migraine attack. An analysis of 750 patients. *Headache*, **18**, 268–71.

Peatfield, R.C. and Clifford Rose, F. (1981). Exacerbation of migraine by treatment with lithium. *Headache*, **21**, 140–2.

Penfield, W. and McNaughton, F. (1940). Dural headache and innervation of the dura mater. *Archives of Neurology and Psychiatry*, **44**, 43–75.

Rao, N.S. and Pearce, J. (1971). Hypothalamic–pituitary–adrenal axis studies in migraine, with special reference to insulin sensitivity. *Brain*, **94**, 289.

Ray, B.S. and Wolff, H.G. (1940). Experimental studies on headache: pain-sensitive structures of the head and their significance in headache. *Archives of Surgery*, **41**, 813–56.

Saxena, P.R., Duncker, D.J., Bom, A.H., Heiligers, J., and Verdouw, P.D. (1986). Effects of MDL 72222 and methiothepin on carotid vascular responses to 5-hydroxytryptamine in the pig: evidence for the presence of vascular 5-hydroxytryptamine$_1$-like receptors. *Naunyn-Schmiedebergs Archiv fuer Pharmakologie*, **333**, 198–204.

Vane, J.R. (1971). Inhibition of prostaglandin synthesis as a mechanism of action for aspirin-like drugs. *Nature New Biology*, **231**, 232–5.

17. Peptidergic mechanisms in human intracranial and extracranial arteries

Lars Edvinsson, Inger Jansen, and Rolf Uddman

Introduction

Migraine attacks are conventionally thought to involve a dysfunction in the regulation of tone in intra- and extracranial blood vessels. A number of agents have been suggested as responsible for the altered vasomotor responses seen in conjunction with migraine attacks (Wolff 1948; Olesen and Edvinsson 1988). Previous histochemical studies have shown that human cerebral arteries are surrounded by adrenergic and cholinergic nerve fibres (Edvinsson *et al.* 1976). In addition, peptide-containing nerve fibres, such as neuropeptide Y (NPY), vasoactive intestinal peptide (VIP), substance P (SP), and calcitonin gene-related peptide (CGRP), have been observed around cerebral blood vessels of laboratory animals (Edvinsson 1985). Few studies have been carried out on human temporal and cerebral arteries (Allen *et al.* 1984; Edvinsson and Ekman 1984; Edvinsson *et al.* 1987*b*, Jansen *et al.* 1986), but none on meningeal arteries. In the present study we have examined the distribution of NPY-, VIP-, SP- and CGRP-immunoreactive fibres around the three types of human cranial arteries and compared the pharmacological effects of the perivascularly located neuropeptides on arterial segments.

Materials and Methods

Immunocytochemistry

Human cerebral (cortex pial) and middle meningeal arteries were removed from macroscopically intact regions during neurosurgical tumour resections. Temporal arteries were obtained during surgery to the middle ear and in conjunction with neurosurgical tumour resections. Vessel segments were fixed in a mixture of 2 per cent formaldehyde and 15 per cent of a saturated aqueous picric acid solution in 0.1 M phosphate buffer, rinsed in cold Tyrode buffer containing 10 per cent sucrose for 48 h, frozen on dry ice and sectioned in a cryostat at 15 μm thickness. They were processed for immunocytochemical demonstration of NPY, VIP, SP, or CGRP by use of an indirect immunofluorescence method (Coons *et al.* 1955). The antisera used have been characterized previously (Table 17.1). Control sections were exposed to antiserum that had been preabsorbed with an excess amount of the antigen (10–100 μg ml^{-1} synthetic or pure natural peptide per ml diluted antiserum). The absolute identity of the immunoreactive sequence is not certain in that cross reactivity with other peptides containing the same immunoreactivity cannot be excluded. It is appropriate therefore, to refer to the immunoreactive material as NPY-like, VIP-like, and so on. For brevity, however, the shorter terms NPY, VIP, *etc.* will be used henceforth.

Vasomotor responses in vitro

Cerebral, middle meningeal and temporal arterial segments were examined with a sensitive *in vitro* system (Högestätt *et al.* 1983). The arterial segments (2–3 mm) were suspended between two L-shaped metal prongs (diameter 0.1–0.2 mm) in small tissue baths containing a buffer solution aerated with 5 per cent CO_2 in O_2, pH 7.4, and kept at 37°C. Mechanical activity was recorded by force displacement transducers (Grass FT03C) connected to a Grass polygraph. The cerebral, middle meningeal, and temporal arteries were given a passive load of 4, 5, and 6 mN, respectively, and allowed to stabilize at this tension for 1.5 h before testing. The contractile capacity of the preparations was first tested by exposure to a buffer solution containing 60 mM potassium; this resulted in strong and reproducible contractions which were 12.0 ± 5.2 mN, 11.6 ± 2.5 mN, and 36.9 ± 5.3 mN (mean ± s.e.m.) for the three types of arteries, respectively. In experiments with NPY, the peptide was either applied alone in increasing concentrations, or when we were examining its potentiating capacity, it was given in a concentration of 10^{-8} M 5 min prior to noradrenaline (NA) administration. When VIP, SP, or human (h) CGRP were tested none of them was able to induce relaxation of vessels at the resting level of tension; therefore, the vessels were precontracted with 3×10^{-6} M prostaglandin $F_{2\alpha}$ ($PGF_{2\alpha}$) which induced strong and stable contractions of cerebral arteries (4.2 ± 1.2 mN), middle meningeal (4.6 ± 0.5 mN), and temporal arteries (11.8 ± 0.8 mN). The data are expressed below as mean EC_{50} or IC_{50} values (concentration of agonist eliciting half maximum contraction or relaxation, respectively) and as E_{max} or I_{max} (mean of the maximum responses), and given as mean values ± s.e.m. of responses from a given number (*n*) of vessel segments (one or two from each patient).

Results and comments

The sympathetic system

Innervation   Varicose NPY immunoreactive fibres were seen in the wall of the cerebral, meningeal, and temporal arteries (Edvinsson *et al.* 1987*b*, Jansen *et al.* 1986). They were located in the adventitia, sometimes in close apposition to the media. In laboratory animals NPY-like fibres surrounding

TABLE 17.1. *Details of the antisera used for immunocytochemistry*

Antigen	Code	Raised against	Raised in	Working dilution	Source	Reference
NPY	8404	Protein conjugated synthetic porcine NPY	Rabbit	1:640	Milab, Malmö, Sweden	Grunditz *et al.* 1984
VIP	7852	Unconjugated pure natural porcine VIP	Rabbit	1:640	Milab, Malmö, Sweden	Grunditz *et al.* 1986
CGRP	8427	Protein conjugated synthetic CGRP	Rabbit	1:1280	Milab, Malmö, Sweden	Sundler *et al.* 1985

NPY, neuropeptide Y; VIP, vasoactive intestinal peptide; CGRP, calcitonin gene-related peptide.

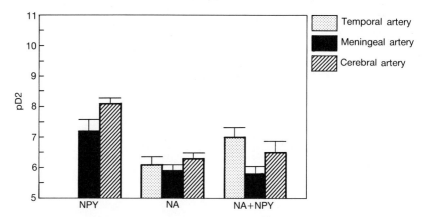

FIG. 17.1. Sensitivity of temporal, middle meningeal, and cerebral arteries to neuropeptide Y (NPY), noradrenaline (NA), and NA in the presence of 3×10^{-8} M NPY. Values given represent mean pD_2 ($-$ log concentration of agonist eliciting half maximum contraction) $\pm$ s.e.m.; $n = 8$–10.

cerebral blood vessels originate in the superior cervical ganglion. Double immunostaining with antibodies against dopamine-β-hydroxylase (used as a marker for noradrenaline-synthesizing capability) and NPY has shown that NPY is co-localized with NA, both in nerve cell bodies in the superior cervical ganglion and in perivascular fibres (Edvinsson *et al.* 1987*a*).

Responses In cerebral and meningeal arteries the administration of NPY elicited concentration-dependent contractions. The maximum contraction induced by NPY was 46.8 ± 13.4 per cent for cerebral, and 71.4 ± 12.1 per cent for meningeal arteries, of that elicited by potassium. The NPY-induced contraction was in both regions somewhat stronger in magnitude when compared with that of NA (26.6 ± 7.7 per cent and 34.5 ± 9.3 per cent, respectively). NPY was markedly more potent [EC_{50}: $(7.0 \pm 2.6) \times 10^{-9}$ M and $(6.3 \pm 2.3) \times 10^{-8}$ M] than NA [EC_{50}: $(4.9 \pm 1.5) \times 10^{-7}$ M and $(1.3 \pm 0.5) \times 10^{-6}$ M] in both cerebral and meningeal arteries respectively (Fig. 17.1). The EC_{50} values for NA in cerebral and meningeal arteries were in the presence of NPY, $(3.8 \pm 1.6) \times 10^{-7}$ M and $(1.6 \pm 0.4) \times 10^{-6}$ M, with E_{max} values of 39.1 ± 2.9 per cent and 40.0 ± 6.2 per cent, respectively.

In human temporal arteries NPY usually did not induce contraction. However, vessel segments from one patient (nine patients tested) exhibited contraction (3.6 ± 1.5 mN) when exposed to NPY. Administration of NA, on the other hand, invariably resulted in strong contractions (86.4 ± 4.8 per cent). Neuropeptide Y (10^{-8} M) significantly potentiated contractions elicited by NA ($10^{-8}-10^{-5}$ M) without changing maximum contraction. The EC_{50} for NA was $(8.1 \pm 1.8) \times 10^{-7}$ M when tested alone and $(1.0 \pm 1.5) \times 10^{-7}$ M in the presence of NPY (Student's *t*-test; $p < 0.01$; Fig. 17.1).

In cerebral as well as in meningeal and temporal arteries, the contractile responses to NA were antagonized by the α_1-adrenoceptor blocker prazosin (10^{-7} M). Neither this antagonist nor the 5-hydroxytryptamine blocker, ketanserin (10^{-7} M), caused any blockade of contractions induced by NPY, nor did they affect the NPY-induced potentiation of NA contraction in temporal arteries, apart from shifting the NA concentration curve towards higher concentrations of NA. The NPY-induced constriction of human cerebral and meningeal arteries was somewhat more pronounced than that noted for NA and occurred at much lower concentrations. In human temporal arteries NPY potentiated adrenergically mediated responses, a result that was not seen in experiments performed on human cerebral and meningeal arteries. Thus, NPY and NA appear to act synergistically in human cerebral and meningeal arteries since no potentiation of the NA-induced contraction was seen. Other studies have shown that NPY-induced contractions in feline cerebral arteries are markedly reduced by calcium antagonists or by calcium depletion, while adrenoceptor or 5-hydroxytryptamine antagonists are without effects (Edvinsson *et al.* 1983). In contrast, the potentiating effect of NPY on peripheral arteries has been shown not to be directly dependent on the extracellular calcium, but is attenuated by the Na^+/K^+ ATPase pump inhibitor, ouabain, and is absent in a sodium-free buffer solution (Wahlestedt *et al.* 1986). The present results revealed that there is a different mode of action of NPY on cerebral and meningeal as compared to temporal arteries. In the cerebrovascular bed NPY may participate with NA in maintaining the upper limit of autoregulation during acute increases in arterial blood pressure. In temporal arteries NPY may serve as a modulator of adrenergically mediated responses.

The parasympathetic system

Innervation A sparse to moderate supply of vasoactive intestinal peptide (VIP)-immunoreactive fibres was seen in the wall of cerebral, meningeal, and temporal arteries. In a previous study the supply of acetylcholinesterase activity in brain vessels appeared fairly rich (Edvinsson *et al.* 1976).

Responses When VIP was given in increasing concentrations to $PGF_{2\alpha}$-contracted arteries, concentration-dependent relaxations occurred (Fig. 17.2). The relaxation was not affected by the β-adrenoceptor antagonist, propranolol (10^{-7} M), the histamine H_2-blocker, cimetidine (10^{-6} M), or the cholinergic antagonist, atropine (10^{-6} M). Recently, it was found that the VIP precursor also contains another peptide, peptide histidine methionine-27 (PHM-27). VIP and PHM-27 are thought to be co-localized with the cholinergic transmitter acetylcholine (Hara *et al.* 1985). In feline

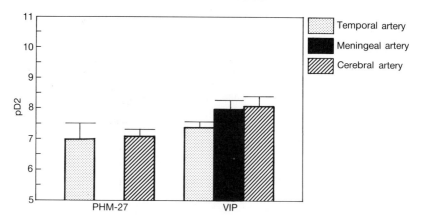

FIG. 17.2. Sensitivity of temporal, middle meningeal, and cerebral arteries to peptide histidine methionine-27 (PHM-27) and vasoactive intestinal peptide (VIP). Values given represent mean pD_2 (relaxation) ± s.e.m.; $n = 6–8$.

cerebral arteries it has been shown that VIP-mediated responses, in contrast to those of acetylcholine, are independent of the removal of the vascular endothelium. These two agents may mediate an increase in the vessel wall adenylate cyclase activity in parallel with producing dilatation (Edvinsson *et al.* 1985).

Sensory nerve fibres

Innervation A moderate supply of substance P (SP)- and calcitonin gene-related peptide (CGRP)-like immunoreactive nerve fibres was located in the adventitia of cranial arteries, sometimes being in close apposition to the media layer.

Responses Studies of isolated, precontracted arterial segments revealed that the cumulative administration of SP or hCGRP resulted in concentration-dependent relaxations; hCGRP was more potent than SP in both cerebral and temporal arteries (Fig. 17.3). Neither SP nor hCGRP were affected by propranolol (10^{-7} M), cimetidine (10^{-6} M), or atropine (10^{-6} M). SP responses, but not hCGRP responses, were antagonized by the SP-antagonist Spantide (10^{-6} M).

Lesion experiments have shown that cerebrovascular SP- and CGRP-immunoreactive fibres originate in the ipsilateral trigeminal ganglion (Liu-Chen *et al.* 1983; Uddman *et al.* 1985). Furthermore, the two peptides are co-localized in trigeminal ganglion cells and in perivascular nerve fibres (Uddman *et al.* 1985). The vasomotor response to CGRP occurs concomitantly with activation of adenylate cyclase, which is in contrast to that of

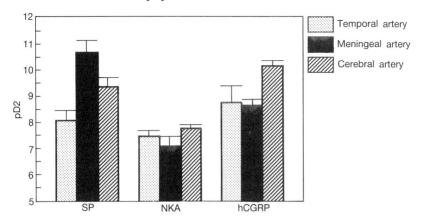

FIG. 17.3. Sensitivity of temporal, middle meningeal, and cerebral arteries to substance P (SP), neurokinin A (NKA), and human calcitonin gene-related peptide (hCGRP). Values given represent mean pD_2 (relaxation) $\pm$ s.e.m.; $n = 6-11$.

SP (Edvinsson *et al.* 1985). On the other hand, SP requires an intact endothelium for the dilator responses. The functional role of the trigemino-cerebrovascular system has been examined in some detail in the feline cerebral circulation (McCulloch *et al.* 1986). Cerebral arterioles respond with vasoconstriction upon administration of, for example, NA to the same degree in sham-operated and trigeminal ganglion-lesioned animals (McCulloch *et al.* 1986). However, the return to base-line levels after constriction is markedly prolonged in lesioned animals. The trigemino-cerebrovascular system may thus have an important role in normalizing the vessel diameter after intense vasoconstriction. This response or 'reflex' may be of particular significance in, for example, classical migraine, where cerebrovascular vasoconstriction is, reportedly, observed (Olesen 1985).

Acknowledgements

Supported by grants from the Swedish Medical Research Council (no. 5958, 6859).

References

Allen, J.M., Todd, N., Crockard, H.A., Schon, F., Yeats, J.C., and Bloom, S.R. (1984). Presence of neuropeptide Y in human circle of Willis and its possible role in cerebral vasospasm. *Lancet*, **ii**, 550–2.

Coons, A.H., Leduc, E.H., and Connolly, J.M. (1955). Studies on antibody production. I: A method for the histochemical demonstration of specific antibody and its application to a study of the hyperimmune rabbit. *Journal of Experimental Medicine*, **102**, 49–60.

Edvinsson, L. (1985). Role of perivascular peptides in the control of the cerebral circulation. *Trends in Neurosciences*, **8**, 126–31.

Edvinsson, L. and Ekman, R. (1984). Distribution and dilatory effect of vasoactive intestinal polypeptide (VIP) in human cerebral arteries. *Peptides*, **5**, 329–31.

Edvinsson, L., Owman, C., and Sjöberg, N.-O. (1976). Autonomic nerves, mast cells, and amine receptors in human brain vessels. An histochemical and pharmacological study. *Brain Research*, **115**, 337–93.

Edvinsson, L., Emson P., McCulloch, J., Tatemoto, K., and Uddman, R. (1983). Neuropeptide Y; Cerebrovascular innervation and vasomotor effects in the cat. *Neuroscience*, **43**, 79–84.

Edvinsson, L., Fredholm, B.B., Hamel, E., Jansen, I., and Verrecchia, C. (1985). Perivascular peptides relax cerebral arteries concomitant with stimulation of cyclic adenosine monophosphate accumulation or release of an endothelium-derived relaxing factor in the cat. *Neuroscience Letters*, **58**, 213–8.

Edvinsson, L., Copeland, J.R., Emson P.C., McCulloch, J., and Uddman, R. (1987*a*). Nerve fibres containing neuropeptide Y in the cerebrovascular bed: Immunocytochemistry, radioimmunoassay, and vasomotor effects. *Journal of Cerebral Blood Flow and Metabolism*, **7**, 45–57.

Edvinsson, L., Ekman, R., Jansen, I., Ottoson, A., and Uddman, R. (1987*b*). Peptide-containing nerve fibres in human cerebral arteries: Immunocytochemistry, radioimmunoassay and in vitro pharmacology. *Annals of Neurology*, **21**, 431–7.

Grunditz, T., Håkanson, R., Rerup, C., Sundler, F., and Uddman, R. (1984). Neuropeptide Y in the thyroid gland: Neuronal localization and enhancement of stimulated thyroid hormone secretion. *Endocrinology*, **115**, 1537–42.

Grunditz, T., Håkanson, R., Hedge, G., Rerup, C., Sundler, F., and Uddman, R. (1986). Peptide histidine isoleucine amide stimulates thyroid hormone secretion and coexists with vasoactive intestinal peptide in intrathyroid nerve fibers from laryngeal ganglia. *Endocrinology*, **118**, 783–90.

Hara, H., Hamill, G.S., and Jacobowitz, D.M. (1985). Origin of cholinergic nerves to the rat major cerebral arteries; Coexistence with vasoactive intestinal polypeptide. *Brain Research*, **14**, 179–88.

Högestätt, E.D., Andersson, K.-E., and Edvinsson, L. (1983). Mechanical properties of rat cerebral arteries as studied by a sensitive device for recording of mechanical activity in isolated small blood vessels. *Acta Physiologica Scandinavica*, **117**, 49–61.

Jansen, I., Uddman, R., Hocherman, M., Ekman, R., Jensen K., Olesen, J., Stjernholm, P., and Edvinsson, L. (1986). Localization and effects of neuropeptide Y, vasoactive intestinal peptide, substance P, and calcitonin gene-related peptide in human temporal arteries. *Annals of Neurology*, **20**, 496–501.

Liu-Chen, L.-Y., Han, D.H., and Moskowitz, M.A. (1983). Pia arachnoid contains substance P originating from trigeminal neurons. *Neuroscience*, **9**, 803–8.

McCulloch, J., Uddman, R., Kingman, T.A., and Edvinsson, L. (1986). Calcitonin gene-related peptide: Functional role in cerebrovascular regulation. *Proceedings of the National Academy of Sciences USA*, **83**, 5731–5.

Olesen, J. (1985). Migraine and regional cerebral blood flow. *Trends in Neurosciences*, **8**, 318–21.

Olesen, J. and Edvinsson, L. (eds) (1988). *Basic mechanisms of headache*. Elsevier, Amsterdam.

Sundler, F., Brodin, E., Ekblad, E., Håkanson, R., and Uddman, R. (1985). Sensory nerve fibers: distribution of subtance P, neurokinin A and calcitonin gene-related peptide. In *Tachykinin antagonists*, (ed. R. Håkanson and F. Sundler), pp. 3–14. Elsevier, Amsterdam.

Uddman, R., Edvinsson, L., Ekman, R., Kingman, T.A., and McCulloch, J. (1985). Innervation of the feline cerebral vasculature by nerve fibres containing calcitonin gene-related peptide: Trigeminal origin and co-existence with substance P. *Neuroscience Letters*, **62**, 131–6.

Wahlestedt, C., Edvinsson, L., Ekblad, E., and Håkanson, R. (1986). Neuropeptide Y potentiates noradrenaline-evoked vasoconstriction: mode of action. *Journal of Pharmacology and Experimental Therapeutics*, **234**, 735–41.

Wolff, H.G. (1948). *Headache and other head pain*. Oxford University Press, New York.

Discussion

SANDLER: We found that the highest activity of benzylamine oxidase was in the meningeal arteries of the brain (Lewinsohn *et al.* 1980). We do not know what the natural substrate for it is; in the rat and in humans too, for that matter, it may well be methylamine (Precious *et al.* 1988). So we ought to add that to your review of mechanisms.

BLAU: Wolff (1963) and others have shown by direct stimulation in patients under local anesthesia that nociceptive endings are present near the *venous* sinuses or the dural *veins*. Because the brain, the veins, and the arteries form a 'closed' system, those veins will pulsate. The concept of vascular headache may therefore be related to the pain endings being found on the veins. In your studies of a calcitonin gene-related peptide (CGRP), the arteries were very dilated but the regional veins remained unchanged. In any flow studies, if the arteries are enlarged surely there must be increased flow in the veins too?

EDVINSSON: If the other stored agent — substance P — is released at the same time, then the veins could dilate in response to substance P.

MOSKOWITZ: We did some extensive horseradish peroxidase tracing on some major cerebral veins, including the sagittal sinus and sigmoid sinus. We found that the first division of the trigeminal ganglion supplied all those vessels (Mayberg *et al.* 1984).

GRYGLEWSKI: What type of antagonism did you find between acetylcholine and neuropeptide Y (NPY)? Might it be that the contractile action of NPY is antagonized by the vasorelaxant action of endothelium-derived relaxing factor (EDRF), which was released by acetylcholine?

EDVINSSON: In the uterine artery preparation, we found that NPY was a poor vasoconstrictor and a modest potentiator of noradrenaline. However, NPY may inhibit acetylcholine-induced and substance P-induced relaxations. The concentration of NPY causing this inhibition is lower than that at which we see contraction in other vessels. Thus, NPY produces a slight contraction and inhibits the action of acetylcholine in this preparation. Other dilatory agents — CGRP and vasoactive intestinal peptide (VIP) — were not modified by NPY (Fallgren *et al.* 1989).

GRYGLEWSKI: If NPY activated voltage-operated calcium channels, then one could expect a release of EDRF. Perhaps in some vascular regions with a special kind of endothelium, NPY was a weak vasoconstrictor.

EDVINSSON: Our data from different vascular regions may have created a complicated picture. NPY has different effects in various parts of the circulation. We know of four different patterns of action that it may have in different regions (Edvinsson et al. 1987).

MOSKOWITZ: You compared the decreases in the levels of substance P and CGRP after trigeminal ganglionectomy. When we did extensive quantitative evaluation of trigeminal lesions, we were disturbed that we could obtain only 50 to 65 per cent depletion (Norregaard and Moskowitz 1985). An explanation may come from the recent work of Loesch and Burnstock (1988), who have demonstrated substance P in rat endothelium. We have measured substance P in human, cow, dog, and rat endothelium, in amounts that could account for a percentage of that remaining fraction. We have done some high-pressure liquid chromatography (HPLC) studies to authenticate the immunoreactivity. We are currently doing Northern blots to determine the presence of the mRNA, to find out whether substance P is synthesized by endothelial cells.

EDVINSSON: It is a similar story for choline acetyltransferase (CAT) in the microvessel endothelium. CAT activity can be detected both in the endothelium and in the smooth muscle cells of the blood vessel wall. To discriminate between the neural (nerve terminals in adventitia) and the non-neural CAT activity (endothelium and muscle cells), one needs to do many types of control experiment. I am personally sceptical about the importance of a storage of every neurotransmitter in the endothelium. The measurable levels of substance P in brain vessels after trigeminal lesions (Uddman et al. 1985) may be due to either bilateral innervation from this ganglion or a bilateral innervation from the second cervical (C_2) dorsal root (Edvinsson et al. 1989).

MOSKOWITZ: We have done similar experiments. If you can describe a bilateral innervation, what were your controls? We found it was essential to control for the spread of horseradish peroxidase (and also true blue axon tracer). Our test of whether the labelling was authentically from the blood vessel was to ligate the blood vessel proximally to the site of application, and we abolished the staining (Mayberg et al. 1984). If you could abolish the staining by this method in your cervical ganglion studies, bilaterally, then I would be convinced about what one could conclude.

FERREIRA: We did some experiments in which we used clonidine to release enkephalin-like peptides in the rat paw, to produce analgesia (Nakamura and Ferreira 1988). Have you found any neurones containing enkephalin-like substances in the cerebral vessels?

EDVINSSON: Rolf Uddman has looked at that in our laboratory. With the antibodies that we have available we were not successful in confirming this. The purity of the antibodies is very influential here. When small levels of the enkephalin-like peptides are present, the tissue levels can be increased by colchicine treatment. This may provide a future avenue for research.

FOZARD: Do you have any evidence that the co-stored NPY has a functional role? Does it have the potential for taking a message across the junction and also for controlling the release of the transmitter?

EDVINSSON: A few years ago, we stimulated the superior cervical ganglion and could see constriction of both arterioles and veins with a pial window technique (Auer et al. 1983). When a high dose of phenoxybenzamine was administered, a block of about 70 per cent of the constriction was seen. The remaining 30 per cent could not be affected by adrenergic blockers. Retrospectively, the result might have been due to an action of released NPY, but an unknown substance stored there could equally well be involved.

References

Auer, L.M., Edvinsson, L., and Johansson, B.B. (1983). Effect of sympathetic nerve stimulation and adrenoceptor blockade on pial arterial and venous calibre and on intracranial pressure in the cat. *Acta Physiologica Scandinavica*, **119**, 213–17.

Edvinsson, L., Håkanson, R., Wahlestedt, C., and Uddman, R. (1987). Effects of neuropeptide Y on the cardiovascular system. *Trends in Pharmacological Sciences*, **8**, 231–5.

Edvinsson, L., Hara. H., and Uddman, R. (1989). Retrograde tracing of nerve fibers to the rat middle cerebral artery with true blue: colocalization with different peptides. *Journal of Cerebral Blood Flow and Metabolism*, **9**, 212–8.

Fallgren, B., Ekblad, E., and Edvinsson, L. (1989). Co-existence of neuropeptides and differential inhibition of vasodilator responses by neuropeptide Y in guinea pig uterine arteries. *Neuroscience Letters*, **100**, 71–6.

Lewinsohn, R., Glover, V., and Sandler, M. (1980). Development of benzylamine oxidase and monoamine oxidase A and B in man. *Biochemical Pharmacology*, **29**, 1221–30.

Loesch, A. and Burnstock, G. (1988). Ultrastructural localization of serotonin and substance P in vascular endothelial cells of rat femoral and mesenteric arteries. *Anatomy and Embryology*, **178**, 137–42.

Mayberg, M.P., Zervas, N.T. and Moskowitz, M.A. (1984). Trigeminal projections to supratentorial pial and dural blood vessels in cats demonstrated by horseradish peroxidase histochemistry. *Journal of Comparative Neurology*, **223**, 46–56.

Nakamura, M. and Ferreira, S.H. (1988). Peripheral analgesic effect of clonidine, mediated by release of endogenous, enkephalin-like substance. *European Journal of Pharmacology*, **146**, 223–8.

Norregaard, T.V. and Moskowitz, M.A. (1985). Substance P and the sensory innervation of intra- and extracranial feline cephalic arteries: implications for vascular pain mechanism in man. *Brain*, **108**, 517–33.

Precious, E., Gunn, C.E., and Lyles, G.A. (1988). Deamination of methylamine by semicarbazide-sensitive amine oxidase in human umbilical artery and rat aorta. *Biochemical Pharmacology*, **37**, 707–13.

Uddman, R., Edvinsson, L., Ekman, R., Kingman, T.A., and McCulloch, J. (1985). Innervation of the feline cerebral vasculature by nerve fibers containing calcitonin gene-related peptide: trigeminal origin and co-existence with substance P. *Neuroscience Letters*, **62**, 131–6.

Wolff, H.G. (1963). *Headache and other head pain*, (2nd edn). pp. 53–95. Oxford University Press, New York.

18. Novel agents affecting enkephalinergic and histaminergic transmissions in brain

J.C. Schwartz, B. Giros, C. Gros, C. Llorens-Cortes, J.M. Arrang, M. Garbarg, and H. Pollard

Introduction

Progress in cephalalgia therapy may be anticipated from the development of novel classes of drugs that affect either the transmission of pain messages or the control of vascular mechanisms in the brain.

A valuable strategy for achieving such an aim consists in identifying new molecular targets that are critically involved in neurotransmitter metabolism or actions.

This line has been followed in recent years in our laboratory to identify the mechanisms responsible for opioid peptide inactivation, and for the control of histamine release from its cerebral neurones. In both cases, relevant molecular targets were identified — that is, two 'neuropeptidases' responsible for enkephalin breakdown (De la Baume *et al.* 1983), and the H_3 autoreceptor responsible for the control of histamine synthesis and release (Arrang *et al.* 1983, 1985). Agents able to interact selectively and potently with these various targets have been rationally designed to help us to study the corresponding control mechanisms. These agents may constitute new drugs to be used in human therapeutics.

Inhibitors of enkephalin-degrading peptidases

It is now well established that the opioid peptides, and particularly the enkephalins, are neurotransmitters involved in the control of pain-transmitting pathways at various levels of the central nervous system.

During the last decade the mechanisms responsible for the inactivation of enkephalins have been clarified. Two ectopeptidases — enzymes of the plasma membranes with their active sites directed towards the extracellular space — seem almost equally responsible for the rapid hydrolysis that follows the release of these pentapeptides from their neurones. Both are zinc-containing metallopeptidases.

The first is enkephalinase (EC 3.4.24.11., membrane metalloendopeptidase; Malfroy *et al.* 1978; Almenoff *et al.* 1981) which cleaves the enkephalins and the heptapeptide Tyr-Gly-Gly-Phe-Met-Arg-Phe at the level of their Gly^3–Phe^4 amide bond. It is localized in synaptic membranes from the central nervous system and its precise cellular distribution, recently unravelled with the aid of monoclonal antibodies (Pollard *et al.* 1987), seems closely parallel to that of proenkephalin A markers. For instance, high levels of the enzyme are detected in areas where enkephalins are believed to modulate pain signals, such as in the external layers of the dorsal horn of the spinal cord, the nucleus of origin of the trigeminal nerve, the periaqueductal grey, and other areas.

The hydrolysis of enkephalins and the heptapeptide generates the characteristic extracellular tripeptide Tyr-Gly-Gly which can be detected as an endogenous compound in the brain (Llorens-Cortes *et al.* 1985). Its level is modified by drugs believed to modify the activity of enkephalinergic neurones.

Thiorphan is the first rationally designed enkephalinase inhibitor (Roques *et al.* 1980) but this compound does not easily cross the blood–brain barrier. To circumvent this difficulty, the pro-drug acetorphan was developed (Lecomte *et al.* 1986). Among other properties, this compound displays antinociceptive activity when administered parenterally at low doses, but it is absolutely devoid of dependence liability. The analgesic activity of acetorphan is low compared to that of the opioids but evidence for analgesia has been demonstrated in humans (Floras *et al.* 1983).

The second enkephalin-degrading peptidase is aminopeptidase M (EC 3.4.11.2), evidence for which was found only recently, in cerebral synaptic membranes (Giros *et al.* 1986). Immunohistochemical studies have also shown it to be abundant in the walls of cerebral microvessels (Solhonne *et al.* 1987). Aminopeptidase M can be inhibited by bestatin, a natural compound of bacterial origin, whose potency is limited, and which does not cross the blood–brain barrier. For this reason, we have recently developed a series of thiol-containing inhibitors of aminopeptidases, some of which are approximately one hundred times more potent than bestatin, without losing their selectivity. Furthermore, we have recently prepared carbaphethiol, a compound that inhibits cerebral aminopeptidases after its parenteral administration at reasonable dosages. Carbaphethiol exerts antinociceptive activity in rodents, when administered alone, and when given in association with acetorphan its antinociceptive activity is remarkable, becoming comparable to that of the exogenous opioids (Gros *et al.* 1988).

Hence, it seems more and more likely that co-inhibition of the two enkephalin-degrading peptidases will provide new approaches to the treatment of pain syndromes.

Agents interacting with histamine H_3 receptors in the brain

Histaminergic neurones localized in the posterior hypothalamus innervate the whole central nervous system, through long axons. Histamine affects target cells (neurones and microvessels) via interaction with well-characterized H_1 and H_2 receptors. However, only H_1 antagonists that cross the blood–brain barrier are used in therapeutics, and they appear to be devoid of any significant efficacy in cephalalgia.

The presynaptic H_3 receptor: definition and design of potent and selective ligands

The third histamine receptor was only recently discovered and differs from the two others both in its pharmacology (hence it is designated as H_3) and in its localization (Arrang et al. 1983). It is exquisitely sensitive to histamine and, even more, to the chiral agonist (R)α-methylhistamine, which is active at nanomolar concentrations, whereas the S-isomer is approximately one-hundredfold less potent. A potent and highly selective antagonist, thioper-amide, has also recently been rationally designed (Arrang et al. 1987). Although H_1 receptor antagonists are ineffective, some H_2 receptor agonists (for example, impromidine) or antagonists (for example, burimamide) are reasonably potent H_3 receptor antagonists. This last feature suggests that some actions of histamine previously categorized as being mediated by H_2 receptors might, in fact, be attributable to H_3 receptor activation.

Histamine inhibits its own depolarization-induced release via stimulation of H_3 receptors in slices of various brain regions as well as in isolated nerve endings, indicating that the H_3 receptors are autoreceptors involved in a local feedback regulation of histaminergic neurones. It should be empha-sized that this action is observed only when endogenous stores of histamine are labelled with the precursor tritiated amino acid and not with pre-formed [^{3}H]histamine, presumably because the latter is not selectively taken up into histaminergic axons. In addition, activation of H_3 receptors inhibits the depolarization-induced stimulation of [^{3}H]histamine synthesis (Arrang et al. 1988).

Radioligand assay and visualization of H_3 receptors

The high apparent affinity of (R)α-methylhistamine in functional studies suggested that the drug might constitute, when radiolabelled, a suitable probe for H_3 receptor assay and visualization.

Indeed, [^{3}H]-labelled (R)α-methylhistamine was found to bind in a re-versible and saturable manner to cerebral cortex membranes with a K_D of 0.5 nM derived from either saturation kinetics or dissociation/association rates and a maximal number of sites representing 30 ± 3 fmol mg^{-1} protein (J.M. Arrang et al., unpublished results). In comparison, H_1 and H_2 recep-tors appear to be significantly more abundant.

In autoradiographic studies performed with the same ligand, H_3 receptors were found to be fairly widespread in rat brain, as previously shown in release studies. The areas showing the highest grain densities were telen-cephalic areas such as the cerebral cortex (particularly in its most rostral part), the striatum, the hippocampus (molecular layer of the dentate gyrus), the lateral septum, the bed nucleus of the stria terminalis, and the olfactory nuclei, to which diffuse projections of the ascending histaminergic neurones have been demonstrated. In contrast, fainter labelling was observed in the cerebellum (all layers), and in the brainstem or mesencephalon (except for a few areas, such as the substantia nigra) which contain a lower density of projections. In the posterior hypothalamus a thin band of dense labelling was observed in the perimamillary area, which is known to contain most histamine perikarya, and which suggests the presence of H_3 receptors on these perikarya. However, in the rest of the hypothalamus, in which levels of L-histidine decarboxylase and histamine are much higher than in the telencephalon, a relatively low labelling was observed. This may indicate that H_3 receptors are not restricted to histaminergic neurones, a hypothesis recently confirmed by lesion studies (H. Pollard *et al.*, unpublished results).

Histamine H_3 receptors control cerebral histamine turnover in vivo

With the recent design of brain-penetrating ligands that selectively interact with H_3 receptors, it has become feasible to test the role of these receptors in the control of histamine turnover in the rat brain *in vivo*.

Whereas the activity of some monoaminergic neurones — for example the dopaminergic neurones — seems, at least partly, to be controlled via neuronal feedback loops that involve postsynaptic receptors, the activity of others such as the noradrenergic neurones seems mainly, if not solely, controlled via autoreceptors.

The [^{3}H]histamine synthesis in the cerebral cortex was unaffected by the administration of a combination of mepyramine, an H_1 receptor antagonist, and zolantidine, an H_2 receptor antagonist which, like the former, easily crosses the blood–brain barrier. In contrast, the administration of (R)α-methylhistamine significantly decreased the histamine turnover, as shown by a series of indexes: the rate of [^{3}H]histamine synthesis from [^{3}H]histidine, its precursor amino acid; the rate of endogenous histamine depletion after administration of a suicide inhibitor of L-histidine decarboxylase; and the steady-state level of telemethylhistamine, a major histamine metabolite (Garbarg *et al.* 1989).

Not only were these actions antagonized by thioperamide but also, when thioperamide was administered alone in rather low dosage, it markedly increased the histamine turnover, as revealed by the same indexes.

These observations indicate that these agents may be useful tools for behavioural investigations into the function of histaminergic neuronal systems in the brain.

Histamine H_3 receptors control histamine release in human brain

It is very likely that histamine plays a neurotransmitter role in the human brain, as in the brains of other species. Its regional distribution and that of L-histidine decarboxylase, its specific synthesizing enzyme, seem to be roughly parallel to those of these markers in rodent brain. Also, H_1 receptors have been characterized in membranes from human brain, and their blockade is likely to account for the sedative effects of many classical H_1 antihistamines (see Schwartz *et al.* 1986). However, no information has become available about histamine release in the human brain.

We have recently studied this problem by using samples of fresh human cerebral cortex obtained during the surgical removal of deep tumours (Arrang *et al.* 1988). Slices were prepared and labelled with [^{3}H]histidine according to a procedure essentially similar to that used with rat brain tissues (Arrang *et al.* 1983). [^{3}H]Histamine was released in response to depolarization elicited by 30 mM K^+, and this release was progressively inhibited, by up to 60 per cent, in the presence of exogenous histamine. The concentration–response curve to the amine was shifted to the right in the presence of thioperamide, leading to a K_i value for the compound of around 10 nM.

These observations identify H_3 receptors as mediating the autoinhibition of histamine release in human brain, and suggest that their pharmacological properties are similar to those of the corresponding receptors in rodents.

Summary

Endogenous enkephalins are inactivated by two metallopeptidases, enkephalinase and aminopeptidase M, for which potent and selective inhibitors were recently designed. When administered parenterally these compounds — acetorphan and carbaphethiol — protect the endogenous opioid peptides from degradation, and elicit naloxone-reversible analgesia.

Histamine is a cerebral neurotransmitter which seems to be involved mainly in the control of arousal and cerebrovascular mechanisms. With the design of potent and selective agents able to interact with the presynaptic H_3 receptor it is now possible to modulate histaminergic transmissions in the brain. The potential usefulness of these novel drugs in the management of cephalalgia remains to be assessed by clinical trials.

References

Almenoff, J., Wilk, S., and Orlowski, M. (1981). Membrane-bound pituitary metalloendopeptidase: apparent identity to enkephalinase. *Biochemical and Biophysical Research Communications*, **102**, 206–14.

Arrang, J.M., Garbarg, M., and Schwartz, J.C. (1983). Autoinhibition of brain histamine release mediated by a novel class (H_3) of histamine receptor. *Nature*, **302**, 832–7.

Arrang, J.M., Garbarg, M., and Schwartz, J.C. (1985). Histamine synthesis and release in CNS: control by autoreceptors (H_3). In *Frontiers in histamine research*, (ed. C.R. Ganellin and J.C. Schwartz) pp. 143–153. Pergamon, Oxford.

Arrang, J.M., Garbarg, M., and Schwartz, J.C. (1987). Autoinhibition of histamine synthesis mediated by presynaptic H₃-receptors. *Neuroscience*, **23**, 149–57.

Arrang, J.M., Devaux, B., Chodkiewicz, J.P., and Schwartz J.C. (1988). H₃-receptors control histamine release in human brain. *Journal of Neurochemistry*, **51**, 105–8.

De la Baume, S., Yi, C.C., Schwartz, J.C., Chaillet, P., Marcais-Collado, M., and Costentin, J. (1983). Participation of both "enkephalinase" and aminopeptidase activities in the metabolism of endogenous enkephalins. *Neuroscience*, **8**, 143–51.

Floras, P., Bidabe, A.M., Caille, J.M., Simonnet, G., Lecomte, J.M., and Sabathie, M. (1983). Double blind study of effects of enkephalinase inhibitor on adverse reactions to myolography. *American Journal of Neuroradiology*, **4**, 653–5.

Garbarg, M., Trung Tuong, M.D., Gros, C., and Schwartz, J.C. (1989). Effects of histamine H₃-receptor ligands on various biochemical indices of histaminergic neuron activity in rat brain. *European Journal of Pharmacology*, **164**, 1–11.

Giros, B., Gros, C., Solhonne, B., and Schwartz, J.C. (1986). Characterization of aminopeptidases responsible for the inactivation of endogenous (Met⁵) enkephalin in brain slices using peptidase inhibitors and aminopeptidase M antibodies. *Molecular Pharmacology*, **29**, 281–7.

Gros, C., Giros, B., Schwartz, J.C., Vlaiculescu, A., Costentin, J., and Lecomte, J.M. (1988). Potent inhibition of cerebral aminopeptidases by carbaphethiol, a parenterally active compound. *Neuropeptides*, **12**, 111–8.

Lecomte, J.M. *et al.* (1986). Pharmacological properties of acetorphan, a parenterally active "enkephalinase" inhibitor. *Journal of Pharmacology and Experimental Therapeutics*, **237**, 937–44.

Llorens-Cortes, C., Gros, C., and Schwartz, J.C. (1985). Study of endogenous Tyr-Gly-Gly, a putative enkephalin metabolite, in mouse brain: validation of a radioimmunoassay localization, and effects of peptidase inhibitors. *European Journal of Pharmacology*, **119**, 183–91.

Malfroy, B., Swerts, J.P., Guyon, A., Roques, B.P., and Schwartz, J.C. (1978). High affinity enkephalin-degrading peptidase in brain is increased after morphine. *Nature*, **276**, 523–6.

Pollard, H., De la Baume, S., Bouthenet, M.L., Schwartz, J.C., Ronco, P., and Verroust, P. (1987). Characterization of two probes for the localisation of enkephalinase in rat brain: [³H]thiorphan and a [¹²⁵I]labeled monoclonal antibody. *European Journal of Pharmacology*, **133**, 155–64.

Roques, B.P. *et al.* (1980). The enkephalinase inhibitor thiorphan shows antinociceptive activity in mice. *Nature*, **288**, 286–8.

Schwartz, J.C., Garbarg, M., and Pollard, H. (1986). Histaminergic transmission in the brain. In *Handbook of physiology, Section 1: The nervous system, Vol. IV: Intrinsic regulatory systems of the brain*, (ed. V.B. Mountcastle, F.E. Bloom, and S.R. Geiger), pp. 257–316. American Physiological Society USA, Philadelphia.

Solhonne, B., Gros, C., Pollard, H., and Schwartz, J.C. (1987). Major localization of aminopeptidase M in rat brain microvessels. *Neuroscience*, **22**, 225–32.

Discussion

VANE: In your work on the relevance of histamine to migraine, have you discovered what the histamine H₃ receptor antagonist does to mast cells?

SCHWARTZ: Other groups have tested the antagonist on several populations of mast cells which, as a group, are very heterogenous. On peritoneal mast cells there is apparently no H_3 receptor able to modulate histamine release induced by immunoglobulin E or compound 48/80 (unpublished observations). In human allergy studies, H_3 receptors appear not to be present on skin mast cells. But we have evidence that these H_3 receptors control histamine synthesis in the rat and guinea-pig lung (Arrang *et al.* 1987). Up to now, the only cell population known to synthesize histamine in the lung is the mast cell. Hence, the H_3 receptors could be present in certain but not all mast-cell populations.

SANDLER: You used the histamine/*tele*methylhistamine ratio to measure turnover. I have always been intrigued by the quantity of *tele*methylhistamine in the brain; there is almost as much there as histamine. Does it have a life of its own? Does it act at any of these receptor sites?

SCHWARTZ: No. It is absolutely inactive at H_1, H_2, and H_3 receptors.

SANDLER: Does it have any other receptors of its own?

SCHWARTZ: No. It is formed in either glial or neuronal cells, or in the liver. There is strong evidence that it is an inactivation product.

LANCE: The H_3 receptor seems to be an autoreceptor regulating the amount of histamine *release*. The *action* of histamine would still be mediated by H_1 and H_2 receptors. We have done extensive clinical trials on both migraine and cluster headache with both chlorpheniramine and cimetidine (Anthony *et al.* 1978) without showing any effect at all on the prophylaxis of either migraine or cluster headache. Does this not mean that, however important this system is in other ways, it is unlikely to be relevant to migraine?

SCHWARTZ: Your results with chlorpheniramine are convincing, but the conclusion is not straightforward with cimetidine, because the drug does not cross the blood–brain barrier. Until very recently there was no H_2 receptor antagonist able to cross the blood–brain barrier. (One has been developed at Smith Kline and French, but as far as I know it has not been used any more in therapeutics). We do not know in which direction a possible role of endogenous histamine should be tested — either blockade or activation. Furthermore, H_3 receptors are not always presynaptically located on histaminergic neurones. Hence, the hypothesis of a role of histamine in migraine cannot be discarded.

ZIEGLER: In general, altering the chemical structure of biogenic amines at the α-position to the nitrogen renders the substance more stable to biodegradation by the monoaminoxidases. Receptor ligands with increased metabolic stability could reach remote receptors, which are neither activated nor labelled by the physiological ligand. The chemically modified substances would then label only another fraction of the same receptor population and not a new type of histamine receptor.

SCHWARTZ: Yes. Monoamine oxidase does not play any direct role in the inactivation of histamine. It acts upon *tele*methylhistamine, which is a substrate for monoaminoxidase B, but not histamine, so this is not a factor in resistance. We have recent evidence that (R)α-methylhistamine can be methylated *in vivo* as well as *in vitro* by histamine *N*-methyltransferase but direct inactivation by monoamine oxidase seems unlikely.

SAXENA: Is there not some evidence that the H_2 receptors in the heart might be different from those in the gastrointestinal tract?

SCHWARTZ: The evidence for the H_2 receptor being different in the heart is not clear. Some people have claimed that there is a *tissue preference* for some compounds — which is quite different — for heart as compared to the gastrointestinal tract. But I am not aware of any direct evidence for a pharmacological difference between the H_2 receptors of the two tissues.

OLESEN: Histamine is known to induce attacks of cluster headache, although with a rather long latency phase of 30 to 60 minutes, and histamine by itself does not cross the blood–brain barrier. Is it known whether the peripheral effects of histamine in any way 'communicate' with the central histaminergic system?

SCHWARTZ: Several possible means of communication are available. A large dose of histamine has a massive cardiovascular effect which might, secondarily, induce changes in neuronal activity or cerebral circulation activity. We were puzzled recently because (R)α-methylhistamine, which is structurally close to histamine, has very clear central effects at dosages which are not very high, in the mg/kg range. We tested whether histaminergic perikarya in the posterior hypothalamus might be located outside the blood–brain barrier by using inulin or other markers, and we were forced to conclude that they are inside the blood–brain barrier. (H. Pollard and J.C. Schwartz, unpublished observations).

SANDLER: You have also described to us the use of enkephalinase inhibitors in an experimental headache model. I understand that the enkephalinase-inhibitory effect of phosphoramidon has been shown by Ukponmwan *et al.* (1986) to be potentiated by phenylethylamine or by deprenyl. Furthermore, this effect was attenuated by deprivation of REM (rapid eye movement) sleep. Could this help us to approach the problem of why sleep helps migraine?

SCHWARTZ: At least in the rat and the mouse the enkephalinase inhibitor, acetorphan, elicits a number of responses on monoaminergic systems involved in the control of sleep. 5-HT neurones are activated whereas noradrenergic neurones show a reduced activity (Lecomte *et al.* 1986). Both effects are naloxone-reversible, indicating that they are, presumably, due to protection of the endogenous opioids.

VANE: What does acetorphan do to mood?

SCHWARTZ: Enkephalinase inhibitors display 'antidepressant' activity in the mouse 'behavioural despair' test (Ben Natan *et al.* 1984). Also, one of these compounds has been studied in human depression, in open trials (J.M. Lecomte, personal communication). The data were promising but this remains to be confirmed in double-blind studies.

VANE: One has heard of people who say they run regularly to get a 'high' on enkephalins. Do your patients experience this?

SCHWARTZ: No. I myself have taken this compound and I did not feel this.

SAXENA: I understand that both thiorphan and bestatin have been shown, in animals, to attenuate the morphine-withdrawal symptoms. On the other hand you tell us that there is no evidence of dependence with the enkephalinase inhibitors. Aren't the two points contradictory?

SCHWARTZ: Some withdrawal symptoms are attenuated by enkephalinase inhibitors, as shown by several studies. I do not know of any such studies with aminopeptidase inhibitors. In collaboration with H. Loo and F. Hartman, we are currently performing a small double-blind trial in our psychiatric hospital. Ten morphine-addicted patients were being treated with clonidine which, as you know, is the reference treatment for withdrawal symptoms; another 10 patients were on acetorphan. We have not seen any significant difference between the two. Acetorphan was better at treating most of the withdrawal symptoms, while clonidine was better on the withdrawal symptoms in the cardiovascular field, such as hypertension. I do not know why enkephalinase inhibitors do not elicit dependence, and neither do I know the molecular processes that give rise to dependence. We do see some but not all opioid-like effects with these compounds.

SAXENA: Secondly, the inhibition of enkephalinase would lead to an increase in endogenous enkephalins in the brain. These substances act on four different types of receptor to elicit various pharmacological responses. Would it not be a better approach to synthesize a selective agonist at one of the receptor sites?

SCHWARTZ: One always has to try several possible approaches. Until now, all the agonists at the *mu*-opiate receptors have been shown to have the same drawback as morphine itself. It seems that for the *mu*-morphine receptor, one cannot find an agonist with the analgesic activity without its also having the various side-effects. There have been claims that stimulation of *kappa*-receptors was much less liable to give dependence than stimulation of the *mu*-receptor. On the other hand, it is also known that stimulation of the *kappa*-receptor does not give as strong an analgesic effect as stimulation of the *mu*-receptor.

DE BELLEROCHE: What worries me about the approach is that you may affect the metabolism of up to about 20 other neuropeptides, because inhibition of the endopeptidase (enkephalinase; EC 3.4.24.11.) will affect other peptides, some of which are involved in analgesia and some in pain pathways. So you have to work out what the net effect is going to be.

SCHWARTZ: From my knowledge of the published work on this enzyme (enkephalinase, EC 3.4.24.11), I know of no other neuropeptide than enkephalins for which there is evidence of physiological inactivation by the enzyme *in vivo*. For example, although this enzyme *in vitro* can cleave cholecystokinin, this does not mean that it is physiologically involved in cholecystokinin inactivation. On the other hand, there is good evidence for another peptidase being involved in the inactivation of endogenous cholecystokinin (Rose *et al.* 1988). Although it is possible that this peptidase can inactivate other neuropeptides, it is, in the central nervous system, very selectively localized on certain neuronal populations. Therefore one should not expect it to have such a broad specificity as suggested by *in vitro* studies with homogenates. Usually, enzymes are less selective than receptors, so drugs acting at receptors are theoretically 'cleaner' than the enzyme inhibitors. However, receptors are involved in many different neuronal processes, and therefore drugs interacting with receptors might raise the same kinds of specificity problems.

DE BELLEROCHE: When you found the peptidase inhibitor to be ineffective, what antinociceptive tests were you using?

SCHWARTZ: Enkephalinase inhibitors lack antinociceptive activity on the tail withdrawal test for mice or rats. We know that this result is not because of insufficient protection of the endogenous enkephalins, because when the latter are totally protected by an association of enkephalinase and aminopeptidase inhibitors, a very strong analgesic effect is observed on some tests (for example, the 'hot plate jump'), whereas on the tail withdrawal test we still do not have any effect. My interpretation of the data is that enkephalin neurones are involved in the control of *some* nociceptive reflexes; in other reflexes, they are not. After administration of naloxone, an opiate receptor antagonist, hyperalgesic responses are observed on the hot-plate jump test but not on the tail withdrawal test. This strengthens my interpretation that enkephalins may control some nociceptive reflexes but not others.

References

Anthony, M., Lord, G.D.A., and Lance, J.W. (1978). Controlled trials of cimeti-dine in migraine and cluster headache. *Headache*, **18**, 261–4.

Arrang, J.M. *et al.* (1987). Highly potent and selective ligands for histamine H₃-receptors. *Nature*, **327**, 117–23.

Ben Natan, L. *et al.* (1984). Involvement of endogenous enkephalins in the mouse 'behavioural despair' test. *European Journal of Pharmacology*, **97**, 301–4.

Lecomte, J.M. *et al.* (1986). Pharmacological properties of acetorphan, a parenteral-ly active enkephalinase inhibitor. *Journal of Pharmacology and Experimental Therapeutics*, **237**, 937–44.

Rose, C., Camus, A., and Schwartz, J.C. (1988). A serine peptidase responsible for the inactivation of endogenous cholecystokinin in brain. *Proceedings of the Nation-al Academy of Sciences, USA*, **85**, 8326–30.

Ukponmwan, O.E., Rupreht, J., and Dzoljic, M. (1986). An analgesic effect of enkephalinase inhibition is modulated by monamine oxidase-B and REM sleep deprivation. *Naunyn-Schmiedeberg's Archives of Pharmacology*, **332**, 376–9.

19. The biochemical basis of migraine predisposition

Vivette Glover and Merton Sandler

Introduction

Most people do not suffer from migraine, whatever the provocation, and even migraine sufferers differ from each other in their susceptibility.

As Latham wrote in 1872,

'The sufferers possess what is called the nervous temperament ... the attacks are produced by prolonged mental work, protracted mental excitement, or any intense strain on the feelings such as grief, anxiety, passion, etc. ... the depression that follows over excitement, a debauch, etc. are all predisposing causes.'

This passage contains two crucial observations. Certain types of individual are more likely to suffer from migraine than others, and an attack is frequently preceded by a period of stress.

Even if there is a final common pathway operating in all migraine attacks, which is quite possible but unproven, it seems clear that predisposition to migraine is multifactorial. Different subjects find their attacks to be triggered by different agents, such as stress, diet, or menstrual cycle, and the nature of the trigger is specific to particular individuals. In others, attack and refractory period seem to follow an endogenous rhythm with no obvious external initiator (see Table 19.1). This variability suggests that there are many 'ways in' to a migraine attack, many possible points of vulnerability in different people. Thus, the genetic basis of migraine predisposition (Davies and Clifford Rose 1986) is also likely to be multifactorial or polygenic. In this paper, we discuss some aspects of the biochemistry of migraine predisposition, and indicate how some of the initiating factors may interact with the central monoamine systems. Professor Lance and others in this volume discuss persuasively how these centres (particularly the raphé nuclei and locus coeruleus) may be involved in the generation of a migraine attack. It is likely that the more we understand about individual vulnerability, the more we may be able to tailor specific treatment to particular patients.

Diet and migraine

Many patients believe that dietary factors such as alcohol, red wine, chocolate, or cheese can provoke migraine attacks (Glover *et al*. 1984; Peatfield *et*

TABLE 19.1. *Major triggers reported by 119 migraine patients attending the Princess Margaret Migraine Clinic*

Trigger factor	Percentage of 119
Stress	45
Dietary factors	33
Menstrual cycle	18 (of women)
None	15

al. 1984). However, there has also been much scepticism, particularly among clinicians, about such reports. We have recently shown, in placebo-controlled trials, that both red wine (Littlewood *et al.* 1988) and chocolate (C. Gibb, P.T.G. Davies, V. Glover, M. Sandler, and F.C. Rose, unpublished work) can initiate migraine attacks in particular individuals, who form a minority of the total population at risk. Both trials were conducted on carefully selected patients who were already convinced about their own individual triggering agent; in the former study, no effect of red wine could be demonstrated in migraine patients who had no history of susceptibility to this agent. The biochemical basis of these effects is still unclear. Despite earlier claims, neither tyramine nor phenylethylamine are likely to be involved, because their concentrations in red wine and chocolate are very low (Schweitzer *et al.* 1975; Hurst and Toomey 1981; Hannah *et al.* 1988). In wine, flavonoid phenols are plausible candidates; they are present in much higher concentration in red than in white wine (Littlewood *et al.* 1988). Even so, there is as yet no direct evidence for their involvement in migraine. Nor is there convincing evidence that allergic mechanisms play some part in dietary migraine (Merrett *et al.* 1983).

Platelet levels of the enzyme, phenolsulphotransferase P (PST P), one of the two forms of an enzyme that conjugates phenols with sulphate (Rein *et al.* 1982), have been found to be significantly decreased in patients with self-reported dietary migraine compared with a non-dietary group (Littlewood *et al.* 1982; Soliman *et al.* 1987), although there is considerable overlap in individual values. If platelet PST P activities reflect those elsewhere in the body, it is plausible that low levels can reduce the body's defences against dietary or environmental phenols because this enzyme provides a major detoxication mechanism (Sandler and Usdin 1981). PST P is under strong genetic control (Reveley *et al.* 1983) and low values might be a manifestation of one of the many possible forms of genetic predisposition to migraine.

Menstrual migraine

Many women report an association between time of menstruation and their migraine attacks although, in others, no such link is observed (Epstein *et al.*

1975; Peatfield 1986). Migraine often remits in pregnancy (Eadie and Tyrer 1985) and recurs *post partum* (Stein *et al.* 1984). One interpretation of these findings is that high levels of oestrogen, or progesterone, or both, protect against migraine, with the sudden fall that occurs at menstruation or parturition provoking an attack in susceptible individuals. Somerville (1971, 1972) has reported that oestrogen injections at the end of the menstrual cycle can postpone an attack, whereas progesterone has no such effect. Dennerstein *et al.* (1978) claim that oestrogen withdrawal is associated with an increase in headache intensity; conversely, oestrogen therapy appears to reduce migraine severity (Chaudhuri and Chaudhuri 1975). As yet, there is no firm evidence that menstrual migraine is linked with abnormal hormone concentrations. Women may well vary in their response to fluctuating hormone levels, rather than to absolute concentrations of the hormones themselves.

Both oestrogen and progesterone have many effects on the neurotransmitter systems of the central nervous system (Deakin 1988). There are receptors for both in many different brain regions but they are especially concentrated in brainstem monoamine-containing cell body groups (Maggi and Perez 1985). Oestrogen appears to affect both dopamine and 5-hydroxytryptamine (5-HT) systems. It has clear actions on dopamine receptors and turnover, and both oestrogen and progesterone augment the number of 5-HT_1 receptors in the cortex (Biegon *et al.* 1983). O'Connor and Feder (1985), working in guinea-pigs, found evidence to suggest that a decline in oestrogen level reduces functional 5-HT neurotransmission. Conceivably, this may form a possible basis for increased vulnerability to menstrual migraine.

Platelet monoamine oxidase (MAO) and migraine

Apart from a transitory decrease during an attack (Sandler *et al.* 1970; Glover *et al.* 1977) mean platelet MAO activity is significantly reduced in migraine patients between attacks, compared with controls (Sicuteri *et al.* 1972; Sandler *et al.* 1974; Bussone *et al.* 1977; Glover *et al.* 1981). The finding is particularly marked in males (Glover *et al.* 1981). Platelet MAO activity is under genetic control (Sandler *et al.* 1981) and it seems possible that the low values represent another vulnerability point for migraine.

We have recently found a direct and significant correlation in migraine patients between platelet MAO activity and anxiety and depression level, as assessed by questionnaire (Glover *et al.* 1987; J.T. Littlewood, A. Prasad, C. Gibb, V. Glover, M. Sandler, R. Joseph and F.C. Rose, unpublished results). Others have observed that high anxiety levels are associated with both extremes of the platelet MAO range (Schalling 1987). High platelet MAO activity has also been found in several studies of depression (Sandler *et al.* 1981). It is, thus, of interest that only low and not high values have been identified in migraine patients. Both anxiety and depression are likely to be biochemically heterogeneous and only certain subtypes appear to be linked with migraine.

Low platelet MAO activity has been noted in certain other clinical states (see Sandler *et al.* 1981 for review). Of most interest, perhaps, in the present context are the low values recorded in the idiopathic pain syndrome (Knorring *et al.* 1984). Oreland *et al.* (1984) have shown that platelet MAO activity correlated with 5-hydroxyindoleacetic acid concentrations in the cerebrospinal fluid, and they suggested that low enzyme activities reflect a hypoactive 5-HT system. There is evidence that 5-HT-depleted rats have an increased sensitivity to pain (Willner 1985). It may well be that a low platelet MAO activity reflects an underactive 5-HT system and is a predisposing factor for migraine for this reason.

Anxiety and depression in migraine

There is now considerable evidence that migraine patients have more anxiety and depression than controls (Diamond 1964; Howarth 1965; Kashiwagi *et al.* 1972; Price and Blackwell 1980). When patients in a migraine clinic are investigated, there is always the concern that the patients are to some extent self-selected and perhaps more neurotic than those in the general population. There have been some thorough investigations of the characteristics of migraine sufferers in the general population which have, in fact, been in good agreement with findings at specialist clinics. The consensus of opinion, however, is that there is little evidence of a migraine *personality* as such (Hundleby and Loucks 1985).

A major study of psychological aspects of migraine patients in the British Civil Service was carried out by Henryk-Gutt and Rees (1973), who showed significantly increased levels of anxiety, compared with controls. Two more recent population studies, one in an English market town (Crisp *et al.* 1977) and another in New Zealand (Paulin *et al.* 1985), found a higher incidence of anxiety and depression in migraine patients than in the general population; in the latter, there was a positive relationship with headache frequency. Price and Blackwell (1980) also found that migraine sufferers, too, show higher levels of trait anxiety, by a variety of rating scales, than normal subjects, as did Howarth (1965).

The association of migraine and depression has been explored in depth rather more recently. Garvey *et al.* (1983) asked 116 patients with major depressive disorder about their headache pattern. They had a headache rate similar to that of controls during their non-depressed phase, but an increased rate during episodes of depression. Merikangas *et al.* (1988) studied the association between migraine and depression in a family study of probands with major depressive disorder, and in community controls and relatives of both groups. They noted a significant association between migraine and depression in both probands and their relatives; they also observed

TABLE 19.2. *SADS-L diagnosis in 40 migraine patients attending the Princess Margaret Migraine Clinic*

Diagnosis	Lifetime	Current
Major depression	16	6
(Endogenous major depression)	15	6
Minor depression	2	1
Anxiety disorders	6	1
Labile personality	3	0
Other	5	1
No psychiatric disorder	17	0

SADS-L, Schedule for affective disorder — Lifetime version.

symptoms of anxiety in depressed patients with migraine. However, while both migraine and depression were strongly familial, their association appeared to be only partly transmissible. One explanation for these results would be if the depression were secondary to the migraine.

In a recent study (J. Jarman, M. Fernandez, V. Glover, M. Sandler, P.T.G. Davies, T. Steiner, C. Thompson and F.C. Rose, unpublished results), we have used the *Schedule for Affective Disorder — Lifetime version* to obtain a more detailed psychiatric profile than had been obtained before of typical migraine patients who attend a specialist clinic. The results are given in Table 19.2. More than half the patients interviewed had a lifetime history of some degree of psychiatric disorder. Major depression was much the commonest diagnosis and, in all but one patient, was of the endogenous type. This finding is in marked contrast with the depression observed in other circumstances; postnatal depression, for example, predominantly corresponds to the neurotic subtype. Given the high anxiety incidence in migraine patients, and their high score on the *Eysenck Personality Questionnaire* (Henryk-Gutt and Rees 1973), it might have been predicted that they, too, would have manifested predominantly neurotic depression. It seems possible that the biological factors that predispose to endogenous depression also predispose to migraine.

The tyramine test in migraine patients

Evidence that the high incidence of endogenous depression of these migraine sufferers was at least partly due to a biological predisposition comes from the results of the tyramine test (J. Jarman, M. Fernandez, V. Glover, M. Sandler, P.T.G. Davies, T. Steiner, C. Thompson and F.C. Rose, unpublished results). Low tyramine sulphate conjugation after an oral load (Sandler *et al.* 1975; Bonham Carter *et al.* 1978) is a trait marker for

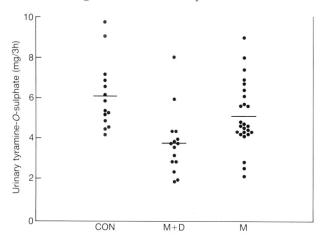

FIG. 19.1. The tyramine test: a biological trait marker for depression in migraine patients. Urinary tyramine sulphate output after an oral load is shown for controls (CON), for migraine patients with a history of endogenous depression (M+D), and for other migraine patients (M). Two-tailed Student's *t*-test showed (M+D) group to be significantly different ($p < 0.01$) from CON group and ($p < 0.05$) from M group. (CON versus M groups were not significantly different).

endogenous depression, compared with the neurotic variant of the illness (Harrison *et al.* 1984; Hale *et al.* 1986). It is also likely to be a genetic marker, because some first-degree relatives of low tyramine sulphate excreters, who themselves have never been depressed, also excreted significantly lower amounts of conjugate than did controls (Hale *et al.* 1986). Despite substantial investigative effort, the biochemical basis for this finding, which appears to be unrelated to phenolsulphotransferase activity (Bonham Carter *et al.* 1981), remains unknown, as does its relationship to other putative markers of endogenous depression.

The migraine patients described in Table 19.2 had significantly lower tyramine sulphate excretion on oral tyramine challenge than controls. Figure 19.1 shows that almost all the migraine patients with a lifetime history of endogenous depression had a low tyramine sulphate output. This study gives strong independent support to the psychiatric diagnosis in these patients. It also has therapeutic implications. There is evidence (Hale *et al.* 1989) that depressed patients with low values in the tyramine test respond better to tricyclic antidepressant medication than those with normal values. It may be that the test will also identify a subgroup of migraine sufferers who respond well to these drugs (Kashiwagi *et al.* 1972; Couch *et al.* 1976).

Paradoxically enough, the tyramine conjugation deficit was first identified in a group of patients classified as having dietary migraine (Youdim *et al.*

1971), although a later attempt at replication proved unsuccessful (S. Bonham Carter and M. Sandler, unpublished results). In the light of the present findings (J. Jarman *et al.*, unpublished results), it seems likely that the earlier group included, by chance, an enrichment of subjects with a lifetime incidence of endogenous depression. The present data fail to show any difference between dietary and non-dietary migraine in the tyramine test.

The tyramine conjugation study also provides evidence against the idea that depression is secondary to migraine in these patients (Merikangas *et al.* 1988), and rather supports the interpretation that a disturbance of particular biochemical systems predisposes to both migraine and depression. Whether monoamine systems are involved has been a subject of much speculation in published work.

Links between monoamine systems, anxiety, depression, and migraine

There is evidence from animal models that in anxiety as well as stress there is increased activity of the sympathetic nervous system, and release of catecholamines both peripherally (Gray 1982) and centrally, where there is increased firing of the locus coeruleus (Stone 1975). There is also evidence for enhanced noradrenergic function, with increased anxiety, in humans (Ballenger *et al.* 1984). As anxiety seems to predispose to migraine, and as stress is a major triggering factor, the release of catecholamines seems to be one possible cause of an attack.

Anthony (1981) noted a significant rise in plasma noradrenaline and dopamine β-hydroxylase levels during a migraine attack. Hsu *et al.* (1977) reported a rise in mean plasma noradrenaline levels three hours before a group of migraine subjects awoke, with a headache already present. Spierings (1985) suggested that activation of the sympathetic system may be a *result* of the headache, but the fact that stress often precedes headache makes it more likely that headache follows activation of catecholamine systems.

The biochemical basis of depression is unclear; despite many provisos (Stone 1983), the current evidence is still, on balance, compatible with early hypotheses that depression is associated with functionally *hypo*active catecholamine systems (Ballenger *et al.* 1984) and/or 5-HT systems (Van Praag 1984) in the brain. It is possible that a hypoactive 5-hydroxytryptaminergic system is also associated with headache. 5-HT is released peripherally during a migraine attack (see Peatfield 1986, for review), and may well be released centrally also. There is evidence that reserpine, which depletes monoamines, causes headache in susceptible individuals (Curzon *et al.* 1969) whereas 5-hydroxytryptophan, the precursor of 5-HT, can alleviate it (Sicuteri 1972; Titus *et al.* 1986).

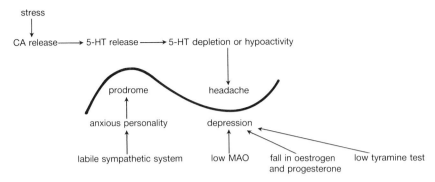

FIG. 19.2. Model of central monoamine changes during a migraine attack: links with predisposing factors. CA, catecholamine (released from the locus coeruleus); 5-HT, 5-hydroxytryptamine (released from the raphé nucleus); MAO, monoamine oxidase.

A migraine attack follows a characteristic pattern: 'The most important emotional colourings during the clinically recognised portion of a common migraine attack are states of anxious and irritable hyperactivity in the early portions of the attack and states of apathy and depression in the bulk of the attack' (Sacks 1973). This progression, too, needs to be explained in biochemical terms.

Gray (1982) has discussed the biochemical effects of stress, and its relationship to anxiety and depression, in a way that may be relevant here. In rat models, after acute anxiety or stress has increased the activity of noradrenergic neurones in the central nervous system (Stone 1975), there may be depletion of noradrenaline from vesicles, and this may correspond to a state of functional exhaustion or depression. This, in turn, may be followed by transneuronal enzyme induction, occuring 16 to 18 hours after the original stimulus, and remaining elevated for a number of days (Thoenen 1975; Fillenz 1977). These three stages of neuronal and biochemical hyperactivity, underactivity, and reaction or recovery are possible biochemical correlates of the prodrome, the headache phase and the refractory period of a migraine attack.

Figure 19.2 shows a model that illustrates this hypothesis. The beginning of a migraine attack is associated with a surge of 5-HT release. 5-HT cells in the dorsal raphé nucleus are innervated by excitatory noradrenergic projections from the locus coeruleus (Willner 1985). The sequence can thus be triggered by stress, and occurs more readily in an anxious personality. This stage is followed by lowered activity of the 5-hydroxytryptaminergic system, possibly owing to 5-HT depletion or altered receptor sensitivity, associated with the headache itself. Low platelet MAO activity and the fall of oestrogen at menstruation may both be associated with a hypoactive 5-HT system which predisposes to this stage, as does a vulnerability to endogenous depression (as indicated by the tyramine test). The refractory period may involve a reactive enzyme or receptor induction. How dietary triggers enter this cycle is, at present, unknown.

The picture is clearly both speculative and an oversimplification and will be testable only by new methods such as positron emission tomography scanning. However, the model may be useful to focus attention on different potential points of vulnerability which, perhaps, need different treatments.

Directions for the future

The biochemical cascade of the type discussed above, or the one earlier envisaged by Sandler (1972) — which involved a dietary triggering agent, release of an intermediate agent from the gut wall to the portal and venous circulation, and a 'spasmogen' released into the arterial circulation from the pulmonary vascular bed — provide one possible scenario, but it can obviously be short-circuited. Recent observations of Brewerton *et al.* (1988) on *m*-chlorophenylpiperazine (*m*-CPP), a triazolopyridine metabolite of trazodone, appear to be important here. Oral administration of this compound was able to produce a typical, common migraine-like headache in 28 out of 52 subjects, eight to 12 hours after its administration. Tryptophan or a placebo failed to initiate attacks. There was a significantly higher headache incidence in the tested subjects who had a history or a family history of migraine and, indeed, 18 out of 20 of these developed severe symptoms. Thus, in this case at least, the postulated biochemical sequence was bypassed and the chemical substance responsible for the end-organ response probably travelled directly to its site of action.

The presence of acute peripheral concomitants of a migraine attack — a second transitory type of platelet MAO deficit present only across the acute episode (Sandler *et al.* 1970; Glover *et al.* 1977), platelet 5-HT release (Curran *et al.* 1965; Anthony *et al.* 1967); liberation of platelet β-thromboglobulin (Gawel *et al.* 1979); and increased platelet aggregability (Hilton and Cumings 1972) — have encouraged speculation that a circulating platelet-damaging agent might be present (Sandler 1978), perhaps being liberated from the pulmonary vascular bed (Sandler 1972). This substance may also be responsible for known blood-vessel calibre changes and, conceivably, for head pain. Where such a humoral agent might interact is, of course, unknown, although in the light of present information it is tempting to nominate the 5-HT$_1$-like receptor system.

m-CPP itself seems to be a 5-HT$_1$ receptor ligand (Brewerton *et al.* 1988). It is noteworthy that most of the drugs that are clinically effective in migraine therapy bind to one or other central 5-HT receptor (Peroutka 1988). Do migraine-initiating foodstuffs bind similarly? It would be of great interest to see whether fractions of red wine, now shown objectively to provoke migraine attacks (Littlewood *et al.* 1988), attach themselves to these receptors. Chocolate, too, is another migraine-provoking agent identified objectively (C. Gibb, P.T.G. Davies, V. Glover, M. Sandler and F.C. Rose, unpublished work) and extracts of it might be similarly investigated.

The approach adopted by Peroutka (1988), to identify possible 5-HT receptor ligands that act as therapeutic agents, exploited their ability to displace other known ligands from human brain membranes. Whether receptor-binding kinetics undergo substantial *post mortem* changes in human brain and, indeed, whether brains from migrainous subjects bind ligands similarly to those from controls, are other urgent questions that must be tackled in the future. And do the antimigraine drugs which bind to 5-HT$_1$-like receptors displace *m*-CPP from its binding sites? We shall try to provide some answers in the near future.

References

Anthony, M. (1981). Biochemical indices of sympathetic activity in migraine. *Cephalalgia*, **1**, 83–9.

Anthony, M., Hinterberger, H.J., and Lance, J.W. (1967). Plasma serotonin in migraine stress. *Archives of Neurology*, **16**, 544–52.

Ballenger, J.C., Post, R.M., Jimerson, D.C., Lake, C.R., and Zuckerman, M. (1984). Neurobiological correlates of depression and anxiety in normal individuals. In *Frontiers of clinical neuroscience*, (ed. R.M. Post and J.C. Ballenger), Vol. 1, pp. 481–501. Williams and Wilkins, Baltimore.

Biegon, A., Reches, A., Snyder, S.L., and McEwan, B.S. (1983). Serotonergic and noradrenergic receptors in the rat brain: modulation by chronic exposure to ovarian hormones. *Life Sciences*, **32**, 2015–21.

Bonham Carter, S., Sandler, M., Goodwin, B.L., Sepping, P., and Bridges, P.K. (1978). Decreased urinary output of tyramine and its metabolites in depression. *British Journal of Psychiatry*, **132**, 125–32.

Bonham Carter, S.M., Glover, V., Sandler, M., Gillman, P.K., and Bridges, P.K. (1981). Human platelet phenolsulphotransferase: separate control of the two forms and activity range in depressive illness. *Clinica Chimica Acta*, **117**, 333–44.

Brewerton, T.D., Murphy, D.L., Mueller, E.A., and Jimerson, D.C. (1988). Induction of migrainelike headaches by the serotonin agonist m-chlorophenylpiperazine. *Clinical Pharmacology and Therapeutics*, **43**, 605–9.

Bussone, G., Giovanni, P., Boiardi, A., and Boeri, R. (1977). A study of the activity of platelet monoamine oxidase in patients with migraine headache or cluster headache. *European Neurology*, **15**, 157–62.

Chaudhuri, T.K. and Chaudhuri, S.T. (1975). Estrogen therapy for migraine. *Headache*, **15**, 139–41.

Couch, J.R., Ziegler, D.K., and Hassanein, R. (1976). Amitriptyline in the prophylaxis of migraine. *Neurology*, **236**, 121–7.

Crisp, A.H., Kalucy, R.S., McGuinness, B., Ralph, P.C., and Harris, G. (1977). Some clinical, social and psychological characteristics of subjects with migraine in the general population. *Postgraduate Medical Journal*, **53**, 691–7.

Curran, D.A., Hinterberger, H., and Lance, J.W. (1965). Total plasma serotonin,

5-hydroxyindoleacetic acid and p-hydroxy-m-methoxy-mandelic acid excretion in normal and migrainous subjects. *Brain*, **88**, 997–1010.

Curzon, G., Barrie, M., and Wilkinson M.I.P. (1969). Relationships between headache and amine changes after administration of reserpine to migrainous patients. *Journal of Neurology Neurosurgery and Psychiatry*, **32**, 555–61.

Davies, P.T.G. and Clifford Rose F. (1986). Migraine genetics. *Trends in Neurosciences*, **9**, 541–2.

Deakin, J.F.W. (1988). Relevance of hormone–CNS interactions to psychological changes in the puerperium. In *Motherhood and mental illness, vol. 2: Causes and consequences*, (ed. R. Kumar and I.F. Brockington), pp. 113–32. Wright, London.

Dennerstein, L., Laby, B., Burrows, G.D., and Hyman, G.J. (1978). Headache and sex hormone therapy. *Headache*, **18**, 146–53.

Diamond, S. (1964). Depressive headaches. *Headache*, **4**, 255–9.

Eadie, M.J. and Tyrer, J.J. (1985). *The biochemistry of migraine*. MTP Press, Lancaster.

Epstein, M.T., Hockaday, J.M., and Hockaday, T.D.R. (1975). Migraine and reproductive hormones throughout the menstrual cycle. *Lancet*, **i**, 543–7.

Fillenz, M. (1977). The factors which provide short-term and long-term control of transmitter release. *Progress in Neurobiology (Oxford)* **8**, 251–78.

Garvey, M.J., Schaffer, C.B., and Tuason, V.B. (1983). Relationship of headaches to depression. *British Journal of Psychiatry*, **143**, 544–7.

Gawel, M., Burkitt, M., and Clifford Rose, R. (1979). The platelet release reaction during migraine attacks. *Headache*, **19**, 323–7.

Glover, V., Sandler, M., Grant, E., Rose, F.C., Orton, D., Wilkinson, M., and Stevens, D. (1977). Transitory decrease in platelet monoamine oxidase activity during migraine attacks. *Lancet*, **i**, 391–3.

Glover, V., Peatfield, R., Zammit-Pace, R., Littlewood, J., Gawel, M., Clifford Rose, F., and Sandler, M., (1981). Platelet monoamine oxidase activity and headache. *Journal of Neurology Neurosurgery and Psychiatry*, **44**, 786–90.

Glover, V., Littlewood, J., Sandler, M., Peatfield, R., Petty, R., and Clifford Rose, F. (1984). Dietary migraine: looking beyond tyramine. In *Progress in migraine research, vol. 2*, (ed. F. Clifford Rose), pp. 113–119. Pitman, London.

Glover, V., Prasad, A., Littlewood, J., Rampling, R., and Sandler, M. (1987). Platelet MAO activity: correlations with anxiety and depression in cancer and migraine patients. *Pharmacology and Toxicology*, **60**, Suppl. 1, 21.

Gray, J.A. (1982). An enquiry into the functions of the septo-hippocampal system. In *The neuropsychology of anxiety*, (ed. D.E. Broadbent et al.), pp. 374–408. Clarendon Press, Oxford.

Hale, A.S., Walker, P.L. Bridges, P.K., and Sandler, M. (1986). Tyramine-conjugation deficit as a trait-marker in endogenous depressive illness. *Journal of Psychiatric Research*, **20**, 251–61.

Hale, A.S., Sandler, M., Hannah, P., and Bridges, P.K. (1989). Tyramine conjugation for prediction of treatment response in depressed patients. *Lancet*, **i**, 234–6.

Hannah, P., Glover, V., and Sandler, M. (1988). Tyramine in wine and beer. *Lancet*, **i**, 879.

Harrison, W.M. et al. (1984). The tyramine challenge test as a marker for melancholia. *Archives of General Psychiatry*, **41**, 681–5.

Henryk-Gutt, R. and Rees, W.L. (1973). Psychological aspects of migraine. *Journal of Psychosomatic Research*, **17**, 141–53.

Hilton, B.P. and Cumings, J.N. (1972). 5-Hydroxytryptamine levels and platelet aggregation responses in subjects with acute migraine headache. *Journal of Neurology Neurosurgery and Psychiatry*, **35**, 505–9.

Howarth, E. (1965). Headache, personality and stress. *British Journal of Psychiatry*, **111**, 1193–7.

Hsu, L.K.G., Crisp, A.H., Kalucy, R.S., Koval, R.S., Chen, C.N., Carruthers, M., and Zilkha, K.J. (1977). Early morning migraine. Nocturnal plasma levels of catecholamine, tryptophan, glucose and free fatty acids and sleep encephalographs. *Lancet*, **i**, 447–51.

Hundleby, J.D. and Loucks, A.D. (1985). Personality characteristics of young adult migraineurs. *Journal of Personality Assessment*, **49**, 497–500.

Hurst, W.J. and Toomey, P.B. (1981). High-performance liquid chromatographic determination of four biogenic amines in chocolate. *Analyst*, **106**, 394–402.

Kashiwagi, T., McClure, J.N., and Wetzel, R.D. (1972). Headache and psychiatric disorders. *Diseases of the Nervous System*, **33**, 659–63.

Knorring, L. von, Perris, C., Oreland, L., Eisemann, M., Eriksson, V., and Perris, H. (1984). Pain as a symptom in depressive disorders and its relationship to platelet monoamine oxidase activity, *Journal of Neural Transmission*, **60**, 1–9.

Latham, P.W. (1872). Nervous or sick-headaches. *British Medical Journal*, **1**, 305–6.

Littlewood, J., Glover, V., Sandler, M., Petty, R., Peatfield, R., and Rose, F.C. (1982). Platelet phenolsulphotransferase deficiency in dietary migraine. *Lancet*, **i**, 983–6.

Littlewood, J.T., Gibb, C., Glover, V., Sandler, M., Davies, P.T.G., and Clifford Rose, F. (1988). Red wine as a cause of migraine. *Lancet*, **i**, 558–9.

Maggi, A. and Perez, J. (1985). Role of female gonadal hormones in the CNS: clinical and experimental aspects. *Life Sciences*, **37**, 893–906.

Merikangas, K.R., Risch, N.J., Merikangas, J.R., Weissman, M.M., and Kidd, K.K. (1988). Migraine and depression: association and familial transmission. *Journal of Psychiatric Research*, **22**, 119–29.

Merrett, J., Peatfield, R.C., Clifford Rose, F., and Merrett, T.G. (1983). Food related antibodies in headache patients. *Journal of Neurology, Neurosurgery and Psychiatry*, **46**, 738–42.

O'Connor, L.H. and Feder, H.H. (1985). Estradiol and progesterone influence L-5-hydroxytryptophan-induced myoclonus in male guinea pigs: sex differences in serotonin-steroid interactions. *Brain Research*, **330**, 121–5.

Oreland, L., Von Knorring, L., and Schalling, D. (1984). Connections between monoamine oxidase, temperament and disease. In *Proceedings of the Ninth International Congress of Pharmacology, Vol. 2*, (ed. W. Paton, J. Mitchell, and P. Turner) pp. 193–202. Macmillan, London.

Paulin, J.M., Waal-Manning, H.J., Simpson, F.O., and Knight, G.K. (1985). The prevalence of headache in a small New Zealand town. *Headache*, **25**, 147–51.

Peatfield, R. (1986). *Headache*. Springer, Berlin.

Peatfield, R., Glover, V., Littlewood, J.T., Sandler, M., and Rose, F.C. (1984). The prevalence of diet-induced migraine. *Cephalalgia*, **4**, 179–83.

Peroutka, S.J. (1988). Antimigraine drug interactions with serotonin receptor subtypes in human brain. *Annals of Neurology*, **23**, 500–4.

Price, K.P. and Blackwell, S. (1980). Trait levels of anxiety and psychological responses to stress in migraineurs and normal controls. *Journal of Clinical Psychology*, **36**, 658–60.

Rein, G., Glover, V., and Sandler, M. (1982). Multiple forms of phenolsulphotransferase in human tissues: selective inhibition by dichloronitrophenol. *Biochemical Pharmacology*, **31**, 1893–7.

Reveley, A.M., Bonham Carter, S.M., Reveley, M.A., and Sandler, M. (1983). A genetic study of platelet phenolsulphotransferase activity. *Journal of Psychiatric Research*, **17**, 303–7.

Sacks, O. (1973). *Migraine. Evolution of a common disorder*. Faber and Faber, London.

Sandler, M. (1972). Migraine; a pulmonary disease? *Lancet*, **i**, 618–9.

Sandler, M. (1978). Implications of the platelet monoamine oxidase deficit during migraine attacks. *Research and Clinical Studies in Headache*, **6**, 65–72.

Sandler, M. and Usdin, E. (ed.) (1981). Phenolsulfotransferase in mental health research. Macmillan, Basingstoke.

Sandler, M., Youdim, M.B.H., Southgate, J., and Hanington, E. (1970). The role of tyramine in migraine: some possible biochemical mechanisms. In *Background to migraine, 3rd Migraine Symposium*, (ed. A.L. Cochrane), pp. 104–115. Heinemann, London.

Sandler, M., Youdim, M.B.H., and Hanington, E. (1974). A phenylethylamine oxidising defect in migraine. *Nature*, **250**, 335–7.

Sandler, M., Bonham Carter, S., Cuthbert, M.F., and Pare, C.M.B. (1975). Is there an increase in monoamine-oxidase activity in depressive illness? *Lancet*, **i**, 1045–9.

Sandler, M., Reveley, M.A., and Glover, V. (1981). Human platelet monoamine oxidase activity in health and disease: a review. *Journal of Clinical Pathology*, **34**, 292–302.

Schalling, D., Asberg, M., Edman, G., and Oreland, L. (1987). Markers for vulnerability to psychopathology: temperament traits associated with platelet MAO activity. *Acta Psychiatrica Scandinavica* **76**, 172–82.

Schweitzer, J.W., Friedhoff, A.J., and Schwartz, R. (1975). Chocolate, β-phenethylamine and migraine re-examined. *Nature*, **257**, 256.

Sicuteri, F. (1972). 5-Hydroxytrytophan in the prophylaxis of migraine. *Pharmacological Research Communications*, **4**, 213–8.

Sicuteri, F., Buffoni, F., Anselmi, B., and Del Bianco, P.L. (1972). An enzyme (MAO) defect on the platelets in migraine. *Research and Clinical Studies in Headache*, **3**, 245–51.

Soliman, H., Pradalier, A., Launay, S.M., Dry, J., and Dreux C. (1987). Decreased phenol and tyramine sulphoconjugation by platelets in dietary migraine. In *Advances in headache research, Proceedings of the 6th International Migraine Symposium, Current problems in neurology*, vol. 4, (ed. F. Clifford Rose), pp. 117–121. John Libbey, London.

Somerville, B.W. (1971). The influence of hormonal change upon migraine in women. *Proceedings of the Australian Association of Neurologists*, **8**, 47–53.

Somerville, B.W. (1972). The role of estradiol withdrawal in the etiology of menstrual migraine. *Neurology*, **22**, 355–66.

Spierings, E.L.H. (1985). Migraine: symptomatology and pathogenesis. *Sandorama, The Physicians' Panorama* (Sandoz Ltd, Basle), **11**, 26–34.

Stein, G., Morton, J., Marsh, A., Collins, W., Branch, C., Desaga, U. and Ebeling, J. (1984). Headaches after childbirth. *Acta Neurologica Scandinavica*, **69**, 74–9.

Stone, E.A. (1975). Stress and catecholamines. In *Catecholamines and behaviour*, (ed. A.J. Friedhoff), Vol. 2, pp. 31–74. Plenum, New York.

Stone, E.A. (1983). Problems with current catecholamine hypotheses of antidepressant agents: speculations leading to a new hypothesis. *Brain and Behavioral Sciences*, **6**, 535–77.

Thoenen, H. (1975). Transsynaptic regulation of neuronal enzyme synthesis. In *Handbook of psychopharmacology*, (ed. L.L. Iversen, S.D. Iversen, and S.H. Snyder), Vol. 3, *Biochemistry of biogenic amines*, pp. 443–75. Plenum, New York.

Titus, F., Davalos, A., Alom, J., and Codina, A. (1986). 5-Hydroxytryptophan versus methysergide in the prophylaxis of migraine. *European Neurology*, **25**, 327–9.

van Praag, H.M. (1984). Depression, suicide and serotonin metabolism in the brain. In *Frontiers of clinical neuroscience*, (ed. R.M. Post and J.C. Ballenger), Vol. 1, pp. 601–18. Williams and Wilkins, Baltimore.

Willner, P. (1985). *Depression: a psychobiological synthesis*. John Wiley, New York.

Youdim, M.B.H., Bonham Carter, S., Sandler, M., Hanington, E., and Wilkinson, M. (1971). Conjugation defect in tyramine-sensitive migraine. *Nature*, **230**, 127–8.

Discussion

LANCE: Somerville (1971), working in my department, showed that an artificially maintained progesterone level does not eliminate a headache. It is the *fall in oestradiol* that seems to trigger premenstrual migraine (Somerville 1972). If the oestradiol level is artificially maintained, the cyclic headache does not occur until the oestradiol is allowed to fall. The same applies to postmenopausal women and anovulatory women: it is the falling phase of oestradiol that triggers the migraine.

GLOVER: A fall in oestradiol also happens in mid-cycle. Premenstrually there is a fall of both oestradiol and progesterone, so perhaps a fall of oestradiol, *superimposed* on a fall of progesterone, could be the trigger for migraine.

LANCE: This is possible, but these women often get mid-cycle headaches too, although not as frequently.

SANDLER: A further point about progesterone and monoamine oxidase activity could be mentioned here. We found that progesterone 'switches on' monoamine oxidase A (Mazumder *et al.* 1980). At peak plasma progesterone concentration, there was a 7- to 10-fold increase in tissue monoamine oxidase activity. When the progesterone level falls rapidly, monoamine oxidase activity switches off. MAOA, of course, metabolizes the classical neurotransmitter monoamines such as noradrenaline and 5-HT.

WELCH: When you did the very interesting *tyramine sulphate excretion test* in patients with endogenous depression did you pay due attention to what stage of the oestrogen cycle these patients were at?

GLOVER: No, we did not do that. But in pregnant patients we found that the response was the same as that out of pregnancy. That result argues strongly against there being much hormonal influence over the results.

WELCH: In your studies on postnatal depression, were all the patients diagnosed as having a reactive depression as opposed to a psychotic depression?

GLOVER: In general, that type of patient's depression is classified as predominantly reactive but not totally. Our own study is still in progress and we have not yet done proper psychiatric interviews. It is of interest in the present context because almost none of the patients with a self-reported history of postnatal depression were low on the tyramine test. This forms some sort of control group for the migraine clinic, and shows very different results.

COPPEN: In your other results (Table 19.2) you showed that 16 out of 40 patients attending the migraine clinic had major depression, and that 15 of those 16 had *endogenous* major depression. That is a very high prevalence. How does that compare with the population studies done by others?

GLOVER: As far as I know there have not been any population studies that have used the same criteria. Every study uses different questionnaires. I recall that usually about a third of depressed patients have an endogenous origin, and two-thirds are reactive. To find 15 out of 16 is very far from typical. But, on the other hand, it may be that migraine is biochemically linked with endogenous depression.

PEATFIELD: To change the subject, when we consider the quantities of tyramine in different foodstuffs we should always bear in mind the size of the normal dietary load — the amount of chocolate eaten in one go, for example.

GLOVER: I agree entirely. In any case, I do not believe that tyramine can be the chemical in chocolate that triggers headache because the levels of tyramine, phenylethylamine, and all other monoamines tested in chocolate are very low.

PEATFIELD: How is the amount of tyramine in different foodstuffs measured? Is it extracted and digested beforehand?

GLOVER: This work was done by Hurst and Toomey (1981), for chocolate. They defatted the chocolate, extracted the monoamines into an ethylacetate acetone mixture and quantified the tyramine by high-pressure liquid chromatography (HPLC).

VANE: Now that tyramine is believed not to be an important trigger for migraine, is *m*-CPP the only pure chemical that has been shown to cause headache in those predisposed to migraine?

GLOVER: No, there are others, such as fenfluramine.

LANCE: Reserpine and zimelidine can also trigger migraine (Syvälahti *et al.* 1979).

GLOVER: *m*-CPP is interesting, even if we do not know yet exactly how it is acting. It may be a receptor agonist that can tell us which receptors are abnormally sensitive in migraine patients.

COPPEN: 5-HT re-uptake inhibitors such as fluvoxamine are used fairly commonly in the UK in the treatment of depression. Fluvoxamine has the side-effect of vomiting. Does this drug also precipitate migraine headache?

PEATFIELD: There are some hints that these agents can exacerbate migraine during the first few weeks of treatment (Syvälahti *et al.* 1979).

VANE: Do these other substances trigger headache in non-migrainous people or only in those who are susceptible to migraine attacks?

GLOVER: Although reserpine can cause a headache in non-migraineurs, it does not cause a migraine attack in them. These drugs trigger migraine only in migraine patients.

CURZON: Does *m*-CPP cause anxiety and thereby cause migraine? Or is there a specific site in the brain that it acts on directly to cause migraine? Have other kinds of anxiogenic drugs been studied from this point of view?

SANDLER: The archetypal anxiogenic drug, of course, which acts in humans as a benzodiazepine receptor inverse agonist is β-carboline-3-carboxylic acid ethylester (β-CCE; Dorow *et al.* 1983). It has not been investigated in a migraine context and headache was not reported after its administration.

GLOVER: These compounds are interesting tools but they are no longer used in humans because they may be dangerous.

PEATFIELD: I do not think we can completely dismiss tyramine as a substance of some interest. Although tyramine is not the triggering factor in any of the foods and drinks that we have studied, it can induce headache in some patients. Hanington (1983) has found this, and I also found this when I was doing blood pressure studies (Peatfield *et al.* 1983). So tyramine is one possible trigger, the first to have been suggested. The real trigger factor must be something quite different, but it may operate via a similar biochemical pathway.

GLOVER: I doubt that it is a trigger factor in the real world, except possibly in cheese.

PEATFIELD: There should be some proper biochemical analysis of chocolate. Chocolate is very complex, containing many lipids, and may well contain some active ingredient, such as a phenolic amine, covalently bound to those lipids. If the biochemical analysis of it involves grinding it up with chloroform, this is very far removed from the way the chocolate is handled *in vivo*.

GLOVER: Chocolate analysis on a mass spectrometer would reveal about 5000 peaks! However, I believe that theobromine is a likely candidate.

PEATFIELD: Have you done any of your *tyramine sulphate excretion tests* on patients with chronic daily headaches? This might reveal some interesting insights into the difference between them and the patients who have episodic attacks of headache, be they migrainous or not according to the new classification developed by Professor Olesen's committee (Headache Classification Committee 1988).

GLOVER: We are starting to study that, and have so far found an even higher incidence of low tyramine sulphoconjugator than among the migraine patients — something like seven out of 10.

COPPEN: Some years ago, we looked at the *tyramine pressor test* in migraine (Ghose *et al.* 1977) and found another similarity between depression and migraine. The tyramine pressor test allows you to estimate how much tyramine is needed to raise the blood pressure by 30 mmHg. We found that depressives were very sensitive to tyramine, and that migraine patients had almost the same hypersensitivity.

SANDLER: There is another aspect to consider in the sensitivity of migraine patients to intravenous tyramine. When Dr Peatfield was working with our group, he looked at a number of patients with low platelet MAO activity and a comparable clinical group with normal platelet activity (Peatfield *et al.* 1983). Those with MAO values one standard deviation or more lower than the mean showed a significantly greater pressor sensitivity to intravenous tyramine. Thus, the platelet MAO deficit may reflect a more generalized decrease in MAO activity in the body.

PEATFIELD: Yes. The interesting thing was that the dietary-induced migraine patients among that group got headaches, while the non-dietary patients did not. Whether a headache developed was not correlated with their calculated tyramine sensitivity, nor with the increase in blood pressure that was produced by the tyramine. We suggested that two separate substances must be released from the nerve endings as a result of tyramine. One of these was rapidly increasing the blood pressure, and the other was giving them a headache after an hour or more. Perhaps some peptide was released as well as noradrenaline, but this is speculation.

COPPEN: In our intravenous tyramine tests on depressive patients we did not observe headaches afterwards. And I do not think the migraine patients had headaches either.

PEATFIELD: We differ about this. I suspect it is just a reflection of the selection of the population.

COPPEN: This demonstration of a high sensitivity to intravenous tyramine has been reproduced several times. It is an interesting finding, and still requires an explanation.

WELCH: Dr Glover, when you found the significant association between red wine and migraine in the patients who believed they had such a dietary trigger, you suggested that flavonoid phenols, rather than the low levels of tyramine, were plausible constituents for triggering the attacks. Can you be sure the behavioural association — taking the chocolate or taking the red wine — is not provoked by the anxiety that also triggers the migriane? Do you have to invoke a chemical?

GLOVER: That was why we did a placebo-controlled study for both the red wine and the chocolate trial, using different chemicals but with similar appearances and tastes.

GROSS: Some patients seem to distinguish between certain types of red wine if they say they are red wine-sensitive. They say that they tend to produce migraines after drinking cheap red wine, but they have relatively little trouble from claret. Is there anything, chemically, that could explain this?

GLOVER: Yes. We have speculated that the flavonoid phenols are involved. They make the difference between red and white wine, and they tend to polymerize as the wine ages. In this polymerized form, perhaps one does not absorb them.

WELCH: Do you believe that migraine is a low 5-HT state?

GLOVER: I think it is possible that low 5-HT predisposes to it.

WELCH: We have been studying the platelet dense body (which contains 5-HT and catecholamine) as a model of vesicular function in the CNS (Pletscher et al. 1984). Between migraine attacks, the platelet dense body is present in large numbers, and the turnover of 5-HT is lower. There is also an impaired secretion of 5-HT as revealed by ATP release. We believe the impaired secretion is because of changes in the cytosolic Ca^{2+} concentration. If these results can be translated to CNS neurones they might suggest a low 5-HT state, based on impaired release. So it is compatible with what you said. We may, therefore, suppose there is a big store of 5-HT in the dense body and a low functional 5-HT state between migraine attacks. When the migraine stimulus comes along — perhaps stress — there could be a massive release of the 5-HT. Some features of migraine could be explained on this basis: changes in the sensory endings, for example. In summary, at the start of a migraine attack there would be a low functional 5-HT state, high 5-HT stores, sudden release of the 5-HT, stimulation of the cortical events, and the painful sensory events would follow. Initially, there would be antinociception because of the release of the same 5-HT. As the 5-HT becomes depleted by the release, a flow of the nociceptive impulses would ensue. This theory explains the biphasic nature of the disease — both the initial prodrome and also the headache.

GLOVER: I think that during a migraine attack the *changes* in the 5-HT system could be important. We should also consider the possibility of changes in 5-HT receptors — up- or down-regulation.

VANE: I have become a little lost in all of this. What was the experimental result on which you based your speculations, Dr Welch?

WELCH: That is the problem! We have pathophysiological data on the platelet dense body in humans. We also have pharmacological evidence of benefit from serotoninergic drugs. Those results would be compatible, both centrally and peripherally, with the system that I have outlined. What one cannot do is to measure the 5-HT metabolism in the central nervous system.

GLOVER: We hope that one day, with PET scanning, that might be possible.

WELCH: That is a long way away. One may be able to measure 5-HT receptors in the cortex by that method, but is will be a long time before one can do dynamic studies.

GROSS: You mentioned, Dr Glover, the problem of why some phenomena, such as stress, will produce migraine in some people but not in others. The extension of that argument is to ask why stress produces migraine in susceptible patients at some time and not at other times. And why is there a reversal so that some patients with migraine develop their problems at the *end* of a so-called stressful situation? Could that be related to the stress producing a constant 'high' of 5-HT, and allowing a 'relaxation' of the 5-HT when the stress is over?

GLOVER: Part of the problem is that one can make a theory fit almost anything!

WELCH: John Fozard in his paper (this volume) said that migraine had to be a 5-HT depletion state, from evidence based on the reserpine studies. The headache occurs as 5-HT is released or shortly after. 5-HT may, indeed, be effective in relieving headache, but there must be an initial 5-HT release. You said, Dr Fozard, that 5-HT is not released centrally, because there is a lot of MAO present, centrally.

FOZARD: No! I said that it was highly likely that 5-HT would reach the outside of the cell in an intact form because it seemed to be packaged within neurones with monoamine oxidase B, for which 5-HT has a relatively low affinity.

GLOVER: But that is just within the serotoninergic fibre. There is plenty of MAOA around in other cells.

PEATFIELD: 5-HT could easily be doing one thing for the nociceptive system and another thing on an inflammatory basis. It could be causing pain by a peripheral action when, paradoxically, it might be antinociceptive via more physiological spinal cord pathways.

CURZON: We always talk about reserpine acting to release 5-HT. There is no doubt that it releases it to monoamine oxidase inside the neurone but is there any evidence that reserpine ever releases 5-HT to receptors, except in the presence of a monoamine oxidase inhibitor? If it does not release 5-HT to receptors, that would simplify considerably the interpretation of reserpine-induced headache.

GLOVER: The sort of MAO inside serotoninergic neurones is MAOB, which does not act on 5-HT, so, theoretically, if 5-HT is released from vesicles inside neurones it should just go straight on out.

FOZARD: David Bouillin (1978) incubated platelets with reserpine *in vitro* and found that what came out is unmetabolized 5-HT. May I please return to Dr Welch's concept of the platelet reflecting what is going on in the CNS (Pletscher *et al.* 1984)? The problem with that idea is that the platelet cannot synthesize 5-HT. Therefore, when 5-HT is lost from the platelet, it will not be replenished unless it is taken up from the plasma. In contrast, the brain neurones have the synthetic machinery for 5-HT. In 5-HT-containing neurones there is also a feedback inhibitory control mechanism operating, so that when the neurone releases its newly synthesized 5-HT, synthesis increases to replace what has been lost. It is, therefore, quite inappropriate to infer from platelet data that there may be a low 5-HT state in the brain. Neurones conserve their transmitters very effectively, and one cannot draw too many analogies between the platelet and the neurone.

SANDLER: I cannot agree that it is simply a question of the wrong kind of MAO in the 5-HT neurone. One simply needs *enough* 5-HT to be present for it to act as a substrate for MAOB. Another point is that I believe that platelets in migraine sufferers have been found to be more sensitive to platelet activating factor than normal platelets.

WELCH: Yes; that is Dr Joseph's work, which won the Wolff prize in 1988 (Joseph *et al.* 1988). We think it is a membrane effect.

VANE: Is this a significant difference, such as 5-fold or 2-fold?

WELCH: He studied platelet activating factor, thrombin and collagen with platelet cytosolic calcium activation being the marker of activity. He compared the migraine patients to stroke patients. Whereas the stroke patients showed a non-specific activation to all three, the migraine patients showed much more activity with platelet activating factor than the others. So it is not non-specific; it was compared with the stroke patients, and with controls.

CURZON: To return to my last point, if 5-HT is released by reserpine, why has nobody ever seen 5-HT syndrome behaviour in animals treated with reserpine? The 5-HT syndrome is a complex of motor behaviours that the rat shows when one gives it a 5-HT releaser — for example, parachloroamphetamine. Only a tiny fraction of the total neuronal 5-HT stores needs to be outside the neurone to produce the syndrome (Adell *et al.* 1989).

GLOVER: How do you suggest reserpine causes headaches?

CURZON: There seem to be two possibilities. Either 5-HT is coming out of the neurone or it is destroyed inside the neurone so that not enough 5-HT can come out.

GLOVER: It seems quite possible that reserpine is just depleting 5-HT so that when the neurone fires there is little release through vesicles.

WELCH: We have already said that reserpine in non-migraine patients does not produce the syndrome. That is the difference. And there is something different about the central serotoninergic metabolism in the migraine patients. I do not think one can draw the parallels with normal rats.

FOZARD: We know that reserpine is not selective for 5-HT. Reserpine given to a rat will deplete its neurones of all those monoamines that are bound within the granular complex; these would include noradrenaline, dopamine, *and* 5-HT. Because there will be concomitant depletion of noradrenaline and dopamine, there may well be a depressant effect which could suppress manifestation of an excitatory behavioural syndrome. It could be as simple as that.

References

Adell, A., Sarna, G.S., Hutson, P.H., and Curzon, G. (1989). An in vivo dialysis and behavioural study of the release of 5-HT by *p*-chloroamphetamine in reserpinized rats. *British Journal of Pharmacology* **97**, 206–12.

Boullin, D.J. (1978). Biochemical indicators of central serotonin function. In *Serotonin in mental abnormalites*, (ed. D.J. Boullin), pp. 1–28. Wiley, Chichester.

Dorow, R., Horowski, R., Paschelke, G., Amin, M., and Braestrup, C. (1983). Severe anxiety induced by FG7142, a β-carboline ligand for benzodiazepine receptors. *Lancet*, ii, 98–9.

Ghose, K., Coppen, A., and Carroll, D. (1977). Intravenous tyramine response in patients with migraine before and during treatment with indoramin. *British Medical Journal*, **1**, 1191–3.

Hanington, E. (1983). Migraine. In *Clinical reactions to food*, (ed. M.H. Lessof), pp. 155–80. Wiley, Chichester.

Headache Classification Committee of the International Headache Society. (Jes Olesen, chairman). (1988). Classification and diagnostic criteria for headache disorders, cranial neuralgias and facial pain. *Cephalalgia*, **8**, Suppl. 7, 1–96.

Hurst, W.J. and Toomey, P.B. (1981). High-performance liquid chromatographic determination of four biogenic amines in chocolate. *Analyst*, **106**, 394–402.

Joseph, R., Welch, K.M.A., Grunfeld, S., Oster, S.B., and D'Andrea, G. (1988). Cytosolic ionized calcium homeostasis in platelets: an abnormal sensitivity to PAF-activation in migraine. *Headache*, **28**, 396–402.

Mazumder, R.C., Glover, V., and Sandler, M. (1980). Progesterone provokes a selective rise of monoamine oxidase A in the female genital tract. *Biochemical Pharmacology*, **29**, 1857–9.

Peatfield, R., Littlewood, J.T., Glover, V., Sandler, M., and Rose, F.C. (1983). Pressor sensitivity to tyramine in patients with headache: relationship to platelet monoamine oxidase and to dietary provocation. *Journal of Neurology, Neurosurgery and Psychiatry*, **46**, 827–31.

Pletscher, A., Affolter, H., Cesuro, A.M., Ezne, P., and Muller, K. (1984). Blood platelets as model for neurons: similarities of the 5-hydroxytryptamine system. In *Progress in tryptophan and serotonin research*, (ed. H.G. Schlossberger, W. Kochen, B. Linzen, and H. Steinbast), pp. 231–9. Walter de Gruyter, Berlin.

Somerville, B.W. (1971). The role of progesterone in menstrual migraine. *Neurology*, **21**, 853–9.

Somerville, B.W. (1972). The role of estradiol withdrawal in the etiology of menstrual migraine. *Neurology*, **22**, 355–65.

Syvälahti, E., Kangasniemi, P., and Ross, S.B. (1979). Migraine headache and blood serotonin levels after administration of zimelidine, a selective inhibitor of serotonin uptake. *Current Therapeutic Research*, **25**, 299–310.

20. Depression and migraine

Kathleen R. Merikangas and Jules Angst

Association between migraine and depression

Clinical descriptions of migraine have noted the frequent occurrence of psychiatric symptoms with the migraine prodrome, with the attack, and during interim periods as well. Liveing (1873) described depression and drowsiness as characteristic concomitants of migraine; Moersch (1923) reported the frequent occurrence of mild mental and physical depression, characterized by a sense of apathy, lack of energy, and fatigue among migraine patients; and Wolff (1937) noted extreme physical fatigue and apathy as characteristic traits of subjects with migraine. A more recent description by Blau (1988) of the symptoms that comprise the migraine prodrome is remarkably similar to the symptoms that characterize the affective disorders: irritability, depression or elation, changes in motor activity, changes in appetite and sleep, and circadian rhythm disturbances.

Despite the consistency of this clinical observation, very few controlled studies have systematically examined the association between migraine and depression. Table 20.1 presents a review of studies from which data can be applied to examine this association. Most of these studies were derived from clinical samples, employed symptom checklists rather than diagnostic assessments of depression, and failed to use adequate control groups. Nevertheless, a significant association between migraine and depression was found in nearly all the studies that have examined this question, irrespective of the source of ascertainment of the index case.

There are several possible artefactual explanations for an association between two or more disorders. Associations may arise as artefacts of either the population stratification or the sampling source. An erroneous association may result from sampling of a particular stratum of the population in which there is an increased risk in the base rates of both conditions. The use of samples derived solely from clinical settings may also lead to erroneous inferences about associations between disorders. Two conditions may appear to be associated because of an increased likelihood of detection of cases with more than one condition. This is known as 'Berkson's bias', which originally resulted from sampling of hospitalized cases (Berkson 1946).

The association between migraine and depression cannot be attributed to increased treatment-seeking among subjects with both conditions, because

TABLE 20.1. *Association between migraine and depression: previous studies*

Source	Number of probands	Association	Controls	Authors
Clinical samples				
Migraine	500	Yes	No	Selby and Lance (1960)
	100	Yes	No	Kashiwagi *et al.* (1972)
	236	Yes	No	Couch *et al.* (1975)
Depression	100	Yes	Yes	Cassidy *et al.* (1957)
	423	Yes	No	Diamond (1964)
	116	No	No	Garvey *et al.* (1984)
	133	Yes	Yes	Merikangas *et al.* (1988)
Community samples				
	727	Yes	–	Crisp *et al.* (1977)
	1139	Yes	–	Paulin *et al.* (1985)
	400	Yes	–	Merikangas *et al.* (1988)

the association between the two conditions was found in community samples as well. Indeed, the association was stronger in unselected community samples than in studies that derived from treatment settings. Moreover, the association between migraine and depression remains after appropriate controls have been made for factors, such as sex or age, that may be expected to confound the relationship.

Epidemiology of migraine and depression

There is a remarkable similarity in the epidemiology of migraine and depression. Both disorders are more common in females and in young adults, and the two conditions have an equal distribution across race and social class. There is also a nearly equal lifetime prevalence of the two disorders with an average across different studies of 10 per cent for migraine and 12 per cent for major depression. The mean age of onset for both conditions occurs in the mid-to-late twenties.

Estimates of the prevalence and incidence of these disorders show a wide variation according to the definition of the syndrome and the method of its ascertainment. Because both migraine and depression rely solely on a clinical description of signs and symptoms, the point at which the diagnostic threshold should be drawn for frequency, duration, and impairment is not known. Operational definitions of both disorders have been established in order to minimize false positives. The studies reviewed here have generally used the definition of the Ad Hoc Committee for the Classification of Migraine (1962); and the Research Diagnostic Criteria (Spitzer *et al.* 1978) for defining major depression. The latter criteria require a two-to-four week

TABLE 20.2. *Association between migraine and depressive symptoms: epidemiological studies (US National Health and Nutrition Evaluation Survey)*

	Sex	Number	X̄ Depression score
Migraine	Female	835	12.14
	Male	144	10.68
Controls	Female	5454	9.16
	Male	3588	7.38

$F_{(4,10020)} = 81.23$, $p < 0.001$.

episode consisting of depressive or irritable mood, accompanied by disturbances of sleep, appetite, concentration, or motor activity, with a significant degree of impairment in the usual level of functioning.

National Health and Nutrition Examination Survey

Data from a recent follow-up to an epidemiological survey of the adult US population, the National Health and Nutrition Examination Survey (NHANES), provided further evidence for an association between migraine and depressive symptoms. The first survey for NHANES collected data from a national probability sample of the civilian non-institutionalized population of the United States between 1971 and 1974. This survey included 20 729 people between the ages of 25 to 74 years. A follow-up of this sample was conducted between 1982 and 1984 (Madans *et al.* 1986; National Center for Health Statistics 1987). Information was obtained on 93 per cent of the original sample.

The Center for Epidemiologic Studies Depression Scale (CES-D) was administered to 10 100 adults in order to estimate the current prevalence of a depressive syndrome. The CES-D is a self-reporting symptom scale which was designed to screen for depression in community surveys (Radloff 1977). The mean scores on the CES-D among subjects who had received a diagnosis of migraine are presented in Table 20.2. After controlling for the effect of age in a covariance analysis, a significant elevation in mean depression scores was found among subjects with migraine. The increased depression score is particularly interesting if one considers that many of these subjects no longer suffer from migraine.

Similar findings obtain if the CES-D scores are classified according to the cut-off score that represents clinically significant depression. Nearly twice as many migraine subjects (28.4 per cent) fell beyond the cut-off score of 15 when compared to subjects without migraine (that is, 15.1 per cent). The odds ratio of 1.4 (95 per cent confidence limits range from 1.3 to 1.6), adjusted for sex and age, indicates that migraine was significantly associated with a depressive syndrome.

Zurich cohort study of young adults

A second source of epidemiological data on the co-occurrence of migraine and major depression is a longitudinal study of young adults selected from the general population of Zurich in Switzerland (Angst *et al.* 1984; K.R. Merikangas, J. Angst, and H. Isler, unpublished results). This cohort was originally assessed in 1978, when the age of the subjects was 19 or 20. A previous report on this sample found a high prevalence of headaches (68 per cent), of which only approximately six per cent were of the migraine type. Although increased rates of anxiety and phobias were found among subjects with headache, the association between psychiatric syndromes and migraine headaches was not assessed (Angst and Dobler-Mikola 1983). Data have been collected from 457 subjects who participated in the most recent interview, in 1986, when they were 27 or 28 years of age. A structured psychiatric interview was administered by experienced clinicians with extensive training in clinical psychiatry. The criteria for migraine were assessed from the diagnostic interview that was conducted in 1986. These questions were developed by a neurologist (Dr H. Isler) who directs the headache clinic at the University Hospital, Zurich, and who has extensive experience in the diagnosis and treatment of headache. The criteria for the classification of headache of the migraine type were derived from those of the Ad Hoc Committee (1962).

Although 45 per cent of the subjects reported the presence of headaches during the previous year, the one-year prevalence of migraine headache was 13.4 per cent. Classical migraine was quite rare in this population, with a one-year prevalence of 4.6 per cent. This rate is comparable to those of other studies which find a low prevalence of classic migraine, or migraine with aura, in comparison with that of common migraine, or migraine without aura. As found in previous reports, females had a three-fold increase in the frequency of migraine as compared to males. The sex ratio approximates the one observed both in clinical samples and among relatives of clinical cases. There was a wide range in the reported age of onset of migraine (from 5 to 25 years), with the average age at onset being in the mid-teens.

The association between migraine headache and major depression is shown in Table 20.3. There was a strong association between migraine and major depression among both males and females. The adjusted risk ratio for migraine and depression was 2.9, indicating that people with migraine had three times the frequency of major depression as the controls. Subjects with migraine also showed higher rates of bipolar spectrum (defined as mania or hypomania), phobia, general anxiety, and panic than control subjects.

TABLE 20.3. *Association between migraine and major depression (Zurich, Switzerland, Cohort Study of Young Adults)**

	Sex	Number	Per cent major depression
Migraine	Female	53	18.6
	Male	19	7.7
Controls	Female	104	11.6
	Male	94	4.0

Adjusted risk ratio = 2.9, p < 0.01.
*K.R. Merikangas, J. Angst, and H. Isler, unpublished results.

However, no association was found between migraine and alcoholism, drug abuse, dysthymia, or obsessive–compulsive disorder. In general, the anxiety disorders were more strongly associated with migraine than were the affective disorders. However, the subjects in this study tended to manifest simultaneously symptoms of both anxiety and depression within episodes. Therefore, it was not possible to classify the subjects into either anxiety or depression alone.

The prospective design of the Zurich cohort study also allowed the onset and the time-course of the two conditions to be assessed. Although there was no association between migraine and major depression when the cohort was aged 21, a significant association emerged when the cohort was re-assessed at 24 to 25 years of age. The onset of migraine preceded that of major depression in 67 per cent of subjects with both conditions. Furthermore, the mean age of onset of migraine (14.9 years) was significantly lower than that of depression (17.0 years) in the latter group. A significant direct correlation was observed for the ages of onset of migraine and depression (r = 0.76, p < 0.01) (K.R. Merikangas, J. Angst, and H. Isler, unpublished results).

The results of the latter two studies, together with the previous studies, confirm that there is a strong association between migraine and major depression in both treated and untreated samples of subjects with either condition. However, these results do not provide evidence about possible mechanisms for the association.

Explanations for the association between migraine and depression

There are two possible explanations for an association between two or more conditions. Either the conditions are aetiologically related, thereby sharing common underlying pathological mechanisms, or they are causally related, with one disorder causing or leading to the development of the second condition. Evidence for these explanations may be derived from the following scientific sources: follow-up studies, which demonstrate the course and precursors of the conditions; neurobiological studies and challenge paradigms, which can identify any common underlying susceptibility and aetiological factors; and family studies, which can investigate the co-aggregation of the two conditions.

If the relationship between migraine and depression were aetiological, with migraine causing depression or the converse, the two disorders would not be expected to breed true in families. Rather, the relatives should manifest an increased risk of the *same disorder as the proband* (the index case), or an increased risk of *the combination of the two syndromes*. If migraine caused depression, relatives of probands with migraine should have an increased risk of major depression, but *only* in the presence of a lifetime history or concomitant expression of migraine. Conversely, if depression causes migraine, rates of migraine would be elevated among relatives of probands with depression, but *only* in combination with depression. Rates of either migraine or depression alone should approximate the population base rates.

A common aetiological mechanism for the association between migraine and depression would be suggested by an increased risk, compared to expected population rates, of pure forms of either disorder being found among the relatives of probands with pure forms of the other condition. Therefore, relatives of probands with 'pure' migraine should have an increased risk of pure depression, and *vice versa*.

Co-aggregation of migraine and depression in families

We have studied the association between migraine and major depression in a group of 133 probands with major depression, a group of 82 normal community controls and their 400 interviewed first-degree relatives. There was a significant association between depression and migraine among both the probands and the relatives. We also found that concomitant symptoms of anxiety were prominent among the depressed subjects with migraine.

The results of the application of a bivariate threshold model to test the relationship between the two conditions is shown in Figure 20.1 (Merikangas *et al.* 1988). Both depression and migraine were strongly familial, with transmissibility coefficients of $G_d = 0.62$ and $G_m = 0.58$, respectively. Although we could not definitively resolve the source of the correlation of the two conditions among the relatives, their association did not appear to be highly transmissible. The best fitting model yielded significant components for the unique transmissibility of each of the two disorders and a significant non-transmissible correlation of $E_{DM} = 0.73$, p < 0.01. Thus, the two conditions did not appear to result from the same underlying aetiological factors, as demonstrated by a lack of cross-transmission of the pure forms of the two conditions among probands and their relatives. Rather,

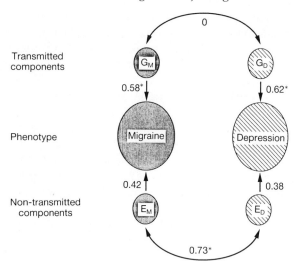

FIG. 20.1. The results of bivariate threshold model of the co-segregation of migraine and depression. G, transmissible component; E, non-transmissible component.

the results suggested either that depression is a sequela of migraine or that the two conditions comprise a distinct subtype of migraine.

The most likely explanation for the above findings is that the combination of the two disorders comprises a subtype of either migraine or depression, in which the symptoms of both disorders are manifest at some point during the longitudinal course. Because disturbances in the same neurochemical systems have been implicated in both disorders, perturbation of a particular system or systems related to migraine may decrease the threshold for depression and precipitate affective symptoms (Mohns 1980).

These findings have both clinical and research implications. Clinicians should systematically assess migraine patients to ascertain the presence of incapacitating major depression or anxiety. The association between migraine and depression, particularly in the light of the finding of this association from prospective data, warrants further study. Future studies that may differentiate pure migraine from migraine associated with an affective disorder could usefully focus on such domains as neurochemistry, treatment response, or brain imaging.

Summary

1. Migraine is strongly associated with depressive symptoms and with a diagnosis of major depression, irrespective of the source of case ascertainment — whether from treatment settings, for either of the two conditions, or from epidemiological samples.

2. Data from prospective studies indicate that the age of onset for migraine and that for depression are highly correlated ($r = 0.76$) with the onset of migraine preceding that of depression by an average of three years in both males and females.

3. An evaluation of possible mechanisms for the association — through analysis of co-aggregation of migraine and depression in families — revealed that the two conditions are not alternative manifestations of the same underlying aetiological factors. Rather, it appears that migraine with depression may represent a subtype of migraine.

4. These findings have important implications for the evaluation and treatment of migraine. A psychiatric assessment, particularly of affective disorders, is strongly indicated by these findings. Choice of treatment may also be influenced by the presence of a chronic or a recurrent depression, or of anxiety syndromes that may lead to significant distress and to social and occupational impairment.

Acknowledgements

This research was supported in part by the United States Public Health Service, Alcohol, Drug Abuse, and Mental Health Administration grants AA07080 and DA50348, by Research Scientist Development Award MH00499 (to Dr Merikangas); and by grant 3.948.085 from the Swiss National Science Foundation (to Dr Angst).

References

'*Ad Hoc*' Committee of the National Institute of Neurological Disease and Blindness: classification of headache (1962). *Archives of Neurology*, **6**, 173–6.

Angst, J., and Dobler-Mikola, A. (1983). Epidemiologic study of headaches in 20-year olds. In *Kopfschmerz 1983: nomenclature and classification of headache syndromes*, (ed. G.S: Barolin, J. Kugler, and D. Soyka), pp. 120–30. Enke, Stuttgart.

Angst, J., Dobler-Mikola, A., and Binder, J. (1984). The Zurich study — a prospective epidemiological study of depressive, neurotic and psychosomatic syndromes. I: Problem, methodology. *European Archives of Psychiatry and Neurological Sciences*, **234**, 13–20.

Berkson, J. (1946). Limitations of the application of fourfold table analysis to hospital data. *Biometrics Bulletin*, **2**: 47–53.

Blau, J.N. (1988). Premonitory symptoms of migraine. In *Basic mechanisms of headache*, (ed. J. Olesen and L. Edvinsson), pp. 345–51. Elsevier, Amsterdam.

Cassidy, W.L., Flanagan, N.B., and Spellman, M.E. (1957). Clinical observations in manic-depressive disease. *Journal of the American Medical Association*, **164**, 1535–46.

Couch, J.R., Ziegler, D.K., and Hassanein, R.S. (1975). Evaluation of the relationship between migraine headache and depression. *Headache*, **15**, 41–50.

Crisp, A.H., Kalucy, R.S., McGuinness, B., Ralph, P.C. and Harris, G. (1977).

Some clinical, social and psychological characteristics of migraine subjects in the general population. *Postgraduate Medical Journal*, **53**, 691–7.

Diamond, J. (1964). Depressive headaches. *Headache*, **4**, 255–8.

Garvey, M.J., Tollefson, G.D., and Schaffer, C.B. (1984). Migraine headaches and depression. *American Journal of Psychiatry*. **141**, 986–8.

Kashiwagi, T., McClure, J.N. and Wetzel, R.D. (1972). Headache and psychiatric disorder. *Diseases of the Nervous System*, **33**, 659–63.

Liveing, E. (1873). *On megrim, sick-headache, and some allied disorders: a contribution to the pathology of nerve storms*. Churchill, London.

Madans, J.H. *et al.* (1986) Ten years after NHANES I: report of initial followup 1982–1984. *Public Health Reports*, **101**, 465–73.

Merikangas, K.R., Risch, N.J., Merikangas, J.R., Weissman, M.M., and Kidd, K.K. (1988). Migraine and depression: association and familial transmission. *Journal of Psychiatric Research*, **22**, 119–29.

Moersch, F.P. (1923). Psychic manifestations in migraine. *American Journal of Psychiatry*, **3**, 697–716.

Mohns, E.P. (1980). The biochemistry of affective disorders and their relationship to headache. In *Wolff's headache and other head pain*. (ed. D. Dalessio) pp. 418–39. Oxford University Press, New York.

National Center for Health Statistics. (1987). *Plan and operation of the NHANES I epidemiologic followup study, 1982–1984, Vital and Health Statistics*, Series 1, No. 122, DHHS Publ No. (Public Health Service) 87–1324.

Paulin, J.M., Waal-Manning, H.J., Simpson, F.O., and Knight, R.G. (1985). The prevalence of headache in a small New Zealand town. *Headache*, **25**, 147–51.

Radloff, L.S. (1977). The CES-D scale: A self-report depressive scale for research in the general population. *Journal of Applied Psychology and Measurement*, **1**, 385–401.

Selby, G. and Lance, J.W. (1960). Observations on 500 cases of migraine and allied vascular headache. *Journal of Neurology, Neurosurgery and Psychiatry*, **23**, 23–32.

Spitzer, R.L., Endicott, J., and Robins, E. (1978). Research diagnostic criteria: rationale and reliability. *Archives of General Psychiatry*, **35**, 773–82.

Wolff, H.G. (1937). Personality features and reactions of subjects with migraine. *Archives of Neurology and Psychiatry*, **37**, 895–921.

Discussion

SANDLER: Your findings about bipolar depression and migraine are particularly interesting. The *tyramine sulphate excretion test* that we have used in depression seems to be fairly specific, in that it reveals a homogenous population of endogenous, *unipolar* depressives (Hale *et al.* 1986). Although some people with bipolar depression tend to have a low tyramine excretion, some have a high one. There is no correlation. The small number of bipolars that we have studied seem to form a different population altogether.

MERIKANGAS: We may be defining bipolar depression differently. The patients I have described are not, strictly, full-blown bipolar depressives. They meet criteria for bipolar II disorder, which requires a history of hypomania rather than mania.

GLOVER: Are you suggesting that there is a different form of depression among these migraine patients from the depression in non-migraineurs?

MERIKANGAS: No; the depression in migraineurs is more often characterized as 'atypical' or retarded. However, this form of depression is quite common in clinical populations, particularly among people with bipolar illness. It may be considered as a depression of young adult life, and it may become more of the so-called melancholic endogenous depression with age. We may not be finding differences at all, depending on the age-dependent expression. Young adults express anxiety, and as the anxiety increases it turns more into depression.

GLOVER: Can you infer how many genes might be involved? Would this fit with a single locus?

MERIKANGAS: Because we did not interview the relatives directly, we did not conduct segregation analyses. Therefore we cannot infer anything about the number of genes involved. My review of the data from previous studies indicates that there is probably a single major locus rather than multiple genes.

COPPEN: In a group of patients with severe bipolar depression would you expect their prevalence of migraine to be significantly higher than that of a unipolar group?

MERIKANGAS: Yes.

COPPEN: We have a large clinic of bipolar depressive patients that we have been seeing for some years now, and your paper encourages me to look seriously at the prevalence of migraine amongst them. Yet, my impression is that the prevalence is relatively low.

MERIKANGAS: I would predict that migraine would be more common among people with bipolar type II than amongst those with bipolar I disorder, or manic depressive psychosis.

WELCH: Some people have observed that migraine that is post-episodic tends to coalesce and become more frequent, almost becoming like the chronic daily headache. Have you studied whether there is any time-locking between the onset of depression and a change in the headache pattern?

MERIKANGAS: No; we did not examine that. Most of these young people did not meet criteria for a diagnosis of chronic daily headache. The prospective data from the Zurich Cohort Study by Jules Angst will tell us more about the onset of depression and the course of migraine.

WELCH: Were they already diagnosed as having migraine at the time you first saw them with depression?

MERIKANGAS: They had already been diagnosed as having migraine, mostly common migraine. Very few of them suffered from 'classical' migraine or 'migraine with aura'. I shall be applying the new diagnostic criteria to these categories in the near future.

WELCH: Was there a change in the frequency or character of the headache after these patients had suffered from depression?

MERIKANGAS: We have no evidence for such a change. These patients were only 28 years old when last seen, so we may need to follow them for another 10 years before such evidence is available.

BLAU: People have always been looking for associations between migraine and other conditions. Epilepsy was the association 'in vogue' in the 1920s; allergy was the association in the '30s and 40s'. But we now believe that migraine is not related to epilepsy or to allergy. I have not seen any association between migraine and depression among the 200 migraine patients that I see each year. I wonder what are your criteria for diagnosing migraine. There is no question that a patient with depression will get headaches, but they are not, in my opinion, migrainous headaches. And, of course, patients with migraine can become depressed. But I would need a lot of convincing to see a relation between migraine ánd depression.

SANDLER: We are perfectly happy that the criteria for diagnosis of migraine were satisfied in our studies (see Glover and Sandler, this volume). Our patients were properly examined by both neurologists and psychiatrists.

GLOVER: Yes. It was the patient's history that was no striking. It was not the current depression. It needed a three-hour psychiatric interview to bring out that they had a lifetime history of endogenous depression.

MERIKANGAS: In our studies, too, we are assessing lifetime histories, rather than current depression alone. Our analyses were conducted blindly, so that the interviewers did not know whether the subject had a history of migraine. Nor were they aware of any family history of either depression or migraine. Thus, the evidence collected blindly from cases and controls, coupled with that derived from epidemiological studies, is quite convincing. In order to determine whether depression exists, one must conduct a psychiatric interview. We found that a large proportion of subjects with clinically significant depression, or anxiety disorder, or both, had not been appropriately assessed or treated for their migraine by their own physicians. Informant reports will often uncover such information on depressive syndromes as well. Co-morbidity for depression may not only affect treatment outcome among migraine patients, but may confound clinical research as well.

References

Hale, A.S., Walker, P.L., Bridges, P.K., and Sandler, M. (1986). Tyramine conjugation deficit as a trait-marker in endogenous depressive illness. *Journal of Psychiatric Research*, **20**, 251–61.

21. Pain, headache, and depression: a discussion

Richard C. Peatfield

Introduction

It is self-evident that any patient with chronic pain is liable to become depressed (Kramlinger *et al.* 1983), and specific treatment for this depression may be justified. Of potentially greater interest is the way in which depressed patients may develop somatic symptoms, of which pain and particularly headache are among the commonest (Singh 1968; Katon *et al.* 1982; Blumer and Heilbronn 1982*a,b*; von Knorring 1983; Merskey 1988). In some non-European cultures, indeed, such somatization is commoner than the more familiar misery, anorexia, and sleep disturbances (Singh 1968; Katon *et al.* 1982). Patients seem to be more likely to experience pains when they are depressed, and are much more likely to seek medical advice about them then.

While structural causes of head, face, and dental pain must always be considered, the vast majority of patients seeking medical advice with such pains (and, indeed, with back pain too) have no demonstrable physical cause, if not for the pain at all, then for pain of the severity expressed in the consultation. Many of these are depressed, though responsiveness of this depression to drug treatment does not correlate consistently with depression rating-scale scores. In the study by Garvey *et al.* (1983) of 116 depressed out-patients, 26 complained of headaches before becoming depressed, and an additional 37 developed headaches only when they became depressed. Other generalized somatic symptoms were commoner among this latter group than among those who experienced headache before their depression.

Biochemical evidence

There is evidence of reduced serotonin (5-HT) turnover in chronic pain patients, which may be reversed by tricyclic drugs (Feinmann 1985). In addition, serotoninergic pathways are known to interact with opioid receptors in the brain and spinal cord (Feinmann 1985). Platelet serotonin uptake is reduced in depression (Tuomisto *et al.* 1979), but seems normal in migraine (Lingjaerde and Monstad 1986). Platelet binding sites for imipramine are reduced in chronic pain patients (Magni *et al.* 1987*a*), including patients whose pain responded to mianserin, even though they were not overtly depressed (Magni *et al.* 1987*b*). Reduced platelet imipramine binding sites have also been found in migraine patients (Geaney *et al.* 1984). The dexamethasone suppression test is significantly abnormal in patients with chronic pain, whether or not they are clinically depressed (France *et al.* 1987). Lowered β-endorphin levels in the cerebrospinal fluid, in contrast, seem to be found in patients experiencing pain, but not in pain-free depressed patients (Nappi *et al.* 1985).

Pharmacological evidence

Tricyclic antidepressants, such as amitriptyline, have been found to be effective both in migraine (Couch and Hassanein 1979; Ziegler *et al.* 1987) and in more chronic 'tension' headaches (Diamond and Baltes 1971; Fogelholm and Murros 1985). Benefit in these trials seems independent of the effect of the drug on depressive symptoms. Fluoxetine, a serotonin uptake inhibitor without 5-HT$_2$ receptor blocking activity (Ogren and Fuxe 1985) is also of value to chronic headache patients (Sjaastad 1983), though its results in migraine treatment are less consistent (Orholm *et al.* 1986).

Patients with atypical facial pain have responded in double-blind trials with phenelzine (Lascelles 1966), and dothiepin (Feinmann *et al.* 1984). The latter study involved careful quantitative psychiatric assessment of the patients. The psychiatric disturbance improved equally in the dothiepin and placebo groups, but pain relief was more frequent and better sustained in the dothiepin group. Psychiatric symptoms, when present, resolved as the pain was relieved, and refractory pain was associated with persistent psychiatric symptoms. The benefit of amitriptyline in post-herpetic neuralgia (Watson *et al.* 1982) and in painful diabetic neuropathy (Max *et al.* 1987) was, again, independent of the prior psychiatric state of the patients, and was not associated with mood improvement. These and other trials, and their mechanisms, are reviewed by Feinmann (1985).

Possible mechanisms

It may be naive to assume that these drugs have an action on the patients' symptom *per se*, rather than on the psychiatric or personality factors that have led the patient to seek medical advice. Tricyclic drugs do have analgesic properties in animal models where psychiatric mechanisms would seem inappropriate (Botney and Fields 1983; Spiegel *et al.* 1983). One wonders if the abnormal transmitters and/or receptors that affect mood and pain are on separate neuronal systems, or whether depression (in part at least) merely means that noxious afferents are being allowed to reach higher centres and, thus, to affect mood. Recent trials suggest that there are patients who do not fulfil research criteria for depression, yet their pain responds to treatment with tricyclic drugs.

References

Blumer, D. and Heilbronn, M. (1982*a*). Chronic pain as a variant of depressive disease — the pain-prone disorder. *Journal of Nervous and Mental Disease*, **170**, 381–406.

Blumer, D. and Heilbronn, M. (1982*b*). Chronic muscle contraction headache and pain-prone disorder. *Headache*, **22**, 180–3.

Botney, M. and Fields, H. (1983). Amitriptyline potentiates morphine analgesia by a direct action on the central nervous system. *Annals of Neurology*, **13**, 160–4.

Couch, J. and Hassanein, R.S. (1979). Amitriptyline in migraine prophylaxis. *Archives of Neurology*, **36**, 695–9.

Diamond, S. and Baltes, B.J. (1971). Chronic tension headache — treated with amitriptyline — a double-blind study. *Headache*, **11**, 110–6.

Feinmann, C. (1985). Pain relief by antidepressants: possible modes of action. *Pain*, **23**, 1–8.

Feinmann, C., Harris, M., and Cawley, R. (1984). Psychogenic facial pain: presentation and treatment. *British Medical Journal*, **288**, 436–8.

Fogelholm, R. and Murros, K. (1985). Maprotiline in chronic tension headache: a double-blind cross-over study. *Headache*, **25**, 273–5.

France, R.D., Krishnan, R.R., Trainor, M., and Pelton, S. (1987). Chronic pain and depression. IV: DST as a discriminator between chronic pain and depression. *Pain*, **28**, 39–44.

Garvey, M.J., Schaffer, C.B., and Tuason, V.B. (1983). Relationship of headaches to depression. *British Journal of Psychiatry*, **143**, 544–7.

Geaney, D.P., Rutterford, M.G., Elliott, J.M., Schachter, M., Peet, K.M.S., and Grahame-Smith, D.G. (1984). Decreased platelet ^{3}H-imipramine binding sites in classical migraine. *Journal of Neurology, Neurosurgery and Psychiatry*, **47**, 720–3.

Katon, W., Kleinman, A., and Rosen, G. (1982). Depression and somatization: a review. *American Journal of Medicine*, **72**, 127–35, and 241–7.

Kramlinger, K.G., Swanson, D.W., and Maruta, T. (1983). Are patients with chronic pain depressed? *American Journal of Psychiatry*, **140**, 747–9.

Lascelles, R.G. (1966). Atypical facial pain and depression. *British Journal of Psychiatry*, **112**, 651–9.

Lingjaerde, O. and Monstad, P. (1986). The uptake, storage, and efflux of serotonin in platelets from migraine patients. *Cephalalgia*, **6**, 135–9.

Magni, G. *et al.* (1987*a*). [^{3}H]Imipramine binding sites are decreased in platelets of chronic pain patients. *Acta Psychiatrica Scandinavica*, **75**, 108–10.

Magni, G. *et al.* (1987*b*). Modifications of [^{3}H]imipramine binding sites in platelets of chronic pain patients treated with mianserin. *Pain*, **30**, 311–20.

Max, M.B. *et al.* (1987). Amitriptyline relieves diabetic neuropathy pain in patients with normal or depressed mood. *Neurology*, **37**, 589–96.

Merskey, H. (1988). Chronic pain syndromes and their treatment. In *Recent advances in clinical neurology*, (ed. C. Kennard), Vol. 5, pp. 87–107. Churchill Livingstone, Edinburgh.

Nappi, G., Facchinetti, F., Martignoni, E., Petraglia, F., Bono, G., and Genazzani, A.R. (1985). CSF β-EP in headache and depression. *Cephalalgia*, **5**, 99–101.

Ogren, S.O. and Fuxe, K. (1985). Effects of antidepressant drugs on cerebral serotonin receptor mechanisms. In *Neuropharmacology of serotonin*, (ed. A.R. Green), pp. 131–80. Oxford University Press, Oxford.

Orholm, M., Honore, P.K., and Seeberg, I. (1986). A randomized general practice group-comparative study of femoxetine and placebo in the prophylaxis of migraine. *Acta Neurologica Scandinavica*, **74**, 235–9.

Singh, G. (1968). The diagnosis of depression. *Punjab Medical Journal*, **18**, 53–9.

Sjaastad, O. (1983). So-called 'tension headache' — the response to a 5-HT uptake inhibitor: femoxetine. *Cephalalgia*, **3**, 53–60.

Spiegel, K., Kalb, R., and Pasternak, G.W. (1983). Analgesic activity of tricyclic antidepressants. *Annals of Neurology*, **13**, 462–5.

Tuomisto, J., Tukiainen, E., and Ahlfors, U.G. (1979). Decreased uptake of 5-hydroxytryptamine in blood platelets from patients with endogenous depression. *Psychopharmacology*, **65**, 141–7.

von Knorring, L., Perris, C., Eisemann, M., Eriksson, U., and Perris, H. (1983). Pain as a symptom in depressive disorders. I: relationship to diagnostic subgroup and depressive symptomatology. *Pain*, **15**, 19–26.

Watson, C.P., Evans, R.J., Reed, K., Merskey, H., Goldsmith, L., and Warsh, J. (1982). Amitriptyline versus placebo in post-herpetic neuralgia. *Neurology*, **32**, 671–3.

Ziegler, D.K., Hurwitz, A., Hassanein, R.S., Kodanaz, H.A., Preskorn, S.H., and Mason, J. (1987). Migraine prophylaxis. A comparison of propranolol and amitriptyline. *Archives of Neurology*, **44**, 486–9.

Discussion

LANCE: In 1964, we did a double-blind controlled trial, showing that amitriptyline was helpful in the treatment of chronic daily headache (Lance and Curran 1964). We found no relation at all between the response of the patient and the presence or absence of depression. There are many reasons other than the relief of depression for the effectiveness of 5-HT re-uptake blockers. Patients with atypical facial pain have, in my opinion, an underlying organic initiating factor. The pain commonly starts after some trauma — for example, a dental extraction. The major site of the pain is often in the nasolabial fold or at a point in the chin opposite the lower gum. These are precisely the same points that act as a trigger for trigeminal neuralgia.

PEATFIELD: I am not asking how the pain starts but why, in biochemical terms, it persists for so long.

LANCE: In post-herpetic neuralgia, the herpes virus destroys part of the inhibitory pathway centrally. There may be unrestrained firing of pain pathways. By analogy with this, a virus may enter the nervous system at, say, the time of a tooth extraction, and 'knock out' specifically a segmental part of the trigeminal pain pathways, thus causing atypical facial pain.

PEATFIELD: So why do you think patients get better on both major forms of antidepressant treatment?

LANCE: For the same reason that post-herpetic neuralgia patients do — that, in all probability, 5-HT builds up in depleted pain-control pathways. Patients with atypical facial pain are often depressed, and antidepressant treatment reduces the pain to the point where they can tolerate it. But I do not think that this therapy is acting only on the psyche. I believe that there is an organic basis to atypical facial pain, which leads to secondary depression.

PEATFIELD: Could that organic basis be the same organic basis of chronic daily headache as well?

LANCE: It could be. I have often seen people who have never had a headache in their lives wake up one morning with a headache that then recurs daily, or with atypical facial pain that persists thereafter, without any obviously related physical or mental factor being present.

PEATFIELD: I wonder if there is a difference between chronic daily headache and atypical facial pain in terms of the biochemical pharmacology. There is clearly a difference in the location of the pain, but we need to know if there is a difference in the biochemical origin of the pain.

LANCE: One cannot answer that.

COPPEN: You mentioned that non-European patients sometimes present with different sorts of somatic symptoms when they have headache. We were the lead centre in the World Health Organization's study on dexamethasone suppression, a biological test in depression, and we had centres in 13 different countries, in which we used the research diagnostic criteria for depression and also the Hamilton Rating Scale for depression (World Health Organization 1987). We found, on the contrary, that these diagnostic scales for measuring depression were readily understood and were applicable amongst different cultures — in Japan, India, Russia, and the USA. The criteria seemed to have a universal application. Secondly, it is very interesting that tricyclic antidepressants now seem to have treatment applications in a wide variety of conditions, including the irritable bowel syndrome, low back pain, and joint pain.

PEATFIELD: Why are they working?

COPPEN: They must work because of some link with 5-HT and its role in pain thresholds or pain perception.

PEATFIELD: We need to consider how not only classical migraine and common migraine but also chronic daily headache may all be related to a pain threshold problem. To what extent can these conditions be interpreted in terms of attacks, with biochemical pathways triggered by specific events?

COPPEN: Interestingly, the dexamethasone suppression test, which is a sensitive measure in depression, is not specific, but is also abnormal, in people with chronic pain syndrome.

PEATFIELD: That is right. You have previously been correlating those results with your own rating scales for depression. Though your rating scales may not be wrong, perhaps there is a further subgroup of people who respond to tricyclics but who are at present outside the rating scale criteria for depression.

References

World Health Organization (1987). The dexamethasone suppression test in depression: a World Health Organization collaborative study. *British Journal of Psychiatry*, **150**, 459–62.

Lance, J.W. and Curran, D.A. (1964). Treatment of chronic tension headache. *Lancet*, **i**, 1236–9.

22. A note on the role of platelets in migraine: a personal view

Richard C. Peatfield

Any hypothetical pathogenesis of migraine has to try to explain the origin of the spreading depression that is believed to underly the classical aura, the occasional cerebral infarcts in classical migraine patients, and the association of migraine with mitral valve prolapse, though this seems to be no commoner in patients with prolonged auras (Pfaffenrath *et al.* 1987). We also need to explain the mechanism of headaches that so often follow a transient ischaemic attack. Two years ago (Peatfield 1987), I advanced the hypothesis that micro-aggregation of platelets is more or less universal, and usually asymptomatic, becoming evident in normal subjects only when large enough to cause the transient ischaemic attack or stroke. I wondered if smaller micro-aggregates would become symptomatic in migraine patients if they caused sufficient ischaemia to trigger spreading depression in the cerebral cortex, when the aggregates were too small to produce primary ischaemic symptoms themselves. Thus, the principal factor causing a patient to have classical migraine (that is, with aura) would be a susceptibility of cortical cells to spreading depression, rather than any particular abnormality of platelet function. This concept would be consistent with Pfaffenrath's observation.

The response to my hypothesis has been interesting — Marie Germaine Bousser drew my attention to a case she described in 1980, of a patient with thrombocythemia, who presented with focal neurological symptoms of gradual onset and also with headache, instead of a more typical transient ischaemic attack (Bousser *et al.* 1980). The attacks ceased when he was given an anti-platelet drug. The editorial that John Edmeads wrote (Edmeads 1987) to accompany my paper (Peatfield 1987) drew attention to the wide scatter of platelet function among migraine patients, and also to the increased aggregation among diabetics, whom we know have a lower prevalence of migraine.

The reason I had submitted such a speculative paper was the difficulty in devising experiments to refute it, and it is reassuring that others clearly feel the same.

Nevertheless I am reluctant to nail all my colours to the platelet hypothesis. Clearly, there is compelling evidence that platelet function is disturbed in many migraine patients (Peatfield 1987; Kozubski *et al.* 1987). Much of the evidence cited against the involvement of platelets is, at best, indirect: the equal efficacy of the pro-aggregant propranolol and the anti-aggregant metoprolol as migraine prophylactic drugs surely tells us only that neither works primarily by influencing platelet function (Steiner *et al.* 1985; Joseph and Welch 1987). This argument has subsequently become more heated (Steiner *et al.* 1987; Hanington 1987).

I persist in believing that much of the pathogenesis of each feature of migraine must relate to feedback loops. There must be two of these to account for the fact that the side affected by aura symptoms is not always the side affected by the headache. Each feedback loop must be able to enhance responses on one side at the expense of the other, and a loop eliminates the need to advance a single *cause* of migraine. As Joseph and Welch (1987) speculate, disturbed platelet function may, indeed, be a consequence of the attack. If platelets then failed to mop up neurotransmitters secreted from nerve endings in cerebral blood vessels and, instead (by the release reaction), re-released them in a deluge (Hanington 1986), this would amplify the pharmacological response induced by the nerve impulse (for example, a sterile inflammatory response) *on a local level*. Modest modifications to global platelet function may not affect an overwhelming disturbance taking place within a small blood vessel. All agree that the amount, for example, of 5-hydroxytryptamine (serotonin) released during a migraine attack is far higher than that stored by platelets under normal circumstances and, yet, that amount is unlikely to produce any generalized circulatory changes (Fozard 1982).

In summary, it may be possible to reconcile antagonistic views on the relevance of disturbed platelet function to the pathogenesis of migraine if abnormal re-release of absorbed neurotransmitters were to play a major role in a feedback loop that resulted in a sterile inflammatory reaction in extracerebral cranial blood vessels, and if platelet aggregates in the cerebral blood vessels were to trigger spreading depression, or even cortical infarcts.

References

Bousser, M.G., Conard, J., Lecrubier, C., and Bousser, J. (1980). Migraine ou accidents ischemiques transitoires au cours d'une thrombocytemie essentielle. Action de la ticlopidine. *Annales de Medecine Interne*, **131**, 87–90.

Edmeads, J. (1987). Platelets (again). *Headache*, **27**, 244–5.

Fozard, J.R. (1982). Serotonin, migraine and platelets. In *Drugs and platelets, Progress in pharmacology*, Vol. 4, (ed. P.A. Van Zwieten and E. Schönbaum), pp. 135–46. Fischer, Stuttgart.

Hanington, E. (1986). Viewpoint — the platelet and migraine. *Headache*, **26**, 411–5.

Hanington, E. (1987). Migraine is a platelet disorder. *Headache*, **27**, 401–2.

Joseph, R. and Welch, K.M.A. (1987). The platelet and migraine: a nonspecific association. *Headache*, **27**, 375–380.

Kozubski, W., Walkowiak, B., Cierniewski, C.S., and Prusinski, A. (1987). Platelet fibrinogen receptors in migraine patients. *Headache*, **27**, 431–4.

Peatfield R.C. (1987). Can transient ischaemic attacks and classical migraine always be distinguished? *Headache*, **27**, 240–3.

Pfaffenrath, V., Pollmann, W., Autenrieth, G., and Rosmanith, U. (1987). Mitral valve prolapse and platelet aggregation in patients with hemiplegic and non-hemiplegic migraine. *Acta Neurologica Scandinavica*, **75**, 253–7.

Steiner, T.J., Joseph, R., and Rose F.C. (1985). Migraine is not a platelet disorder. *Headache*, **25**, 434–40.

Steiner, T.J., Rose, F.C., and Joseph, R. (1987). Migraine is not a platelet disorder. *Headache*, **27**, 400.

Discussion

OLESEN: On the question of ipsilateral aura and headache, we saw similar figures in our retrospective studies when we analysed the location of aura symptoms and headache. Although I have been looking for three or four years, with single-photon emission computed tomography (SPECT), for a patient who presents with spontaneous ipsilateral headache and aura symptoms, I have not yet found one, amongst approximately 25 patients. Headaches artificially produced by intracarotid injection of contrast material are ipsilateral, while aura symptoms are contralateral (that is, from the ipsilateral hemisphere). The patients with spontaneous attacks always have headache on the side where they have a low blood flow and, of course, contralateral aura symptoms. We are still analysing this statistically, but several patients who claimed to have both ipsilateral headache and ipsilateral aura symptoms were not diagnosed in that way when we did the tomography. It seems that there is an inherent tendency for patients to recall that aura symptoms and headache are on the same side because it makes sense to them. But it does not make sense for us who know the anatomical connections. I personally doubt that such 'ipsilateral' cases exist.

PEATFIELD: I must accept that.

OLESEN: If my point of view is correct, it makes it easier for us to speculate about what is going on pathophysiologically.

WELCH: Dr Peatfield, if you conceive that there is a threshold for the depolarizing event — whether it is spreading depression or not — many stimuli may act to set off that event. We can look at the migrainous attack as a response of the brain and the vasculature to some challenge; so it is not inconceivable that a small platelet embolus might set this off. We should consider, here, the presence of a lupus anticoagulant in patients who present with migraine. This is an antiphospholipid group of antibodies that cause a platelet consumptive disorder. The first association of classical migraine with anticardiolipin antibody was presented by Hart *et al.* (1984) in a large series of young stroke patients. We have also reported a couple of cases (Levine *et al.* 1987). The predominant problem for these patients is that they develop stroke. It is likely that some of the previously reported patients with classical migraine, migrainous infarction, or young stroke with migraine have had an anticardiolipin or similar antibody, which has caused the stroke; the migrainous processes may be unrelated to the stroke. We should re-assess the concept of migrainous infarction, and unless we can exclude anticardiolipin antibodies we cannot say for certain that this is true migrainous infarction.

PEATFIELD: What is the pathogenesis of the classical migraine aura in those patients?

WELCH: We can only speculate. Is it related to a release of 5-HT? If the platelets are aggregable, is it related to platelet clumping? The anticardiolipin antibodies are not only directed against the platelet membrane, but also against the endothelial membrane, and possibly against the neuronal membrane. This relationship does not provide complete evidence for the platelet hypothesis, but it should increasingly be considered as contributing to it.

SANDLER: Montalban *et al.* (1988) have recently disputed that the anticardiolipin antibody is involved in migraine-related strokes.

WELCH: Nevertheless, patients with migraine-related strokes need to have the anticardiolipin antibody excluded as a factor in their disease. One cannot dispute the presence of an anticardiolipin antibody, but not all migraine-related strokes are necessarily related to it.

PEATFIELD: Do patients with a lupus anticoagulant have a long history of classical migraine?

WELCH: We have seen one patient who did. In another patient the migrainous auras were very varied: it was not a stereotype.

PEATFIELD: One could argue that as the lupus anticoagulant levels slowly build up, the volume of the platelet clumps increases until an infarction develops in the cortex.

WELCH: We look at it differently: there is an abnormality of platelet consumption, aggregation, and release. Periodically this is responsible for the transient symptoms. But the two patients we reported (Levine *et al.* 1987) did *not* have migrainous infarction. (Some cases of migrainous infarction *have* been reported to have an anticardiolipin antibody.)

PEATFIELD: Can you distinguish the ones with the antibodies from other patients with classical migraine by any other means?

WELCH: No.

MOSKOWITZ: We have heard a lot about 5-HT and platelets in our discussions. In my opinion, the 5-HT metabolite in urine — 5-hydroxyindoleacetic acid — has nothing to do with the nervous system, because the gut and the platelets must be the major source. Do we really have any experimental or clinical evidence to implicate the raphé system in the pathophysiology of migraine headache, other than by inference? The only evidence I know of relates to electrical stimulation of the periaqueductal grey, which inhibits the firing of nucleus caudalis cells that respond to stimulation of the vasculature (Strassman *et al.* 1986).

PEATFIELD: Raskin and his colleagues (1987) found that stimulation of the periaqueductal grey with implanted electrodes sometimes *caused* headache.

References

Hart, R.C. *et al.* (1984). Cerebral infarction associated with lupus anticoagulants. Preliminary report. *Stroke*, **15**, 114–8.

Levine, S.R., Joseph, R., D'Andrea, G., and Welch, K.M.A. (1987). Migraine and the lupus anticoagulant. Case reports and review of the literature. *Cephalalgia*, **7**, 93–9.

Montalban, J., Titus, F., Ordi, J., and Barquinero, J. (1988). Anticardiolipin antibodies and migraine-related strokes. *Archives of Neurology*, **45**, 601.

Raskin, N.H., Hosobuchi, Y., and Lamb, S. (1987). Headache may arise from perturbation of brain. *Headache*, **27**, 416–20.

Strassman, A., Mason, P., Moskowitz, M.A., and Maciewicz, R. (1986). Response of brainstem trigeminal neurons to electrical stimulation of the dura. *Brain Research*, **379**, 242–50.

23. Differential abnormalities in signal transduction in migraine and cluster headache

J. de Belleroche

Introduction

Over the past few years we have used a biochemical approach to study the pathogenesis of migraine by looking at transduction mechanisms which would be common to many agents that are putative trigger factors (for example, hormonal, stress-related, and dietary) in migraine and would also be common targets for a wide range of drug treatments. Hormones, dietary factors, neurogenic agents such as neurotransmitters, neuropeptides, and other neuromodulators and vasoactive agents are all implicated, most of which would mediate their actions through receptors in the cell membrane. Receptor activation is associated with the generation of second messengers — cyclic AMP (cAMP) from adenylate cyclase, and inositol trisphosphate and diacylglycerol from the polyphosphoinositide system (Fig. 23.1). The second messengers in turn produce their effects by activation of protein kinases (for example, cAMP and diacylglycerol) or by mobilization of calcium (for example, inositol trisphosphate); (Berridge and Irvine 1984; Nishizuka 1984). A number of prophylactic treatments would affect these pathways: for example, propranolol blocks the generation of cAMP in response to noradrenaline at β-adrenoceptors; and methysergide blocks the generation of inositol trisphosphate and diacylglycerol at 5-HT$_2$ receptors. Furthermore, in addition to the diversity of agents that channel into each pathway, there is considerable interaction *between* pathways, through which a tight regulation of cellular activity is possible.

Abnormalities in membrane function in cluster headache

In earlier work, we have shown significant biochemical abnormalities in cluster headache. These abnormalities affect membrane phospholipids, cholesterol, and choline transport (de Belleroche *et al.* 1984, 1985). Even in between cluster attacks, receptor-activated cAMP production in the lymphocytes of cluster-headache patients shows a significant reduction in response, in the absence of a change in receptor number or affinity (de Belleroche *et*

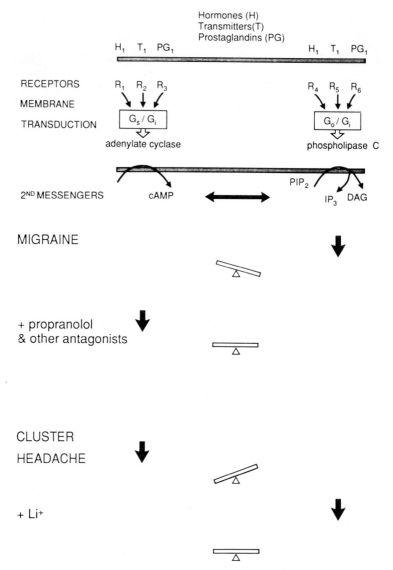

FIG. 23.1. Abnormalities in membrane transduction systems in migraine and cluster headache: treatments that may maintain the balance between these pathways. cAMP, cyclic AMP; PIP$_2$, phosphatidyl inositol bisphosphate; IP$_3$, inositol trisphosphate; DAG, diacylglycerol. G$_s$, G$_i$, and G$_o$ represent guanine nucleotide binding proteins involved in membrane transduction.

al. 1986). These results indicate a defect in coupling between the receptor and adenylate cyclase, a process which depends highly on multiple membrane components. No such effect is seen in migraine patients (Kilfeather *et al.* 1984). The results with cluster-headache patients are consistent with the treatment of this condition since, unlike migraine, it does not respond to propranolol which would block the already depressed adenylate cyclase response. Furthermore, cluster headache is often very effectively treated with lithium, which would damp down the polyphosphoinositide (PPI) system. Migraine, on the other hand, is successfully treated with propranolol but is exacerbated by lithium (Peatfield and Clifford Rose 1981). This led us to hypothesize that the PPI system was affected in migraine.

The polyphosphoinositide system in migraine

We investigated the receptor-mediated activation of the PPI system by using neutrophils as the test system. Chemotactic factor (CF) — formylmethionyl-leucyl-phenylalanine — which causes chemotaxis, aggregation, exocytosis of granules, and a burst in respiratory activity in neutrophils, is known to cause a rapid increase in the hydrolysis of phosphatidyl inositol bisphosphate within a few seconds, with the generation of inositol trisphosphate and diacylglycerol (Takenawa *et al.* 1985; Cockroft *et al.* 1985). This rapid response is thought to be the key intermediate process in the activation of neutrophils, and it leads to the subsequent release of lysosomal enzymes and arachidonic acid, and to the production of superoxide ions.

Neutrophils were purified from fresh blood by differential centrifugation, followed by density-gradient centrifugation on percoll, preincubation with [^{3}H]inositol for two hours, to label inositol phospholipids, and the neutrophils were then challenged with various concentrations of CF (1 nM to 10 μM). Inositol phosphates were fractionated by anion-exchange chromatography (Berridge *et al.* 1982). We have previously characterized the response to CF stimulation in human neutrophils (Das *et al.* 1987). The response is a dose- and time-dependent increase in [^{3}H]inositol phosphate (in the presence of Li^+ to inhibit inositol phosphatase), which is derived from inositol trisphosphate. This method has been well substantiated and is used widely as a measure of the receptor-mediated activation of phosphatidyl inositol bisphosphate turnover.

In neutrophils from control subjects, the maximal stimulation of [^{3}H]inositol phosphate production occurs at approximately 100 nM CF, with an EC_{50} (effective concentration for 50 per cent stimulation) of 13 nM. However, in neutrophils obtained from common migraine subjects (Fig. 23.2) outside an attack, a significant depression in response, compared to controls, is obtained of 58 per cent at 10^{-7} M CF (p < 0.04), and of 52 per cent at 10^{-6} M CF (p < 0.05). The control group were all females, to match the patient group, and of a similar age range.

Neutrophils obtained from cluster-headache patients within a cluster period were not significantly different from control patients (Fig. 23.2). In this case the control group were all male smokers, to match the patient group, and covered a similar age range. In cluster headache patients who had been treated with lithium carbonate for five to seven days (0.8 to 1.6 g per day, to maintain a plasma concentration of approximately 0.7 mM at the time of sampling) a significant depression of the maximal response of approximately 60 per cent was obtained at 10^{-6} M CF ($p < 0.013$) compared to controls or to untreated acute subjects ($p < 0.02$).

Differential modulation of the polyphosphoinositide system in migraine and cluster headache

These results indicate that distinctive abnormalities in membrane transduction, in migraine and cluster headache, affect the PPI system and adenylate cyclase, respectively. The transduction process involves many components — for example, CF receptor, G protein, inositol phospholipids, other phospholipids, phospholipase C, and many regulatory factors that modulate this pathway, all of which provide potential sites at which an abnormality may occur in migraine, so giving rise to the reduced responsiveness. Chronic treatment with lithium is known to block an early stage in this process in the brain — the agonist(carbachol and isoproterenol)-stimulated binding of GTP to the G protein (Avissar *et al.* 1988) — and this is borne out by the present results, where a substantial reduction in the maximal response is seen in lithium-treated cluster-headache patients.

Closely associated with the increased turnover of phosphatidyl inositol bisphosphate upon activation of neutrophils is the release of arachidonic acid, which acts as a precursor for the eicosanoids that are important in platelet and vascular function. This arises from the action of phosholipase A_2 on phosphatidyl inositol bisphosphate. We have previously shown a high level of the arachidonic acid product, leukotriene B_4, during the headache phase. This high level significantly declines after the attack (Selmaj *et al.* 1986). This finding may be relevant to the pain of this headache since, apart from being a potent chemotactic factor, leukotriene B_4 also produces inflammation and hyperalgesia (Lewis *et al.* 1981; Leine *et al.* 1984).

A balance between adenylate cyclase and phosphoinositide transduction

The results obtained with lithium, which is clinically effective in cluster headache, indicate that it may have its therapeutic effect by damping down the PPI system in line with the adenylate cyclase system which is reduced in this condition. A similar balance may be necessary for successful treatment

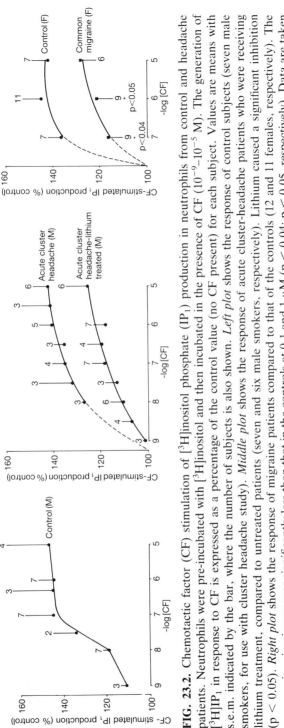

FIG. 23.2. Chemotactic factor (CF) stimulation of [³H]inositol phosphate (IP₁) production in neutrophils from control and headache patients. Neutrophils were pre-incubated with [³H]inositol and then incubated in the presence of CF (10^{-9}–10^{-5} M). The generation of [³H]IP₁ in response to CF is expressed as a percentage of the control value (no CF present) for each subject. Values are means with s.e.m. indicated by the bar, where the number of subjects is also shown. *Left plot* shows the response of control subjects (seven male smokers, for use with cluster headache study). *Middle plot* shows the response of acute cluster-headache patients who were receiving lithium treatment, compared to untreated patients (seven and six male smokers, respectively). Lithium caused a significant inhibition ($p < 0.05$). *Right plot* shows the response of migraine patients compared to that of the controls (12 and 11 females, respectively). The response in migraineurs was significantly less than that in the controls at 0.1 and 1 μM ($p < 0.04$; $p < 0.05$; respectively). Data are taken from de Belleroche *et al.* (1988).

J. de Belleroche

in migraine. Here, the defective PPI system may be balanced by the use of β-blockers and other antagonists that reduce cAMP generation.

Acknowledgements

We are grateful to the Migraine Trust for funding this project.

References

Avissar, S., Schrieber, G., Danan, A., and Belmaker, R.H. (1988). Lithium inhibits adrenergic and cholinergic increases in GTP binding in rat cortex. *Nature*, **331**, 440–3.

Berridge, M.J., and Irvine, R.F. (1984). Inositol trisphosphate, a novel second messenger in cellular signal transduction. *Nature*, **312**, 315–21.

Berridge, M.J., Downes, C.P., and Hanley, M.R. (1982). Lithium amplified agonist dependent phosphatidylinositol responses in brain and salivary glands. *Biochemical Journal*, **206**, 587–95.

Cockroft, S., Barrowman, M.M., and Gomperts, B.D. (1985). Breakdown and synthesis of polyphosphoinositides in f-met-leu-phe-stimulated neutrophils. *FEBS (Federation of European Biochemical Societies) Letters*, **181**, 259–63.

Das, I., de Belleroche, J., and Hirsch, S. (1987). Inhibitory action of spermidine on formyl-methyionyl leucyl phenylalanine stimulated phosphate production in human neutrophils. *Life Sciences*, **41**, 1037–41.

de Belleroche *et al.* (1984). Erythrocyte choline concentrations and cluster headache. *British Medical Journal*, **288**, 268–70.

de Belleroche, J., Clifford Rose, F., Das, I., and Cook, G.E. (1985) Metabolic abnormality in cluster headache. *Headache*, **24**, 310–2.

de Belleroche, J., Kilfeather, S., Das, I., and Clifford Rose, F. (1986). Abnormal membrane composition and membrane dependent transduction mechanisms in cluster headache. *Cephalalgia*, **6**, 147–53.

de Belleroche, J., Morris, R., Davies, P.T.G., and Clifford Rose, F. (1988). Differential changes in receptor-mediated transduction in migraine and cluster headache: studies on polymorphonuclear leucocytes. *Headache*, **28**, 409–13.

Kilfeather, S., Gorgolewska, G., Massarella, A., Ansell, E., and Turner, P. (1984). Beta-adrenoceptor and epoprostenol (prostacyclin) responsiveness of lymphocytes in migraine patients. *Postgraduate Medical Journal*, **60**, 391–3.

Leine, J.D., Lau, W., Kwiat, G., Goetzel, E.J. (1984). Leukotriene B4 produces hyperalgesia that is dependent on polymorphonuclear leukocytes. Science, **225**, 743–5.

Lewis, R.A., Soter, N.A., Corey, E.J., Austen, K.F. (1981). Local effects of synthetic leukotrienes on monkey and human skin. *Clinical Research*, **29**, 492A.

Nishizuka, Y. (1984). Turnover of inositol phospholipids and signal transduction. *Science*, **225**, 1365–70.

Peatfield, R.C., and Clifford Rose, F. (1981). Exacerbation of migraine by treatment with lithium. *Headache*, **21**, 140–2.

Selmaj, K., de Belleroche, J., Das, I., and Clifford Rose, F. (1986). Leukotriene B4 generation by polymorphonuclear leukocytes: possible involvement in the pathogenesis of headache. *Headache*, **26**, 460–4.

Takenawa, T., Ishitoya, J., Homma, Y., Kato, M., and Nagain, Y. (1985). Role of enhanced inositol phospholipid metabolism in neutrophil activation. *Biochemical Pharmacology*, **34**, 1931–5.

Discussion

WELCH: Have you looked at classical migraine patients?

DE BELLEROCHE: We are currently attempting this. We cannot yet say whether there is a trend towards reduced responsiveness in these patients. These coupling systems are widespread not just in neutrophils and lymphocytes, and we are currently looking at the effects of thrombin and 5-HT stimulation on transduction in the platelets of migraine patients.

WELCH: Are any of the processes that you have described magnesium-dependent?

DE BELLEROCHE: Magnesium may be involved in these systems, through effects on ligand binding, enzyme activity, or as a consequence of fluctuations in calcium concentration in the cell.

FOZARD: Do you need to 'home in' on the second messenger systems for your conclusions? Could it not equally be some sort of receptor problem? Are there not enough there? Is there a depletion of receptor sites? If another receptor stimulus to the same second messenger system were to be inhibited to the same extent, that would tend to support a change due to effects beyond the receptor.

DE BELLEROCHE: We are looking at other agents like thrombin and 5-HT that stimulate polyphosphoinositide (PPI) turnover. If responsiveness to these agents is similarly affected then we will know that the site of the defect is in the coupling to the second messenger system. We have looked at prostacyclin, high and low affinity binding sites, and β adrenoceptor number. There is no indication of any differences in receptor number or affinity in these systems. It seems to be coupling that is mainly affected.

GLOVER: Have people looked for similar changes in any other conditions? How specific are the changes likely to be to migraine?

DE BELLEROCHE: We have done something along these lines and have found trends and differences in the adenylate cyclase response with age (Kilfeather *et al.* 1986). We have tried to age-match our subjects and to use an age range over which little change occurs. In contrast to the decrease in adenylate cyclase responses with age, there may be an increase in the PPI system with age. Altered responsiveness can also be obtained experimentally after cholinergic denervation in the cerebral cortex. In this case there is a significant and sustained doubling in muscarinic responsiveness, without any increase in receptor number or affinity (Reed and de Belleroche 1988). We know that the system has compensatory processes that can be manipulated.

FERREIRA: Did you find that the levels of leukotriene B4 were associated with headache?

DE BELLEROCHE: The levels of leukotriene B4 correlated with the duration of headache in the cluster headache patients.

FERREIRA: I would expect that aspirin-induced asthma patients would be much worse if they were treated with aspirin-like drugs. Did you find that?

DE BELLEROCHE: Yes, They do not respond to aspirin. But steroids have sometimes been used.

WELCH: I believe that cluster headache patients sometimes respond to indomethacin when they are resistant to other forms of treatment.

DE BELLEROCHE: This is not generally found in our clinic but, on the other hand, chronic paroxysmal headache (CPH) does respond well to indomethacin.

ZIEGLER: Can lithium treatment achieve *intra*cellular lithium levels sufficient to inhibit the breakdown of inositol phosphates?

DE BELLEROCHE: Lithium probably produces that response by reducing the coupling between the agonist-stimulated binding of GTP to the G protein (Avissar *et al.* 1988). This produces an inhibitory effect on the system, as would the inhibition of the phosphatase.

ZIEGLER: Then the effect of lithium is not an intracellular one, but one occurring at the outside of the cell membrane?

DE BELLEROCHE: Yes. It has been shown after *in vivo* lithium treatment. The net effect would be the same as phosphatase inhibition but I suspect that the membrane effect is the more important therapeutically.

MOSKOWITZ: Would you not expect chronic lithium treatment to block the availability of inositol for reincorporation into the membrane, resulting in a relative deficiency of inositol-containing phospholipids? When you apply labelled inositol, do you find as much inositol incorporated into the membrane in lithium-treated patients?

DE BELLEROCHE: We find the same amounts incorporated in both groups. This is because, in order to measure the inositol phosphate we have high lithium concentrations present, to inhibit the phosphatase.

WELCH: Have these cluster headache patients ever had lithium treatment before?

DE BELLEROCHE: Because of our previous studies of the levels of choline and phosphatidylcholine in cluster headache patients (de Belleroche *et al.* 1984, 1985), we realised that effects of lithium can be very long-lasting. So the patients we categorize as acute untreated will not have had lithium for at least three months, as part of the protocol.

PEATFIELD: Because we never see aspirin-induced headache, can we argue that the leukotrienes cannot be part of the pathogenesis? As I understand it, aspirin-induced asthma is believed to arise because the prostaglandin precursors are sent down the leukotriene pathway rather than the prostaglandin pathway. Can we argue that leukotrienes cannot possibly be anything to do with headache because this never seems to happen in clinical practice?

GRYGLEWSKI: No, I do not think it is the case. Leukotrienes have nothing to do with aspirin-induced asthma and their levels are not increased in patients who have had an attack precipitated by aspirin (Niżankowska 1988; Niżankowska *et al.* 1988).

FERREIRA: Does a lipoxygenase inhibitor block the asthma induced by aspirin?

GRYGLEWSKI: No; at least piroprost is ineffective.

PEATFIELD: What is the pathogenesis of aspirin-induced asthma then?

GRYGLEWSKI: I think it is a selective inhibition of the generation of PGE_2 in the large airways, while the generation of thromboxane A_2 in the parenchyma remains intact. Viral infections of upper airways are closely associated with the development of aspirin-sensitive asthma (Szczeklik 1988). This might be the reason for a higher susceptibility of the upper airways to the inhibitory action of each of the 14 investigated cyclooxygenase inhibitors that can induce asthma (Szczeklik *et al.* 1977). We want to treat aspirin-sensitive patients with thromboxane synthetase inhibitors or with thromboxane A_2 or prostaglandin endoperoxide H_2 receptor antagonists, rather than with lipoxygenase inhibitors.

References

Avissar, S., Schrieber, G., Danon, A., and Belmaker, R.H. (1988). Lithium inhibits adrenergic and cholinergic increases in GTP binding in rat cortex. *Nature*, **331**, 440–3.

de Belleroche, J. *et al.* (1984). Erythrocyte choline concentrations and cluster headache. *British Medical Journal*, **288**, 268–70.

de Belleroche, J., Clifford Rose, F., Das, I., and Cook, G.E. (1985). Metabolic abnormality in cluster headache. *Headache*, **24**, 310–2.

Kilfeather, S.A., Dawson, K., de Belleroche, J. (1986). Lymphocytes, beta-adrenoceptors and multiple prostaglandin receptors—effects of ageing and smoking. *British Journal of Pharmacology*, **87**, 113P.

Niżankowska, E. *et al.* (1988). An abnormality of arachidonic acid metabolism is not a generalized phenomenon in patients with aspirin-induced asthma. *Eicosanoids*, **1**, 45–8.

Niżankowska, E. (1988). Eicosanoids in aspirin-induced asthma. Unpublished Ph.D thesis. Copernicus Academy of Medicine, Cracow, Poland.

Reed, L.J. and de Belleroche, J. (1988). Increased polyphosphoinositide responsiveness in the cerebral cortex induced by cholinergic denervation. *Journal of Neurochemistry*, **50**, 1566–71.

Szczeklik, A. (1988). Aspirin-induced asthma as a viral disease. *Clinical Allergy*, **18**, 15–20.

Szczeklik, A., Gryglewski, R.J., and Czerniawska-Mysik, G. (1977). Clinical patterns of hypersensitivity to non-steroidal anti-inflammatory drugs and their pathogenesis. *Journal of Allergy and Clinical Immunology*, **60**, 276–84.

24. The current status of migraine therapy

F. Clifford Rose

Introduction

A precise diagnosis for migraine is always required (Clifford Rose 1986), since drugs that help one headache syndrome may adversely affect another (Peatfield and Clifford Rose 1981a).

Ideally, drug therapy should be resorted to only if non-drug management is ineffective. Obvious provocative factors, for example, red wine, late nights, or missing meals should be avoided (Peatfield and Clifford Rose 1981b). Treatment of patients with migraine is traditionally divided into management of the acute attack and prevention (Clifford Rose and Peatfield 1988).

A recent method of preventing the attack has been tried on patients with premonitory symptoms, for example, irritability, excitement, euphoria, or food cravings that occur as long as 24 hours before the attack; these patients have been given domperidone, a dopamine D2 receptor antagonist, which is anti-emetic (that is, relieving nausea and vomiting) and gastro-kinetic (that is, stimulating the stomach and opening the pyloric spincter so that oral medication can be absorbed by the small gut). With premonitory symptoms of more than six hours, it can be effective in preventing migraine attacks.

There is still no general agreement as to how migraine is best treated, largely because the many drugs used have not been scientifically evaluated by methodologically sound clinical trials (Steiner and Clifford Rose 1988).

The acute attack

The general principles of treatment are bed rest (since activity aggravates the headache) in a quiet darkened room, since there is increased sensitivity to stimuli such as light (photophobia), sound (phonophobia), smell (osmophobia), and touch (haptophobia). Following sleep, improvement occurs; the longer and deeper the sleep, the greater the improvement. The basic management consists of analgesics, antinauseants, sedatives, and ergot (Peatfield *et al.* 1986).

Analgesics

Aspirin, although an effective analgesic, may cause gastric symptoms, including haemorrhage. Effervescent preparations are probably better absorbed. Paracetamol (acetaminophen) is better in this regard and is often given with other drugs, for example, codeine plus an antihistamine (as in Migraleve) or with a sedative and a sympathomimetic agent (as in Midrid). Because of gastric stasis, analgesic medication given orally is not effective during the acute attack, unless taken very early before the onset of nausea. Diclofenac (Voltarol) is a non-steroidal anti-inflammatory drug (NSAID) that is effective in an acute migraine attack (Del Bene *et al.* 1987) and it is the only NSAID that can be given parenterally. It can also be given as a suppository, as can other NSAIDs, for example, indomethacin (Indocid). More recently, naproxen has been shown to be effective (Sargent *et al.* 1988), and the published work on NSAIDs in migraine has recently been reviewed (Pradalier *et al.* 1988). There are a huge number of remedies that can be bought over the counter which combine analgesics with other drugs, but such 'polypharmacy' is to be deprecated, not least because overconsumption often leads to 'analgesic headaches'.

Antinauseants

As well as an analgesic, an antinauseant is required, for example, metoclopramide, which is effective orally if given early in the attack; it also promotes normal gastro-intestinal activity so that drugs can be absorbed from the small intestine. In a study to compare effervescent aspirin alone against the same combined with metoclopramide, there was no statistical difference in absorption, indicating that metoclopramide will make a difference to absorption only when given before (usually 30 minutes before) the analgesic is given. Some proprietary oral preparations combine metoclopramide with an analgesic, either paracetamol (Paramax) or aspirin (Migravess). Metoclopramide is more effective when given parenterally but can also be given as a suppository. Because it is a dopamine antagonist, its side-effects include extrapyramidal symptoms, particularly in children, in whom it is best avoided. Although both this drug and domperidone are dopamine receptor antagonists, domperidone does not cause extrapyramidal symptoms, presumably because it does not cross the blood–brain barrier.

Sedation

Since many acute migraine attacks resolve with sleep, it is sometimes advisable to give a benzodiazapine such as diazepam but, because of the danger of habituation, this treatment is not suitable for frequent attacks. In order to encourage sleep, any medication containing caffeine, a central nervous system stimulant, is best avoided.

Ergot

Although ergotamine preparations have been used for 60 years, most patients can recover from an attack without their use. These drugs are best avoided unless attacks are infrequent. The bioavailability of ergotamine is remarkably variable. As with other drugs, it is poorly absorbed during a migraine attack, but can be given sublingually (Lingraine), by suppository (Cafergot) or by inhalation (Medihaler). Oral preparations are given with caffeine (Cafergot) and sometimes also with an antihistamine (Migril) and with other drugs. Such 'polypharmacy' is ill-advised and too frequent consumption leads to habituation and 'ergotamine headaches'. As sleep is so beneficial, any vaso-active effect of caffeine is outweighed by its excitatory action. Ergotamine itself can aggravate nausea and cause vomiting. Whilst the severe complication of gangrene is very rarely seen, ergotamine habituation is not infrequent and gives daily headache as well as nausea (Clifford Rose and Wilkinson 1976); its withdrawal can be so upsetting that patients may require admission to hospital for sedation to withstand the withdrawal effects.

Dihydroergotamine, a hydrogenated ergotamine, was introduced in 1945 because it had less adverse reactions than ergotamine, and possibly because its vasoconstrictor effect was less. It has been used for acute attacks, given either parenterally or by nasal spray, but its efficacy using the latter route has been questioned (Tulunay *et al.* 1987).

Preventative treatment

Prophylactic therapy is recommended for those having more than two migraine attacks per month. This is not a rigid rule since a monthly attack that lasts several days would also merit consideration. With the wide range of effective drugs now available, failure to respond is either due to inadequate dosage or to misdiagnosis (Clifford Rose and Peatfield 1988).

β-blockers

Adrenoceptors are classified into α and β (Ahlquist 1948), the α-receptors being mainly excitatory and producing vasoconstriction, whilst the β-receptors are mainly inhibitory and produce vasodilatation. Drugs that antagonize the latter action are called β-blockers and the first to be used in migraine was propranolol. The β-receptors are subdivided into β-1 and β-2, the latter occurring more prominently in smooth muscles of arterioles and bronchioles. In asthma, β-2 blockade should be avoided, so β-1 blockers are used but, even then, caution is required because selectivity between β-1 and β-2 receptors is only relative. β-1 blockers are also preferred in those migraine patients who have Raynaud's syndrome (Zahavi *et al.* 1984).

The efficacy of propranolol was discovered by accident since, while being given for angina, it was found to be effective against migraine (Rabkin *et al.* 1966). Since then it has been shown to have an efficacy of 55–84 per cent, with a dose ranging from 80–240 mg day^{-1}. Of the many β-blockers now available (Table 24.1), only some are effective in migraine.

Whilst the most widely used β-blocker is propranolol (Kangasniemi *et al.* 1982; Steardo *et al.* 1982; Weerasuriya *et al.* 1982), atenolol has been recommended because of its anti-platelet action (Gawel *et al.* 1979; Joseph *et al.* 1985a,b,c, 1986, 1988). Because individual patients vary in their response to β-blockers, which also vary in their cardioselectivity (β-1 activity), care should be taken in the choice between propranolol, atenolol, metoprolol, timolol, and nadolol (Kangasniemi *et al.* 1987). Many placebo-controlled trials of β-blockers have been done, either against propranolol (Table 24.2) or other β-blockers (Table 24.3). For reasons of compliance, once-daily therapy is advantageous but long-acting β-blockers are now also available (Table 24.4), and a recent study showed no difference between flunarizine and long-acting propranolol (Dahlöf 1989). Why β-blockers work is unknown. It cannot simply be due to β-blockade because not all β-blockers work. Furthermore, the dextro-rotatory isomer of propranolol has no β-blocking activity and yet has been shown to be effective in migraine (Stensrud and Sjaastad 1976). Those that are effective share only one property in common — the absence of intrinsic sympathetic activity, that is, they are not partial agonists. They take time to work, but their benefit often outlasts the period of treatment.

Side-effects

Fatigue is the most common side-effect, occurring in about 20 per cent of patients. The reason for this is unknown, but it tends to wear off in a few weeks. β-blockers vary in their lipid solubility, which determines their penetration into the CNS and, hence, their CNS side-effects, for example, drowsiness, nightmares, depression, and even hallucinations. Bradycardia should rarely be a reason for stopping β-blockers as it is unrelated to the incidence of fatigue or cold extremities.

Only 70 per cent of migraine sufferers will respond to β-blockers and, although it has been suggested (Schoenen 1987) that electrophysiological tests (contingent negative variation) may be able to determine which patient is likely to respond, this has not been confirmed (Diener *et al.* 1989).

Antiserotoninergic drugs

The next most commonly used prophylactic drugs are anti-serotoninergic. Pizotifen is the safest but has the disadvantages of sedation and increasing appetite, with consequent weight gain, a side-effect particularly disagreeable in the sex and age groups in which migraine is most common (Steiner *et al.*

TABLE 24.1. *β-blockers currently available*

Generic name	Proprietary name	Cardioselective	5-HT action*	BBB†	Partial agonist	Efficacy in migraine
atenolol	Tenormin	Yes	0	0	No	+
metoprolol	{ Betaloc Lopresor	Yes	?	+	No	+
nadolol	Corgard	No	?	+	No	+
practolol	Eraldin	Yes	0	0	Yes	(+?)
propranolol	Inderal	No	+	+	No	+
timolol	Blocadren	No	?	+	No	+
acebutolol	Sectral	Yes	?	0	Yes	−
alprenolol	Aptin	No	++	+	Yes	−
betaxolol	Kerlone	No	?	?	Yes	?
oxprenolol	Trasicor	No	++	+	Yes	−
penbutolol	Lasipressin	No	?	?	Yes	?
pindolol	Visken	No	++	+	Yes	−
sotalol	{ Betacardone Sotacor	No	?	?	No	?

*Drugs that mimic 5-HT (5-hydroxytryptamine; serotonin) normally (+) or with a considerable effect (++).

†BBB, indicates whether the drug passes the blood-brain barrier (+).

Other symbols: 0, no action; ?, evidence unclear; (+?), may be effective; −, not tested.

TABLE 24.2. *Double-blind, placebo-controlled trials with propranolol for migraine prophylaxis*

Authors (year)	Daily dose (mg)	Period of trial (months)	No. of patients	Patients improved (per cent)
Weber and Reinmuth (1972)	80	12	19	79
Malvea et al. (1973)	120	6	29	55
Ludvigsson (1974)	60 or 120	13	28[†]	93 (of those completing)
Widerøe and Vigander (1974)	160	12	26	81
Borgesen et al. (1974)	120	12	30	60
Nair (1975)	80	8	20	
Diamond and Medina (1976)	80 or 160		62	55
Stensrud and Sjaastad (1976)	160*	4	20	*DL ≥ D > placebo
Forssman et al. (1983)	240	12	32	69
Bernik and Maia (1978)	160	8	46	94
Diamond et al. (1982)	Up to 160	6–24	148	54
Palferman et al. (1983)	120		10 + 12[‡]	

*Mixture (DL) of dextro (D) and laevo (L) rotation isomers or D isomer alone. Both isomers superior to placebo; DL marginally better than D.
[†]Children.
[‡]Mixed group: 10 with migraine; 12 with other headaches.

TABLE 24.3. *Double-blind, placebo-controlled trials with β-blockers other than propranolol*

Name (year)	Drugs used		Daily dose (mg per day)	No. of patients	Comments
Sjaastad and Stensrud (1972)	pindolol:		7.5–15	24	No better than placebo
Ekbom and Lundberg (1972)	pindolol:		7.5–15	26	No better than placebo
Ekbom (1975)	alprenolol:		400	28	No better than placebo
Ekbom and Zetterman (1977)	oxprenolol:		240	30	No better than placebo
Nanda et al. (1978)	acebutolol:		400–800	33	No better than placebo
Briggs and Millac (1979)	timolol:		20	13	Timolol significantly better than placebo
Ryan et al. (1983)	nadolol:		80–240	80	Nadolol (160–240 mg) more effective than 80 mg dose or placebo

Study	Drug (mg)	n	Results
Forssman et al. (1983)	atenolol: 100	20	75% improvement
Andersson et al. (1983)	metoprolol: 200	62	33% improvement (metoprolol); 11% (placebo)
Tfelt-Hansen et al. (1984)	propranolol: 160 timolol: 20 placebo	80	No difference between propranolol (60% improvement) and timolol (55%); both better than placebo (30%)
Ryan and Ryan (1984)	nadolol: 80–160 propranolol: 160	45	Improvement, especially nadolol (80mg)
Kangasniemi and Hedman (1984)	metoprolol: 200 propranolol: 160	33	No difference between the two drugs
Stellar et al. (1984)	timolol: 20–30 placebo	98	Timolol more effective than placebo
Farias da Silva et al. (1979)	propranolol: 30–90 pindolol: 7.5–15	47	Propranolol (82% improved); superior to pindolol (60%)

TABLE 24.4. *Calcium blockers used in the prophylactic treatment of migraine*

Category	General type	Examples
Class I	dihydropyridines	nifedipine
		nimodipine
Class II	hydrophilic bases	verapamil
		diltiazem
Class III	diphenylalkalamines	flunarizine

1980). Since its half-life is nearly 24 hours, pizotifen need be given only once daily and, because of its sedative effect, preferably at night.

Methysergide is probably more efficacious then pizotifen, but it is not the drug of first choice because of the danger of retroperitoneal fibrosis; yet there is no evidence that this occurs when the methysergide treatment pattern is broken for a month every few months. Because retroperitoneal fibrosis is a life-threatening complication, it is easy to understand why methysergide is not more widely used.

Calcium blockers

The rationale for the use of calcium antagonists was based on the vascular hypothesis. When cells are hypoxic, calcium enters into them and, hence, a calcium-entry blocker should prove useful. Since extracellular calcium increases with vasoconstriction, calcium antagonists should also prove useful against vasospasm. Calcium antagonists are not a homogeneous group and they have been subdivided on the basis of their physicochemical and functional properties (Table 24.4).

Class I are dihydropyridines and include nifedipine and nimodipine (Stewart *et al.* 1988). The largest trials of these in migraine have shown no significant differences against a placebo.

Class II are hydrophilic bases such as verapamil and diltiazem, which are not widely used for migraine.

Class III are the diphenylalkalamines which include flunarizine. There have been many trials of these drugs (Sorensen *et al.* 1986), and both the frequency and the severity of migraine attacks are diminished by them. This class of calcium blockers is equally effective against classical migraine (with aura) as well as common migraine (without aura). The most widely used of this group for migraine prophylaxis is flunarizine (Sorensen *et al.* 1986), but there is doubt about whether its efficacy is caused by a calcium-blocking effect. Although widely used, calcium blockers are probably no more effective than antiserotoninergic or β-blocking drugs.

Other pharmacological approaches

Antidepressants

Amitriptyline, a tricyclic antidepressant, is the drug of choice in tension headache and is indicated when patients have both migraine and tension headache (combined headache).

It has been tried in migraine and found to be effective (Gomersall and Stuart 1973), irrespective of the patients' psychiatric state (Couch *et al.* 1976). It may work through its antiserotoninergic effect or analgesic properties, but has been shown to be synergistic with propranolol (Mathew 1981).

Hormonal

The fact that migraine is commoner in women, worse with menstruation, aggravated by the contraceptive pill and often better during pregnancy confirms the hormonal influence over migraine attacks (Clifford Rose 1985).

Menstrual migraine is now defined as attacks on the first day of the cycle plus or minus one or two days. These sufferers almost invariably do not get attacks during pregnancy. Owing to oestrogen withdrawal these attacks can be prevented by an oestradiol ointment rubbed into the skin.

Feverfew used to be given as the leaves of the plant *Tanacetum parthenium*, in a sandwich, but has now been produced as quantified tablets. A recent trial has shown its efficacy (Murphy *et al.* 1989).

References

Ahlquist, R.P. (1948). A study of the adrenotropic receptors. *American Journal of Physiology*, **153**, 586.

Andersson, P.G. *et al.* (1983). Prophylactic treatment of classical and non-classical migraine with metoprolol — a comparison with placebo. *Cephalalgia*, **3**, 207–12.

Bernik, V. and Maia, E. (1978). The use of propranolol on prophylaxis of migraine: a double-blind clinical trial comparing propranolol with an analgesic drug (acetaminophen) and placebo. *Folha Medica*, **77**, 501–8.

Borgesen, S.E., Nielsen, J.L., and Moller, C.E. (1974). Propranolol in migraine. *Lancet*, **ii**, 58.

Briggs, R.S. and Millac, P.A. (1979). Timolol in migraine prophylaxis. *Headache*, **19**, 379–81.

Clifford Rose, F. (1985). Migraine prophylaxis. In *Updating in headache*, (ed. V. Pfaffenrath, P.O. Lundberg, and O. Sjaastad), pp. 177–80. Springer, Berlin.

Clifford Rose, F. (1986). Headache: definitions and classification. In *Handbook of clinical neurology*, Vol. 4, *Headache*, (ed. F. Clifford Rose), pp. 1–12. Elsevier, Amsterdam.

Clifford Rose, F. and Peatfield, R. (1988). Prophylactic therapy. In *The management of headache*, (ed. F. Clifford Rose), pp. 81–96. Raven, New York.

Clifford Rose, F. and Wilkinson, M. (1976). Letter: Ergotamine tartrate overdose. *British Medical Journal*, **1**, 525.

Couch, J.R., Ziegler, D.K., and Hassanein, R. (1976). Amitryptiline in the prophylaxis of migraine. *Neurology*, **26**, 121–7.

Dahlöf, C. (1989). Flunarizine versus long-acting propranolol in the prophylactic treatment of migraine. A double-blind study with parallel groups. In *Further advances in headache research*, (ed. F. Clifford Rose), pp. 281–90. Smith-Gordon, London.

Del Bene, E., Poggioni, M., and Garagiola, U. (1987). Diclofenac sodium in the treatment of acute migraine attack: a double-blind clinical trial. In *Advances in headache research*, (ed. F. Clifford Rose), pp. 103–7. John Libbey, London.

Diamond, S. and Medina, J.L. (1976). Double blind study of propranolol for migraine prophylaxis. *Headache*, **16**, 24–7.

Diamond, S., Kindrow, L., Stevens, J., and Shapir, D.B. (1982). Long term study of propranolol in the treatment of migraine. *Headache*, **2**, 268–71.

Diener, H.C., Scholz, E., and Gerber, W.D. (1989). Central effects of drugs evaluated by visual evoked potentials in *Further advances in headache research*, (ed. F. Clifford Rose), pp. 63–8. Smith-Gordon, London.

Ekbom, K. (1975). Alprenolol for migraine prophylaxis. *Headache*, **15**, 129–32.

Ekbom, K. and Lundberg, P.O. (1972). Clinical trial of LB-46 an adrenergic beta-receptor blocking agent in migraine prophylaxis. *Headache*, **12**, 15–7.

Ekbom, K. and Zetterman, M. (1977). Oxprenolol in the treatment of migraine. *Acta Neurologica Scandinavica*, **56**, 181–4.

Farias da Silva, W., Van der Linden, A.M., and Diegues Serva, W.A. (1979). Prophylaxis of migraine. *Revista Brasiliera de Medicina*, **36**, 442–8.

Forssman, B., Lindblad, C.J., and Zbornikova, V. (1983). Atenolol for migraine prophylaxis. *Headache*, **23**, 188–90.

Gawel, M., Burkitt, M., and Clifford Rose, F. (1979). The platelet release reaction during migraine attacks. *Headache*, **19**, 323–7.

Gomersall, J.D. and Stuart, A. (1973). Amitryptiline in migraine prophylaxis. *Journal of Neurology, Neurosurgery and Psychiatry*, **36**, 684–90.

Joseph, R., Steiner, T.J., Das, I., Schultz, L.U.C., and Clifford Rose, F. (1985a). Beta-blockers used in migraine prophylaxis elevate plasma thromboxane levels. *Cephalalgia*, Suppl. **3**, 416–7.

Joseph, R., Steiner, T.J., Poole, C.J.M., Littlewood, J., and Clifford Rose, F. (1985b). Thromboxane synthetase inhibition: potential therapy in migraine. *Headache*, **25**, 204–7.

Joseph, R., Steiner, T.J., Schultz, L.U.C., and Clifford Rose, F. (1985c). Does the mode of action of β-receptor blockers in migraine involve alteration of platelet function? In *Migraine: clinical and research advances*, (ed. F. Clifford Rose), pp. 115–20. Karger, Basle.

Joseph, R., Steiner, T.J., Sitsapesan, M., Das, I., Hadar, U., and Clifford Rose, F. (1986). Platelet release reaction in migraine may be beneficial. *Neurology*, **36**, Suppl. 1, 100.

Joseph, R., Steiner, T.J., Schultz, L.U.C., and Clifford Rose, F. (1988). A controlled study in migraine of selective beta-blockade and platelets: a case for preferring $beta_1$-adrenoceptor blockers for migraine prophylaxis. *Stroke*, **19**, 704–8.

Kangasniemi, P., Nyrke, T., Lang, H., and Peterson, E. (1982). Propranolol and femoxitene, a 5-HT uptake inhibitor, in migraine prophylaxis. *Acta Neurologica Scandinavica*, **65**, Suppl. 90, 74.

Kangasniemi, P. and Hedman, C. (1984). Metoprolol and propranolol in the prophylactic treatment of classical and common migraine: a double-blind study. *Cephalalgia*, **4**, 91–6.

Kangasniemi, P. *et al.* (1987). Classic migraine: effective prophylaxis with metoprolol. *Cephalalgia*, **7**, 231–8.

Ludvigsson, J. (1974). Propranolol used in prophylaxis of migraine in children. *Acta Neurologica Scandinavica*, **50**, 109–15.

Malvea, B.P., Gwon, N., and Graham, J. (1973). Propranolol prophylaxis of migraine. *Headache*, **12**, 163–7.

Mathew, N.T. (1981). Prophylaxis of migraine and mixed headache: a randomised controlled study. *Headache*, **21**, 105–9.

Murphy, J.J., Heptinstall, S., and Mitchell, J.R.A. (1989). A trial of feverfew for the prophylaxis of migraine. In *Further advances in headache research*, (ed. F. Clifford Rose), pp. 235–42. Smith-Gordon, London.

Nair, K.G. (1975). A pilot study of the value of propranolol in migraine. *Journal of Postgraduate Medicine*, **21**, 111–3.

Nanda, R.N., Johnson, R.H., Gray, J., Keogh, H.J., and Melville, I.D. (1978). A double blind trial of acebutalol for migraine prophylaxis. *Headache*, **18**, 20–2.

Palferman, T.G., Gibberd, F.B., and Simmonds, J.P. (1983). Prophylactic propranolol in the treatment of headache. *British Journal of Clinical Practice*, **37**, 28–9.

Peatfield, R.C. and Clifford Rose, F. (1981*a*). Exacerbation of migraine by treatment with lithium. *Headache*, **21**, 140–2.

Peatfield, R.C. and Clifford Rose, F. (1981*b*). Treatment of migraine and cluster headache. *Practitioner*, **225**, 1321–5.

Peatfield, R.C., Fozard, J.R., and Clifford Rose, F. (1986). Drug treatment of migraine. In *Handbook of clinical neurology*, Vol. 4, *Headache* (ed. F. Clifford Rose), pp. 173–216. Elsevier, Amsterdam.

Pradalier, A., Clapin, A., and Dry, J. (1988). Treatment review: non-steroid antiinflammatory drugs in the treatment and long-term prevention of migraine attacks. *Headache*, **28**, 550–7.

Rabkin, R., Stables, D.P., Levin, N.W., Suzman, M.M. (1966). The prophylactic value of propranolol in angina pectoris. *American Journal of Cardiology*, **18**, 370–83.

Ryan, R.E. Sr., and Ryan, R.E. Jr. (1984). A comparison study of nadolol and propranolol. *Headache*, **24**, 165–6.

Ryan, R.E. Sr., Ryan, R.E. Jr., and Sudilovsky, A. (1983). Nadolol: its use in the prophylactic treatment of migraine. *Headache*, **23**, 26–31.

Sargent, J.D. *et al.* (1988). Aborting a migraine attack: naproxen sodium versus ergotamine plus caffeine. *Headache*, **28**, 263–6.

Schoenen, J. (1987). Sympathetic hyperarousal in migraine? Evaluation by contingent negative variation and psychomotor testing. Effects of beta-blockers. In *Advances in headache research*, (ed. F. Clifford Rose), pp. 155–60. John Libbey, London.

Sjaastad, O. and Stensrud, P. (1972). Clinical trial of a beta-receptor blocking agent (LB 46) in migraine prophylaxis. *Acta Neurologica Scandinavica*, **48**, 124–8.

Sorensen, P.S., Hansen, K., and Olesen, J. (1986). A placebo-controlled, double-blind cross-over trial of flunarizine in common migraine. *Cephalalgia*, **6**, 7–14.

Steardo, L., Bonuso, S., Di Stasio, E., and Marano, E. (1982). Selective and non-selective beta-blockers: are both effective in prophylaxis of migraine? A clinical trial versus methysergide. *Acta Neurologica (Naples)*, **37**, 196–204.

Steiner, T.J. and Clifford Rose, F. (1988). Problems encountered in the assessment of treatment of headache. In *Headache: problems in management*, (ed. A. Hopkins), pp. 305–48. W.B. Saunders, London.

Steiner, T.J., Guha, P., Capildeo, R., and Clifford Rose, F. (1980). Migraine in patients attending a migraine clinic: an analysis by computer of age, sex and family history. *Headache*, **20**, 190–5.

Stellar, S., Ahrens, S.P., Meibohm, A.R., and Reines, S.A. (1984). Migraine prevention with timolol. JAMA (*Journal of the American Medical Association*), **252**, 2576–80.

Stensrud, P. and Sjaastad, O. (1976). Short-term clinical trial of propranolol in racemic form (Inderal), D-propranolol and placebo in migraine. *Acta Neurologica Scandinavica*, **53**, 229–32.

Stewart, D.J., Gelston, A., and Hakim, A. (1988). Effect of prophylactic administration of nimodipine in patients with migraine. *Headache*, **28**, 260–2.

Tfelt-Hansen, P., Standnes, B., Kangasniemi, P., Hakkarainen, H., and Olesen, J. (1984). Timolol vs propranolol vs placebo in common migraine prophylaxis: a double-blind multicenter trial. *Acta Neurologica Scandinavica*, **69**, 1–8.

Tulunay, F.C., Karan, O., Aydin, N., Culcuoglu, A., and Guvenir, A. (1987). Dihydroergotamine nasal spray during migraine attacks. A double-blind cross-over study with placebo. *Cephalalgia*, **7**, 131–4.

Weber, R.B. and Reinmuth, O.M. (1972). The treatment of migraine with propranolol. *Neurology*, **22**, 366–9.

Weerasuriya, K., Patel, L., and Turner, P. (1982). Beta-adrenoceptor blockade and migraine. *Cephalalgia*, **2**, 33–45.

Widerøe, T.-E. and Vigander, T. (1974). Propranolol in the treatment of migraine. *British Medical Journal*, **2**, 699–701.

Zahavi, I., Chagnac, A., Hering, R., Davidovich, S., and Kuritzky, A. (1984). Prevalence of Raynaud's phenomenon in patients with migraine. *Archives of Internal Medicine*, **144**, 742–4.

Discussion

SANDLER: How much are monoamine oxidase inhibitors (Anthony and Lance 1969) used in therapy nowadays?

ROSE: We tend to reserve it until we have tried other treatments, because of the need for a special dietary regimen but it is certainly effective. Sometimes we use both propranolol and a tricyclic antidepressant.

WELCH: Have you observed any side-effects in the form of movement disorders, after metoclopramide treatment?

ROSE: Only in children. I do not advise giving it to children, but I have not seen this in adults. One should always give as small a dose as possible, nevertheless.

OLESEN: In a couple of cases we have given metoclopramide to patients who already received neuroleptics, and they developed acute dystonia.

SAXENA: I think that pharmacologists can learn from the use of drugs by clinicians. However, the lack of a proper model for migraine is not unique since there are several diseases for which no proper animal experimental model exists. I agree with J.H. Gaddum, who once said that the best model for man is man, and the best model for cat is cat. Nevertheless, even a guinea-pig ileum can be utilized to develop a drug for hypertension in the same way as, for example, the dog saphenous vein can be used in developing a drug for migraine.

ROSE: I think that animal studies are absolutely essential, but one cannot necessarily extrapolate from them to humans. The problem is in doing clinical trials. An open study of ten patients that fails to produce a response will sometimes not be pursued. We need more methodologically sound clinical trials.

SAXENA: You said, and I agree, that β-adrenoceptor antagonists with an intrinsic sympathomimetic action are not effective in migraine therapy. Pindolol is one such antagonist. Yet in your list it was mentioned as an effective drug.

ROSE: All the available clinical trial results for pindolol come from one open study.

COPPEN: In our work with Pauline Munro on a clinical trial for migraine (Munro *et al.* 1985). we noticed a surprisingly high incidence of placebo response. I know from my work on antidepressant trials that properly controlled placebo trials are essential, not least when we wish to compare the actions of several drugs. Open trials are completely misleading especially with the sort of illness that migraine is.

ROSE: Everyone would agree, scientifically, that one of the first trials on a new drug should be a placebo-controlled trial. But there are ethical problems. If there is an effective drug, can one give less than the best possible treatment — that is, by administering a placebo? I am unsure whether a placebo-controlled trial has ever been done in epilepsy, for ethical reasons. Yet we need to know whether any of the standard anticonvulsants is more effective than placebo.

COPPEN: We have the same problem with antidepressants, or indeed whenever we are faced with a condition for which there is no standard drug with an established efficacy.

ROSE: It has not been possible in the United States to do a prophylactic trial of a new drug for stroke treatment against placebo because everyone there accepts that aspirin is an effective stroke-preventative treatment. Results have been variable, and those that show an efficacy for aspirin tend to be the trials with larger numbers of patients.

ZIEGLER: Your list of antinauseants or anti-emetics included metoclopramide, cyclizine, cinnarizine, meclozine, and promethazine. With the exception of metoclopramide, these drugs retard gastric emptying. Do you prefer metoclopramide because it promotes motility in the upper gastrointestinal tract? The other drugs mentioned do not share this property. Is it reasonable to use cyclizine, meclozine, or promethazine?

ROSE: We have not done any trials comparing one with the other, but our standard drug is metoclopramide. At the Princess Margaret Migraine Clinic, we do not advocate any particular drug, but we undertake clinical trials. For example, I do not think propranolol is the best β-blocker to use as a migraine prophylactic. The one we tend to use, atenolol, is not registered for its antimigraine properties.

ZIEGLER: Are there any theoretical reasons for using an antihistaminic drug in migraine?

ROSE: No.

BLAU: Different formulations of drugs can cause their own problems in the treatment of migraine. We have to bear in mind that drug absorption can be affected by the type and time of meals. Furthermore some tablets are themselves nauseating, and an effervescent formulation may, in some, potentiate nausea or, in others, help to reduce it. The nasal preparation, or skin absorption, could provide ways forward here. The effectiveness of a drug sometimes owes less to the measured blood level of the drug and more to the patient's psychological state at the time of administration. We must beware of the line of reasoning that says: 'the patient's pneumonia responded to penicillin; therefore the patient was penicillin-deficient'. For example, because the patient responds to a β-blocker, we need not necessarily invoke that β-blockade is acting via blood vessels. We known that propranolol works on the heart, on hypertension, and on muscle, stopping benign essential tremor; besides, it has effects on the nervous system where it promotes dreaming, it relaxes performers, or it makes people tired. Indeed, propranolol could relieve migraine because of its sedative effect rather than by a direct vascular effect. On another point, when it comes to clinical trials we should be meticulous about selection of cases to include in a trial. We should be concerned that migraine patients do not become trial patients, used repeatedly for drug trials. A study conducted in the proper manner with more care and time will produce a more valid result.

HUMPHREY: I agree that it is essential to have the best possible trials, and many published trials have not been conducted properly. We also need to find selective drugs, although I appreciate that there is no such thing as the totally selective drug. Amitryptiline may be useful clinically, but its mixed pharmacology makes it very difficult for people to dissect out its mechanism of action clinically.

FOZARD: Whether or not a drug acts selectively can often depend on the dose used. I do not know how amitryptiline works, but I do know it has the clinical effect of improving migraine. Its action may be related to 5-HT receptors or may not, but all we can do is to put available information in the melting pot with number of different observations and hope to see a common denominator. Then I can formulate a hypothesis and theoretically, on that basis, I can make a compound that will have a degree of selectivity to satisfy the clinician. This is how the compound GR43175 has arisen. Dr Humphrey's group identified a particular 5-HT receptor, defined it, and made a compound with a good degree of selectivity for it over a clearly defined dose range; and it works in migraine. But, currently, it cannot tell us much about the pathology of migraine, because we do not yet know how it works.

OLESEN: There is one class of drugs that has undoubtedly proved better than a placebo, and that is the β-blocker.

ROSE: I agree, but only about 70 per cent of migraine patients respond to it. We need to know why the other 30 per cent do not respond.

OLESEN: I believe that the use of a placebo is not yet an ethical problem in migraine, because it is not such a severe, life-threatening disorder. The ethical issue is too often used an an excuse for not doing proper trials with placebo controls. The real problem is in trying to compare different drugs. If one is going to see a difference between, say, a β-blocker and a new prophylactic drug, it would take a very large number of patients.

COPPEN: Suppose a new drug came along to rival, say, propranolol and was shown, like propranolol, to be more effective than a placebo. If the new drug were no more effective than the standard drug, and if its side-effects and disadvantages were comparable, then I think we should have to have a good reason for introducing the new drug.

OLESEN: The point is that one may need hundreds of patients to show, for instance, a 30 per cent difference between the two drugs. But that is hard to fund and organize. I have not seen any published study demonstrating a convincing difference between two prophylactic agents for migraine treatment.

SAXENA: Why should it be necessary to show a difference between two effective drugs? I can understand that if an established drug is effective with only 30 per cent of patients then you would like a new drug to be effective in 70 per cent of patients, but why should you necessarily show a difference between two effective drugs?

OLESEN: If a new drug does not have any serious side-effects, it is useful to have it alongside the old one, even if it is no more effective. It would also be useful to have more drugs for our daily practice because some patients prefer one drug while others prefer another.

ROSE: The future direction is more likely to be with acute treatment rather than with prophylaxis. Nevertheless most of the currently available prophylactics, *in the correct dose*, will control most migraine patients: 70 per cent respond to propranolol, 60 per cent to pizotifen, and most of the rest to methysergide. There are very few patients with migraine alone who will not respond to one of these. If they do not, there are other influential factors such as depression or too much medication.

BLAU: In addition to the correct dosage being critical, so too is the correct duration of treatment before efficacy is assessed, and the correct frequency of dosage. Furthermore, not infrequently a patient told to take a drug prophylactically will use it as acute therapy. There is another important question: why does acute therapy not work prophylactically?

PEATFIELD: A lot of it does. And there is a hint in a published report (Featherstone 1983) that propranolol will work in both ways.

LANCE: I would suggest that two sorts of patients should be excluded from clinical trials — one is the broadly smiling migraineur, who nevertheless claims 'Yes, my headache is really terrible today, doctor', and the other is the one who defies the doctor to cure him, and has no faith in doctors at all. Another point is that the use of headache indices can be extremely deceptive in trials. For example, in a so-called positive trial, where the headache index in a patient has come down from, say, 9.7 to 6.3, the raw data may show that the patient is still having three or four severe headaches a month. From their point of view they are no better, whatever the statistical analysis may be able to say. In the old days we used to divide patients into those who became headache-free or virtually headache-free, those who were better than half improved and those who experienced no change or were worse. Those are very clearly defined criteria. The patients who become headache-free are thrilled; those who are better than half improved are pleased; and the others are not. One can immediately tell from these criteria whether a drug is going to be of clinical use or not.

References

Anthony, M. and Lance, J.W. (1969). Monoamine oxidase inhibition in the treatment of migraine. *Archives of Neurology*, **21**, 263–8.

Featherstone, H.J. (1983). Low-dose propranolol therapy for aborting migraine. *Western Journal of Medicine*, **138**, 416–7.

Munro, P., Swade, C., and Coppen, A. (1985). Mianserin in the prophylaxis of migraine: a double-blind study. *Acta Psychiatrica Scandinavica*, **72**, Suppl. 320, 98–103.

25. Treatment: where are we going?

Albrecht Ziegler

Introduction

It is remarkable that, as a pharmacologist, I have been asked to answer the question: where are we going? Two reasons may have influenced this decision. First, a major impact on migraine research is anticipated from insights into the mode of action of the drugs used to relieve migraine symptoms. I cannot share this opinion without reservations. The knowledge about mechanisms of drug action in migraine is still very poor or even non-existing (as for ergotamine, methysergide, pizotifen, propranolol, and flunarizine). To use the effects of drugs to elucidate pathophysiological processes may mean describing an unknown relation by an unknown variable. Alternatively, perhaps no neurologist was available and naïve enough to take up the challenge. I am not afraid to be called naïve since naïvety not only means simple-mindedness but also impartiality. It could be advantageous to be free from prejudice about the bewildering amount of available information on migraine.

Where are we going? The gift of prophecy would be needed to answer this. Prophecy is not a science, and therefore developments in migraine cannot be forecast. Rather, the opposite holds true, as shown by the example of innovative contributions to pharmacological advances, which were mostly the result of serendipitous discoveries and not of deliberately planned research.

When, five years ago, I was asked to comment on future directions in migraine research, I placed my hopes on drugs that might be used as substitutes for ergotamine, as a first-line therapy for migraine attacks. At that time this hope was not unfounded, because a couple of laboratories were rumoured to be actively developing a 5-hydroxytryptamine (5-HT, serotonin) agonist, which would allow a migraine attack to be treated without ergotamine. We are currently confronted with the results of these activities, and it seems that the new 5-HT$_1$-receptor agonist has lost at least some of the side-effects that burden the therapy with ergotamine.

In contrast to five years ago, there is no similar glimmer of hope for a new development now, which could help to answer the question: where are we going? And this is despite the intensive research activities currently taking place. If one looks through relevant journals on headaches, there is no longer the detailed discussion that there was five years ago about such topics as the metabolism of biogenic amines, or the sensitivity of cerebral and peripheral blood vessels, or the reactivity of blood platelets, or the regulation of fatty acid turnover and the synthesis of prostaglandins, or the control of the blood–brain barrier, or the formation of endogenous opioid-like substances. The concept of a variety of receptors for 5-HT, and their complex distribution in the vascular tree and central nervous system as well as in the endothelium, with its complex physiological rôle are supposed to help explain the complexity of migraine.

One cannot help thinking that each new system or function that simply becomes accessible to biochemical or physiological exploration will be accepted by some people as a candidate for explaining alone, or in combination with other systems or concepts, the symptoms of migraine.

Where are we going? We are already proceeding further into a jungle of elaborate and highly sophisticated hypotheses that allow us to explain almost everything about migraine. The major disadvantage of this position is that the available instruments of research are too weak, or the pathological situation is too complex or too inconsistent, to allow a definite falsification to be made of at least some of the existing hypotheses.

What may be done to thin out and open the thicket in which we are entangled? As might be anticipated, my suggestions are pharmacological ones, and I intend to focus attention here on the specificity and appropriateness of the drugs used as tools in migraine research.

Ergotamine and its target structure

Does ergotamine penetrate the blood–brain barrier?

This secale alkaloid has taken on the function of a tool, since it is believed to be rather specific in aborting migraine attacks. There is some evidence that the therapeutic effect is brought about by an interference either with the serotoninergic control of the tone of the cerebrovascular bed or with serotoninergic neurones that control pain appreciation (for example, those in the descending pain-control system). In both cases ergotamine has to penetrate the blood–brain barrier to reach its target structures, for example, the synapses of serotoninergic neurones that innervate the smooth muscle of the cerebral vessels, or the synapses within the descending pain-control system. To my knowledge there is no experimental information available about the uptake of ergotamine into tissue protected by the blood–brain barrier. The chemical nature of ergotamine makes it very unlikely that the drug easily penetrates lipophilic barriers. This view is supported by the rather poor enteral absorption of ergotamine, which at its best amounts to 30 per cent of the dose applied. Furthermore, the drug is readily metabolized to products even less likely to cross lipophilic barriers. I doubt whether an acute, single dose of ergotamine can yield pharmacologically relevant concentrations of the drug in the tissue surrounded by the blood–brain barrier. This is because ergotamine is not only an alkaloid (lysergic acid moiety) but also an oligopeptide. Peptides, however, are not able to penetrate lipophilic barriers. This assumption is supported by the spectrum of observed responses to ergotamine in the human, which are not characterized by any direct central effects.

Can we, therefore, interpret the relief of migraine as a result of ergotamine's interaction at 5-HT$_1$-receptors located at the postsynaptic membranes of neurones that supply the cerebrovascular bed? The same question applies to the effects of ergotamine and dihydroergotamine on the electrical activity of cells in the central connections of pain afferents from cerebral vessels (Lance et al., this volume; G.A. Lambert, A.S. Zagami, N. Bogduk, R.W. Adams, and J.W. Lance, unpublished results) or to the blockade, by ergotamine, of a capsaicin-induced neurogenic inflammation (Moskowitz et al. 1988).

If it holds true that ergotamine cannot penetrate the blood–brain barrier, its target structure must be in direct contact with the blood.

For both ergotamine and 5-HT, a site of action directly accessible from the bloodstream has to be assumed; this is because although 5-HT is not taken up across the blood–brain barrier, it is nevertheless effective in easing or abolishing migraine headache (Kimball et al. 1960; Anthony et al. 1969) when given intravenously. The recently introduced 5-HT$_1$-receptor agonist GR43175 seems to be effective in treating migraine but is, at least in animal experiments, excluded from uptake into the central nervous system (Dallas et al. 1988).

Interestingly, intravenously applied 5-HT, bradykinin, histamine, and substance P produce vasodilatation and plasma extravasation, probably by an action of these drugs at endothelial receptors (Furchgott 1984; Stephenson and Summers 1987). It is tempting to speculate that ergotamine could cause its effect by acting at the luminal membrane of endothelial cells, either to inhibit the liberation of endothelium-derived relaxing factors or by stimulating the secretion of endothelin.

Information is needed about the precise tissue distribution of ergotamine in animals, and on the concentration that can be achieved in the central nervous system after a single intravenous dose of, say, one microgram per kilogram body weight.

Ergotamine and its putative endothelial site of action

Ergotamine is known as a partial agonist and an antagonist at α-adrenoceptors and also at certain 5-HT receptors. This characterization is based on experiments on isolated, perfused blood vessels and in intact animals. Several points cast doubt on this characterization.

1. The rate of the vasoconstrictor response to ergotamine differs from that of the response to classical vasoconstrictors such as noradrenaline

(norepinephrine). In isolated vessels, which are sensitive to both stimuli, the response to noradrenaline reaches its maximum within three minutes, whereas it takes 30 to 40 minutes to complete the ergotamine contraction (Mikkelsen *et al.* 1981; Glusa and Markwardt 1982). It is hard to understand why a receptor-mediated response should take such a long time.

2. Isolated vessels or intact animals treated with ergotamine become sensitized not only to noradrenaline but also to other vasoconstricting stimuli, for example, 5-HT and histamine.

3. Vasoconstriction induced by ergotamine outlasts by far the α-adrenolytic effect of ergotamine.

It has been suggested that ergotamine might be bound with high affinity to the glycocalix lining the luminal membrane of endothelial cells (Ziegler 1985). This assumption is based on the experiments of Nimmerfall and Rosentaler (1980), who studied the binding of ergotamine to goblet-cell mucin. Goblet-cell mucin is formed by proteoglycans and sialoconjugates, which are also found as constituents of the endothelial cell coat. The cell coat may function as a sieving meshwork, as a locally differentiated charge barrier, or to provide specific binding sites and receptors for plasma molecules, which become either absorbed to the cell coat, internalized into the cell itself, or selectively transported across the cell. Binding of ergotamine could alter the function of endothelial cells, for example, by making them more susceptible to activating stimuli or by enhancing the secondary signal that reaches the vascular muscle cell.

An endothelial site of action could explain the slow onset of action, the discrepancies between the time course of the vasoconstrictor effect and that of the α-adrenolytic effect, and a sensitization that seems to be independent from the stimulus.

I cannot decide whether the experimental observations of Lance *et al.* (this volume) and G.A. Lambert *et al.* (unpublished results) allow us to exclude an endothelial site of action for ergotamine. M.A. Moskowitz and his group consider an endothelial site of action to be likely for the ergot alkaloids (Markowitz *et al.* 1988).

Whatever its result, a re-investigation of the pharmacological effects of ergotamine would provide a sounder basis for using ergotamine as a tool in migraine research.

Calcium antagonists in the prophylactic treatment of migraine

When considering the prophylactic treatment of migraine, the overwhelming majority of researchers mention the calcium antagonists as a group. Even when the heterogeneous nature of the members in this group is recognized, this classification still seems to be more misleading than helpful. The problem is caused by the term calcium antagonism, which does not allow us to define a group of substances with a common mode of action, since cellular Ca^{2+}-movements can be affected by a variety of interventions.

It is obvious that the dihydropyridines, for example, nifedipin, have nothing in common with flunarizine. Flunarizine possesses neither the properties of a vasodilator nor is it used as an antihypertensive or anti-anginal drug. It does not alter the electrical properties of the heart in the way that verapamil does. There is no electrophysiological documentation of an inhibition of the 'slow, inward' Ca^{2+} current by flunarizine. I wonder why the pharmacological properties of the only so-called calcium antagonist that has proved to be effective in the prophylactic treatment of migraine are neither mentioned nor taken into account. Flunarizine displays α-adrenolytic, antihistamine, anti-5-HT, and antidopamine activities. It is characterized by a high lipophilicity and seems to accumulate in tissues during prolonged treatment. The migraine-prophylactic effect needs several days to develop. Since the specific pharmacodynamic properties as well as the peculiar pharmacokinetics of flunarizine seem to be of relevance for its introduction in the prophylactic treatment of migraine, one should be cautious with the term calcium antagonist, since it might cause unjustified conclusions concerning the efficacy of other so-called calcium antagonists and one should be even more cautious in modelling new concepts for the aetiology of migraine from a more or less arbitrary label given to a drug.

Even if the whole group of so-called calcium antagonists proved to be effective (Solomon 1985) these drugs would not be suitable for elucidating the pathophysiological processes that underly migraine (Meyer et al. 1985), and one would be inclined to believe that any pharmacological treatment could yield some relief in migraine.

Patients' compliance in the prophylactic treatment of migraine

When drugs are being evaluated for their suitability in the prophylactic treatment of migraine it is presumed that the patient has taken the prescribed drug in the prescribed dose at the prescribed interval. In other fields of drug therapy it is known that the patients compliance may be rather poor. This holds true not only for diseases without any concomitant acute suffering but also for those that impair the patient's well-being and, in which, for example, a strong pain should guarantee the patient's compliance. During the headache-free interval there is no stimulus to make the patient keep strictly to the prescribed interval of drug intake. This problem is especially relevant in migraine interval therapy, since this drug treatment includes outpatients, for whom there is no possibility of the medication being controlled by the nursing staff.

In order to maintain their compliance, patients are asked to keep a headache diary, and to include in their reports not only the number and duration of headache periods but also the number of swallowed tablets. To my knowledge, nobody has succeeded in obtaining information about the reliability of those entries in the patient's diary. Headache diaries do not provide a solution to the problem. The value of headache diaries for keeping track of the nature and intensity of the migraine headache itself has been questioned (Bruyn 1985), and the same criticisms apply when such a diary is used for monitoring drug compliance.

Where are we going?

In this paper I have dealt with problems that lie on the borderline between the pathophysiology, the pharmacotherapy, and the pharmacology of migraine. Our hopes must centre on this border, because an intimate and reliable knowledge of these fields will offer a clue towards an optimal therapeutic strategy. Nevertheless, we know it will take a long time before this academic approach will be succcessful. In the first instance, we should concentrate on the drugs that have been developed as alternatives to ergotamine. It is to be hoped that these new drugs will be free of the inherent drawback of ergotamine — its deleterious side-effects when given too frequently. Satisfying results in clinical practice could render the prophylactic treatment of migraine superfluous. It could be a real advantage to avoid prophylactic treatment, which always has to meet the high standards required of any long-term medication. Furthermore, such treatment includes periods of unnecessary exposure of the patient to a drug, since the treatment is continued during the symptom-free interval. Investigating the efficiency of any prophylactic treatment involves problems that do not arise in treatment of acute attacks.

References

Anthony, M., Hinterberger, H., and Lance, J.W. (1969). The possible relationship of serotonin to the migraine syndrome. *Research and Clinical Studies in Headache*, **2**, 29–59.

Bruyn, G.W. (1985). Prevalence and incidence of migraine — a critical review. In *Migraine and β-blockade*, (ed. J.D. Carroll, V. Pfaffenrath, and O. Sjaastad), pp. 237–40. AB Hässle, Mölndal.

Dallas, F.A.A., Dixon, C.M., McCulloch, R.J., and Saynor, D.A. (1988). The kinetics of ^{14}C-GR 43175 in rat and dog. *Proceedings of the 7th Migraine Trust International Symposium, London, 5th to 7th Sept 1988*.

Furchgott, R.F. (1984). The role of endothelium in the response of vascular smooth muscle to drugs. *Annual Reviews of Pharmacology and Toxicology*, **24**, 175–97.

Glusa, E. and Markwardt, F. (1982). Dual effect of dihydroergotamine and dihydroergotoxin in isolated human femoral veins and arteries *Pharmacology*, **24**, 287–93.

Kimball, R.W., Friedman, A.P., and Vallejo, E. (1960). Effect of serotonin in migraine patients. *Neurology*, **10**, 107–11.

Markowitz, S., Saito, K., and Moskowitz, M.A. (1988). Neurogenically mediated plasma extravasation in dura mater: effect of ergot alkaloids. A possible mechanism of action of vascular headache. *Cephalalgia*, **8**, 83–92.

Meyer, J.S., Nance, M., Walker, M., Zetusky, W.J., and Dowell, R.E. (1985). Migraine and cluster headache treatment with calcium antagonists supports a vascular pathogenesis. *Headache*, **25**, 358–67.

Mikkelsen, E., Pedersen, O.L., Ostergaard, I.L., and Pedersen, S.E. (1981). Effect of ergotamine on isolated human vessels. *Archives Internationales de Pharmacodynamie et Therapie*, **252**, 241–52.

Moskowitz, M.A., Henrikson, B.M., Markowitz, S., and Saito, K. (1988). Intra- and extracraniovascular nociceptive mechanisms and the pathogenesis of head pain. In *Basic mechanisms of headache*, (ed. J. Olesen and L. Edvinsson), pp. 429–37. Elsevier, Amsterdam.

Nimmerfall, F. and Rosentaler, J. (1980). Significance of the goblet-cell mucin layer, the outermost luminal barrier to passage through the gut wall. *Biochemical and Biophysical Research Communications*, **94**, 960–6.

Stephenson, J.A. and Summers, R.J. (1987). Autoradiographic analysis of receptors on vascular endothelium. *European Journal of Pharmacology*, **134**, 35–43.

Solomon, G.D. (1985). Comparative efficacy of calcium antagonist drugs in the prophylaxis of migraine. *Headache*, **25**, 368–71.

Ziegler, A. (1985). Future directions: aspects of beta-adrenoceptor blocking agents and other prophylactic therapies. In *Migraine and β-blockade*, (ed. J.D. Carroll, V. Pfaffenrath, and O. Sjaastad), pp. 237–240. AB Hässle, Mölndal.

Discussion

COPPEN: Reports on clinical trials of prophylactic treatment rarely mention patient compliance. I agree entirely with your comments on compliance. In our long-term studies (over 25 years) of psychiatric patients with affective disorders, we have found that even with motivated patients and doctors it takes about six months before the patients learn to take a simple drug like lithium. We have always measured the lithium concentration in the patient's blood, *before* they see the doctor. A basic requirement for testing compliance with any compound is for there to be a simple way of measuring its plasma concentrations; otherwise one cannot carry out a rational trial. It would be a great waste of pharmacological effort if the end result is that only a third of the patients will take the drug, and only for some of the time.

OLESEN: On another point, I agree with you, Professor Ziegler, that flunarizine may not be typical of the so-called calcium antagonists or calcium blockers. Use of the general terms can obscure different modes of action. It is a problem that flunarizine is the only well-documented drug in this whole class. In the past the group of calcium blockers has been considered to be effective as a whole. Some reports of double-blind trials with verapamil may be misleading because too few patients were involved, and there were too many dropouts. Two very good trials with nimodipine showed that it had a positive effect in migraine; although, in my opinion, two trials are not enough to have a drug accepted as effective (see Olesen 1986). This caution has proved to be well-founded because, recently, the big European multi-centre trial on nimodipine ended. It included 200 patients who had migraine without aura. There was a separate trial, with the same protocol, for migraine with aura. Both trials were totally negative. We cannot be sure that flunarizine is effective because of its so-called calcium antagonistic properties. In the WHO committee on calcium blockers, we had heated discussions about whether flunarizine was or was not a calcium antagonist or calcium uptake inhibitor. There were strong views on both sides.

ZIEGLER: I will call flunarizine a calcium antagonist if, in the same breath, you allow me to call, say, phenobarbitone and carbachol calcium antagonists, too! That is to say, if we require a drug only to produce a negative inotropic response and to reduce the concentrations of free calcium ions within the cytosol, in order to define it as a calcium antagonist, then flunarizine *may* be called a calcium antagonist. But by these criteria three-quarters of the drugs mentioned in pharmacology textbooks can be classified as calcium antagonists. I am aware of the interesting experimental results obtained with flunarizine by Godfraind and Dieu (1981). I do not, however, share the published interpretation. Similar experimental results may be obtained with chlorpromazine or phenobarbitone; nevertheless we would not include these drugs within the group of calcium antagonists.

HUMPHREY: It is surprising that such a diversity of compounds can act as prophylactics. Even disregarding the poor quality of some of the drug trials, I find it impossible to come to terms with why these drugs work. It is conceivable that we are often dealing with *active* placebos, and therefore we can never do a placebo-*controlled* study. We know that the migraineur is in a very fine balance. He or she has a low threshold to migraine, and various influences can readily trigger off an attack. We know how powerful the influence of the doctor can be. If the patient believes that he or she is receiving effective medication, that in itself has a powerful influence on the psyche, which therefore reduces the number of attacks.

SANDLER: This is the placebo effect anyway, is it not? Can you subdivide it?

HUMPHREY: No; I am considering here an *active* placebo, which has some pharmacological actions (that is, cardiovascular or sedative) that are unrelated to the specific treatment of migraine.

ZIEGLER: The problem of an 'active' placebo can be eliminated only by repeating the trial several times or by prolonging the observation period within a trial. It has been shown, for example, that chenodesoxycholic acid was active as a migraine prophylactic in a double-blind controlled study lasting four weeks (Lévy *et al.* 1978). Patients treated with this bile acid experience side-effects and are, thus, continuously aware of being treated. I doubt that this sort of treatment is efficient when it is continued for several months.

OLESEN: I agree with Dr Humphrey. There is no question that if a migraine patient is given an active drug as a placebo the patient will have a greater placebo response than if something entirely inert were being taken. The International Headache Society's committee on drug trials has not yet resolved what to do about it. Let me explain this. If a placebo is used which causes certain activities in the body — such as atropine, which causes a dry mouth — but which is not believed to work in migraine, then after the trial people might say that the reason why there is no difference between atropine and flunarizine is that atropine *does* have an effect on migraine; that would be very hard to disprove. It is a remarkable thing that even today the hypothesis remains tenable that all drugs so far shown to be effective in migraine are effective only because of this unspecific placebo-like action. We cannot disprove that hypothesis.

SANDLER: I share doubts about whether pharmacological developments will provide all the answers. Their usefulness may lie mainly in the experiments they suggest. Make no mistake that it is to direct biological experimentation that we need to turn our minds. But how do we gain access to suitable material? For Parkinson's disease at least, there are brain banks — but they store not only Parkinsonian brains but control brains too. That control group might well provide material for the study of migraine if the brain bank team were to include in their protocol a question about the subjects' lifetime history of migraine. It might be possible to carry out receptor binding studies on human material in this way. We could also try to explore the nature of migraine vulnerability. Membrane transport deficits or differences, for example, may explain why some patients have migraine while others do not.

BLAU: I support this idea of using a brain bank. At Guy's Hospital Medical School, London, the multiple sclerosis brain bank would be an even better source of material for the study of migraine because some of the brains are from young women, whose medical history would have been carefully recorded throughout the years when migraine may have struck them.

LANCE: You mentioned, Professor Ziegler, that the vasoconstrictor action of ergotamine took 30 to 40 minutes to develop. Do you mean the latency to the peak of constriction? In our monkey experiments we found that the constriction induced by intravenous ergotamine (3.6 μg/kg) reached its peak 2–11 minutes after administration and was well maintained for two hours in the monkey extracranial vasculature, *in vivo*. Furthermore, in humans, intravenous dihydroergotamine or intramuscular ergotamine are effective in a matter of minutes.

ZIEGLER: I meant the time necessary to attain maximal responses. When dihydroergotamine was infused over two minutes into the cephalic vein of dogs, the maximal response was reached (depending on the dose applied) between 30 and 90 minutes later (Müller-Schweinitzer and Rosenthaler 1987). When the drug was applied as a short-term infusion (lasting 10 minutes) into the superficial hand vein of humans, the rate of vasoconstriction depended on the dose applied, and a maximal response was reached 20 to 60 minutes after the end of the infusion (Aellig 1974). These are exciting results because by the time of the maximal response, dihydroergotamine will be diluted throughout the blood volume. There must be an effect initiated before then, but which develops slowly, on a secondary level; that is, it no longer depends on the presence of the drug in the blood.

LANCE: In our monkey experiments we showed that the constrictor effect of ergotamine on the extracranial vasculature was three times as great as its effect on the cerebral circulation (Spira *et al.* 1976). When there was a marked constrictor effect on the extracranial vessels there was no significant change in systemic blood pressure. We are dealing with the cranial vessels *in vivo*, rather than with some peripheral vein, or an *in vitro* preparation.

SAXENA: We did similar experiments, and found a reasonably quickly developing vasoconstrictor action of ergotamine (Saxena and de Vlaam-Schluter 1974). Peak effect was in five to ten minutes but certainly not in half an hour. However, the effect of ergotamine lasts for a longer time.

FOZARD: Ergotamine has nanomolar affinities at a number of 5-HT receptors, at which it can either be a full or a partial agonist, depending on the tissue. It also has activity in nanomolar concentrations at adrenoceptors. Whether or not ergotamine shows a fast or a slow response onset may depend on which particular receptor site is being activated in the different experimental conditions.

HUMPHREY: There is a misunderstanding here. It is just a question of the effect of ergotamine coming to equilibrium. If you administer ergotamine into isolated blood vessels, it takes over an hour to come to equilibrium. If you inject it as a bolus *in vivo*, you do not get equilibrium; you just get a slowly developing vasoconstriction and then the drug becomes dissipated throughout the circulation. Nobody denies that the *onset* of action is quick in both experiments but pharmacological equilibrium requires a long time even *in vitro*.

OLESEN: P. Tfelt-Hansen has shown that there is an early adrenoceptor-mediated response in the human, when ergotamine is given intravenously: it will increase blood pressure, predominantly by acting on the arterioles. But the effect on the large arteries is a very slow process. In the human extremities, it takes a maximum of three hours. It may be different in the cranium.

SAXENA: Ergotamine does have a nanomolar affinity for 5-HT recognition sites. However, the vasoconstrictor action of ergotamine is not blocked by drugs that antagonize α_1, α_2, 5-HT$_1$-like or 5-HT$_2$ receptors (Saxena *et al.* 1983; Bom *et al.* 1989).

FOZARD: May I make my earlier point again? Unless one is consistently referring to the same interaction between ergotamine and the same membrane receptor, one cannot make comparisons. So few of these responses to ergotamine have been thoroughly characterized in terms of the particular receptor involved.

ZIEGLER: This discussion makes the point of my contribution even more clear: one should question the appropriateness of drugs like ergotamine and flunarizine as tools in migraine research.

References

Aellig, W.H. (1974). Investigation of the venoconstrictor effect of 8'-hydroxydihydroergotamine, the main metabolite of dihydroergotamine in man. *European Journal of Clinical Pharmacology*, **26**, 239–42.

Bom, A.H., Heiligers, J.P.C., Saxena, P.R., and Verdouw, P.D. (1989). Reduction of cephalic arteriovenous shunting by ergotamine is not mediated by 5-HT$_1$-like or 5-HT$_2$ receptors. *British Journal of Pharmacology*, in press.

Godfraind, T., and Dieu, D. (1981). The inhibition by flunarizine of the norepinephrine-evoked contraction and calcium influx in rat aorta and mesenteric arteries. *Journal of Pharmacology and Experimental Therapeutics*, **217**, 510–5.

Lévy, V.G., Nusinovici, V., Rosner, D., and Darius, F. (1978). Chenodesoxycholic acid in the prevention of migraine. *New England Journal of Medicine*, **298**, 630.

Müller-Schweinitzer, E. and Rosenthaler, J. (1987). Dihydroergotamine: pharmacokinetics, pharmacodynamics, and mechanism of venoconstrictor action in beagle dogs. *Journal of Cardiovascular Pharmacology*, **9**, 686–93.

Olesen, J. (1986). The role of calcium entry blockers in the prophylaxis of migraine. *Neurology*, Suppl. 1, 72–9.

Saxena, P.R., and de Vlaam-Schluter, G.M. (1974). Role of some biogenic substances in migraine and relevant mechanism in antimigraine action of ergotamine. Studies in an animal experimental model for migraine. *Headache*, **13**, 142–63.

Saxena, P.R., Koedam, N.A., Heiligers, J., and Hof, R.P. (1983). Ergotamine-induced constriction of cranial arteriovenous anastomoses in dogs pretreated with phentolamine and pizotifen. *Cephalalgia*, **3**, 71–81.

Spira, P.J., Mylecharane, E.J., and Lance, J.W. (1976). The effects of humoral agents and artimigraine drugs on the cranial circulation of the monkey. *Research and Clinical Studies in Headache*, **4**, 37–75.

26. General discussion II

Introduction

WELCH: There have now been defined four stages in migraine: the prodromal stage, the aural stage, the headache stage, and the refractory period. We shall need, over the next few years, to examine the mechanisms of all four stages. The symptoms of the first stage seem to be neurological in origin. We have to find out what metabolic shifts or membranal changes are occurring in this prodromal phase before the migraine is activated. The central nervous system effects are worth pursuing. Our magnetoencephalography studies have to be examined more fully: is it spreading depression or a depolarizing event, and so on. Rao and Wolff (1940) stimulated intracranial structures under local anaesthetic to try to localize the source of pain but Dr Moskowitz is now helping us to understand the mechanisms of this trigeminovascular pain system. There are now attempts to identify what is activating migraine: is it a psychological event that directly activates, cortically, the changes in slow-wave activity, or do we have to propose sub-cortical changes that modulate those cortical activities? How can we get from a primary cortical event to the headache? Some of the trigeminovascular ablative work that Dr Moskowitz is doing is answering that. What we must do in the next few years is to put the whole picture together.

Migraine, seizure, and photophobia

BLAU: Perhaps we can introduce a clinical definition of migraine:

migraine = headache + autonomic disturbances.

If this hypothesis is right, we ought to study headache more. In a recent study of 100 patients with epilepsy, we (Schon and Blau 1987) found that 51 patients had the commonly experienced post-epileptic headache. Of these 51 patients, nine were migraineurs, and eight of those nine were provoked into their typical migraine attacks. That is interesting in the light of Raskin's (1988) view that perturbation of the brain causes migraine.

MOSKOWITZ: Was aura precipitated after the seizure? That would be remarkable because of the presumed relationship between spreading depression and hyperpolarization. I would expect seizure threshold to be quite high.

BLAU: No, they did not have an aura, but the headache had the same quality as their usual migraine headache. In addition, they had vomiting and photophobia; that is, the migraine attacks were normal, lasting several hours. I want to draw attention here to the 43 patients who did not have migraine. A proportion (27 out of 43) of those had headaches lasting 6–72 hours; 11 of the 43 had vomiting; 14 had photophobia, and three reported that when their headache had gone, it returned if they coughed, sneezed, or bent down. That is very much like the clinical picture of migraine. The patients had various sorts of seizures, but those with major seizures were more liable to headache than those who had minor epileptic attacks. In our study we have unearthed a large number of people who are prone to a headache that bears a *close resemblance* to clinical migraine. We need to find out the difference between the ordinary, long, severe headaches that occur in a variety of circumstances, such as after exercise or alcohol, and the migraine headache. Perhaps the group that we classify as migraineurs are at the end of a headache spectrum that we need to study.

MOSKOWITZ: Earlier we described a mechanism for seizure-induced activation of the trigeminal system, as reflected by changes in flow, which are inferential with regard to pain (Moskowitz *et al.*, this volume). One of the two mechanisms for inducing the asymmetry was seizure. One does not need to invoke Raskin's hypothesis to explain this relationship. An increase in potassium and neurotransmitter levels in the extracellular space could activate the pain fibres that surround blood vessels. Of course, it could be more complicated than that, but it need not be.

BLAU: It would be interesting to see whether neural firing could be shown to be dose-related to a noise or light stimulus so that it ultimately would fire with a seizure periodicity.

GARDNER-MEDWIN: It would be helpful to know whether migraine attacks are distinct from seizures in their correlation with disturbances of platelet and plasma 5-HT physiology. Perhaps seizures also cause these disturbances.

MOSKOWITZ: Dr Blau, what is your understanding of the neural mechanisms of photophobia?

BLAU: I like to start with what is physiological. Many of us have experienced the unpleasant effect of bright sunlight when we come out of the cinema in the afternoon; plenty of people wear protective glasses on ski slopes; and, of course, there is snow blindness. These reactions are, in my view, biologically protective and normal. Within the range of normality, too, would be those who are visually sensitive and have to wear dark glasses sooner than others. A greater degree of severity, and what I would call real 'photophobia' is pathological, as in meningitis, encephalitis, or in measles and other conditions where the brain and/or meninges are involved. Many of the migraine symptoms could reflect a generally heightened irritability of the nervous system: that is, the patient is more sensitive to light, noise, smell, touch, and vibration. And, typically with migraine, withdrawal into solitude is the patient's biological response.

MOSKOWITZ: Interestingly, work published in the mid-1930s described three necessary components to the development of photophobia. The first is (obviously) the light, the second is sight, and the third is an intact trigeminal nerve (Lebensohn 1934).

LANCE: Peter Drummond in our laboratory has compared photophobia with pupillary size under varying degrees of illumination, and in the presence or absence of migrainous and tension headache (Drummond 1986). His results show that there are two components to photophobia. One is unilateral, felt in the eye on the side of the headache, and appears to be a trigeminal irritation phenomenon. The other component is a more diffuse, background disinhibition, that Dr Blau referred to, and is associated with hyperacusis, sensitivity to smell, and so on. The second component can also be experienced by tension headache patients.

Migraine and tension headache

GLOVER: I should like to know more about the relationship between tension headache and migraine. There is great effort to separate them diagnostically, but why should we think of them separately instead of as part of a continuum?

LANCE: Peter Drummond and I did a survey in which we tried to divide patients, on clinical grounds, into those with cluster headache, classical migraine (migraine with aura), common migraine (without aura), and tension headache (Drummond and Lance 1984). Independently we had a computer select certain criteria as well, to divide these people into diagnostic categories. For cluster headache and for migraine with aura, our decisions on diagnosis correlated well with the computer categories. However, the categories of migraine and tension headache were extremely difficult: neither we nor the computer could distinguish the precise point of demarcation. For example, initially a patient may have a right-sided headache with nausea, vomiting and photophobia once a month. This headache may become more frequent, say, two or three times a week, and then daily. The nausea and vomiting may have gone, or perhaps a little nausea or photophobia may remain, but the headache can stay precisely in the same spot, on the right side. Why should a migraine be reclassified as a tension headache when the headache is in exactly the same place as it was when we considered it as typical common migraine? My personal view is that we are dealing here with two ends of a headache spectrum.

BLAU: This is a very important point. We may have no difficulty, clinically, in distinguishing tension headache from migraine, because the patients present two different pictures. The migraine patient, between attacks, feels perfectly well: one often hears 'I forget all about it'. The patient with tension headache, however, may have the headache virtually every day, and all day, experienced as a band of pressure all around the head. Analgesics usually provide no relief at all with tension headache. If migraine affects 10 per cent of the population and tension headache is common, there will be some patients with both the intermittent migraine and the superimposed, fairly constant tension headache. Perhaps some of your patients have both, Professor Lance.

LANCE: There is no doubt that one can distinguish clinically between most patients in the two groups, but it is the middle ground, as in my hypothetical instance just now, that remains muddied.

BLAU: I cannot answer that specific instance. However, there is a third variety of headache, after migraine and tension headache. The third sort is a localized head pain, often found in middle age, and consistently in the same place. Sometimes it is provoked by specific stimuli and, unlike tension headache, it will respond to analgesics in 20 to 30 minutes (J.N. Blau, in press). The advent of the EMG has confused the diagnostic picture, here, because the accompanying and measurable muscular contractions have caused it to be called 'muscular contraction headache'. This has led us into a vicious circle of mechanisms and conditions.

GROSS: The localized occipital headache that may be found to occur with increasing regularity may be a form of greater occipital neuralgia. A proportion of them will respond to local injections of corticosteroids and local anaesthetic, particularly when there is localized tenderness in the occipital area.

GLOVER: How good is the evidence that tension headache and migraine have different responses to drugs?

BLAU: In my clinical experience, the localized head pain that I have just described responds to aspirin or paracetamol in 20 to 30 minutes, the relief lasting three to four hours; the tension headache is not influenced by analgesics; and the migraine, as we have heard here, is improved in a proportion of cases by various antimigraine preparations.

MOSKOWITZ: Perhaps ergotamine would relieve some of your tension headache patients. Have you tried it?

BLAU: No.

PEATFIELD: It would be nice to see some systematic, double-blind results of treatment, based on your proposed simple classification, Dr Blau, into three main sorts of headache.

OLESEN: There is no systematic study of the same drug being used to treat the different types of headache. Since flunarizine has been proved to be effective in migraine, I maintain that it would be worthwhile to do a tension headache study with flunarizine. For the millions of patients who suffer from tension headache, it would be important, and it would perhaps teach us something about headache mechanisms.

MOSKOWITZ: There may be a common mechanism by which the ergotamine compounds are working, because they also work in cluster headache, which is very different from common or classical migraine. They may well work in tension headache, too.

LANCE: I believe that we are dealing with a continuum. At one end are the chronic daily headaches, a considerable proportion of which (60 per cent or so) will respond to tricyclic antidepressants, particularly amitryptiline. At the other end of the scale are the typical migrainous headaches that will respond more to methysergide. In between them is a grey area of headaches, and I think we would all agree about their responsiveness to propranolol, pizotifen, and so on. In general, the more frequent the headache, the better the response to amitryptiline. We found in our survey (Drummond and Lance 1984) that all the features associated with migraine became progressively less prominent as the headache became more and more frequent. For example, 60 per cent of monthly headaches were unilateral but only 15 per cent of daily headaches were unilateral. It was the same picture with photophobia, nausea and the other symptoms that we consider to be migrainous. Therefore I find it hard to believe that there is not a common pathophysiology, but I concede the point made by Dr Blau about identifying typical cases.

MOSKOWITZ: We have found no evidence for neurogenic inflammation in temporal muscle, after electrical stimulation and capsaicin treatments (S. Markowitz and M.A. Moskowitz, unpublished results), but our Evans blue staining revealed that the fascia around the muscle had taken up the stain, showing that the connective tissue surrounding the muscle was the site of plasma extravasation. This may be relevant to tension headache, to the sensitivity of the muscle, and to the apparent negativity of the electromyograph studies that Professor Olesen has reported.

BLAU: There is, undoubtedly, a pain of muscle activity. I would suspect that it is in the *fascia* of the muscles, as Dr Moskowitz has just implied, but it could also arise in joints. These localized pains respond to local treatment — to physiotherapy, analgesics, heat, massage, or acupuncture. But this is totally different from the tension headache that I described earlier as a band around the head. Of course the headache will respond to amitryptiline if the patient is depressed; it will respond to anxiolytics if the patient is anxious; but if there is an external source of anxiety —

mortgage, maths homework, bullying at school — the headache will not often respond to pharmacological drugs.

GLOVER: It seems that there could be several different basic mechanisms underlying what goes wrong, and different patients may have different combinations of them. Or perhaps there is a progression to different end-points, so that even with a common pathological basis, one patient's headache would show up more as a tension headache case, while another would develop into migraine.

SANDLER: This is rather like the protean manifestations of syphilis or tuberculosis, before the discovery of the causal microorganism.

BLAU: But surely we would not hold on to the ideas of 200 years ago when all abdominal pain — from the duodenum, the fallopian tubes, the kidneys, or the bladder — was considered to be due to one cause?

MOSKOWITZ: One certainly cannot distinguish between those visceral sites by the *quality* of the pain, but only by its location.

OLESEN: The question of whether migraine and tension headache are two ends of a spectrum, or two different syndromes with overlapping symptoms is very difficult. We have seen a patient with a highly typical migrainous visual aura, and an arteriovenous malformation. Not one of our other patients with aura had anything demonstrably wrong in the cranium. The symptoms were the same, but the aetiology was totally different. Furthermore, in some of the inherited diseases, the phenotype can be extremely different but the genotype is the same. So it is very complicated. We discussed this in the Headache Classification Committee (1988). By and large, my inclination is that we should try to separate them. There are many reasons why the symptoms could be similar, amongst a large intermediate group of patients. One reason, as Professor Ferreira has discussed (this volume), is the memory of pain. One can easily understand how repeated attacks of migraine could gradually create, over the years, a continuous sensation of pain.

References

Cruickshank, J.M. and Neil-Dwyer, G. (1985). Beta-blocker brain concentrations in man. *European Journal of Clinical Pharmacology*, **28**, (Suppl.), 21–23.

Drummond, P.D. (1986). Quantitative assessment of photophobia in migraine and tension headache. *Headache*, **26**, 465–9.

Drummond, P.D. and Lance, J.W. (1984). Clinical diagnosis and computer analysis of headache symptoms. *Journal of Neurology, Neurosurgery and Psychiatry*, **47**, 128–33.

Headache Classification Committee of the International Headache Society. (Jes Olesen, chairman) (1988). Classification and diagnostic criteria for headache disorders, cranial neuralgias and facial pain. *Cephalalgia*, **8**, Suppl. 7, 1–96.

Lebensohn, J.E. (1934). The nature of photophobia. *Archives of Ophthalmology*, **12**, 380–90.

Raskin, N.H. (1988). On the origin of head pain. *Headache*, **28**, 254–7.

Ray, B.S., Wolff, H.G. (1940). Experimental studies on headache: pain-sensitive structures of the head and their significance in headache. *Archives of Surgery*, **41**, 813–56.

Schon, F. and Blau, J.N. (1987). Post-epileptic headache and migraine. *Journal of Neurology, Neurosurgery and Psychiatry*, **50**, 1148–52.

27. The neurovascular basis of migraine: some concluding thoughts

James W. Lance

In early studies of dysphasia, neurologists drew diagrams connecting little bits of the brain with one another to explain their thoughts. Great scorn was poured on these people as 'the diagram-makers'. We have returned to this approach in the understanding of dysphasia, and people readily use diagrams to help clarify various concepts about language function.

With this in mind, I submit a simple schema (Fig. 27.1) which may help to summarize our thoughts on the amalgamation of the neural and vascular hypotheses about migraine. First of all, we are dealing with an inherited susceptibility, not an autosomal dominant or recessive characteristic, but a migrainous threshold. This is analogous to the epileptic threshold, whereby some patients may have one fit in their lives while others have regular attacks and some only after a specific provocation. Similarly, some people might have one migrainous attack in their lives, while others are subject to frequent episodes, and some react only to particular stimuli.

The migrainous threshold itself is of polygenic inheritance and difficult to quantify. It may depend, for example, on the relative distribution of monoamine transmitters or endorphins, or on the imbalance of transduction systems. The advances in knowledge of the biochemistry, physiology, and pharmacology of migraine give us more and more systems to experiment with, more and more that could potentially go wrong.

Then we have the concept which Nat Blau put forward at the beginning of this volume — that many forms of migraine clearly arise within the brain itself. There may be changes in mood and other premonitory symptoms, such as somnolence and hunger, that indicate an origin in the hypothalamus. There must be 'internal clocks' that regulate the onset of a migrainous attack. The most obvious is the link with the menstrual cycle, but many people have headaches at weekly intervals or at other predetermined periods irrespective of the degree of stress they are undergoing at the time. There is, thus, a cyclical variation in this somewhat fragile, delicately balanced, inherited brain.

Superimposed on this fluctuating susceptibility are precipitating factors such as fatigue, stress, and afferent stimuli that act through cerebral mech-

MIGRAINE THRESHOLD

Polygenic inheritance

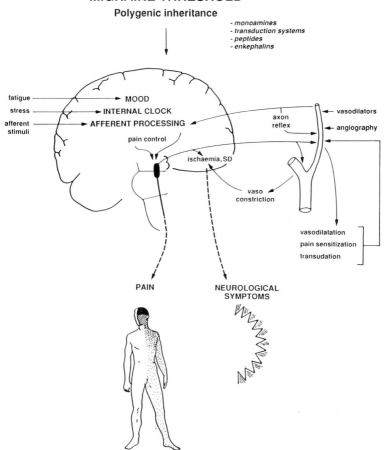

FIG. 27.1. A schema for the neurovascular basis of migraine. An inherited 'migraine threshold' renders the subject susceptible to fluctuations in hypothalamic function (signalled by alteration of mood or craving for sweet foods), environmental changes, fatigue, stress, or excessive afferent stimulation (including input from cranial vessels). Brainstem monoaminergic nuclei influence cerebral and extracranial bloodflow by direct and indirect projections. cortical ischaemia, often accompanied by spreading depression (SD), is associated with focal neurological symptoms. The release of 5-hydroxytryptamine (5-HT, serotonin) and vasodilator peptides induces a sterile inflammatory response, in blood vessels, which feeds pain-producing impulses back to the nervous system and may produce further vascular responses by an axon reflex. Depression of the endogenous pain control system may be an additional factor in increasing the discharge frequency of trigeminothalamic (and sometimes spinothalamic) neurones so that migrainous pain is experienced in the head with radiation to the neck (often), shoulder and arm (occasionally), or leg (rarely). Pharmacotherapy is aimed at interrupting this vicious circle in the central nervous system, or peripherally in the cranial vasculature.

anisms. For example, exposure to flickering light may lead to a person experiencing visual disturbance and headache within a matter of minutes if he or she is a migrainous patient. Very often, the type of aura bears a direct relation to the nature of the afferent stimuli that impinge on the nervous system, which must surely mean a disturbance of afferent processing, a failure of normal inhibitory mechanisms. This breakdown of perceptual restraint may underlie the sensitivity to light, sound, smell, and touch that is such a common feature of the migraine attack. Whether disinhibition of the pain control pathway, or a segment of it, plays a part in migraine headache remains to be seen.

This is the neural side of the picture, but we also have to consider the vascular side because we know that vasodilator substances or the injection of contrast medium for cerebral angiography may induce migrainous headache. This may be caused by a direct effect on the vessels or be mediated by afferent discharges from the vascular system. We have heard Mike Moskowitz's concept of the part that the axon reflex may play in vascular dilatation, pain sensitization and transudation, with the liberation of peptides and prostaglandins (see Markowitz *et al.* 1987, 1988, 1989). Vascular changes may also be induced by projections from the brainstem.

Let us look again at the central area. Our own work in the monkey has demonstrated that stimulation of locus coeruleus constricts the intracranial circulation and dilates the extracranial circulation, while the raphé nuclei can induce dilatation in both circulations. These monoaminergic nuclei are also involved in the endogenous pain-control mechanism. There is, thus, a temptation to think in terms of a wave of excessive monoaminergic activity followed by a phase of depletion.

The migraine attack may start in the brain and affect the vascular system secondarily. Feedback from vessels to the brain completes a vicious circle. In the internal carotid circulation, the phase of constriction is associated with neurological symptoms. There may be a diffuse ischaemia of the brain or a progressive, slow march of oligaemia that correlates with spreading depression.

What is the origin of the headache itself? Migrainous pain, while centred on the head, is often referred to the neck, or to the lower part of the face — we recognize facial migraine ('lower-half headache') — and sometimes to the shoulder and the arm. Some patients give a clear history of referral of pain down the entire side of the body, as illustrated in Fig. 27.1. This would imply to me that there is an unrestrained discharge of neurones not only in the trigeminal system but also in the spinothalamic system. This extends the concept of the origin of migrainous pain to thalamic level. Headache is often associated with hyperalgesia and hyperaesthesia, and we have heard that there can be a pain memory, so to speak, implanted by prostaglandins with repetitive stimulation.

If we accept the schema in Fig. 27.1 as a vague outline of the interaction between neural and vascular factors, where do we go? What are the recommendations? What should we be doing over the next few years?

The first thing is to observe patients carefully to assess whether *the site of the headache* is on the side one would expect from the nature of the neurological symptoms. I have always accepted my patients' histories. After patients have experienced a visual or sensory aura, let us say, on the right side of the body, half of them state that the ensuing headache is felt on the left side and the other half say it appears on the right. Jes Olesen has observed patients during attacks while studying cerebral blood flow and, irrespective of what they have said in the past, he has found that their headache has been contralateral to the neurological symptoms they have just experienced. If this is so, it would help to validate the hypothesis put forward by Mike Moskowitz that the axon reflex and sterile inflammatory response associated with the cerebral disturbance could give rise to headache (see Markowitz *et al.* 1987, 1988, 1989). I have criticized this view in the past on the grounds that the headache is, as often as not, stated to occur on the side inappropriate for the production of the aura. We shall have to check this with patients during each headache to see if we can attribute aura and headache to one localized response, or whether we have to postulate a brainstem mechanism that can produce neurological symptoms on one side followed by headache on the other side.

The development of new pharmacological tools is obviously important. The more *specific pharmacological probes* we have, the more we can extrapolate to the pathophysiology of migraine after we have determined precisely what these pharmacological tools will do. The clinical effects of new drugs, such as the $5HT_1$ agonist GR43175, will have to be applied to our concept of the mechanism of migraine.

We could study the human trigeminal system more effectively, but we have to study *small-fibre activity*. The present method of studying evoked responses depends, of course, on potentials conducted in large fibres. When we talk about pain, we are interested in fibres of small diameter in which volleys become dispersed and unrecordable because of their low conduction velocity. We need to devise new techniques to assess trigeminal activity during and between migraine attacks, possibly by quantification of reflexes that employ the trigeminal nerve as their afferent limb.

How can we test brainstem activity, the raphé nuclei, locus coeruleus and reticular formation? Ingenious studies by Jean Schoenen in Belgium have shown that the *contingent negative variation* is affected in migraine, that it depends on a noradrenergic input (which could well originate from locus coeruleus) to the cerebral cortex, and that it can be altered by β-blockers. This is a method of determining what is going wrong *physiologically* in humans, who are the primary source of our study, not the monkey, cat, or rat.

Finally, is it possible that the sort of work that we are doing might lead to some more accurate *surgical approach*? We have been quite excited by the dorsolateral area of the second cervical segment that we have found, in the cat, to be involved in the transmission of vascular afferents. If it proves to bear any great relevance to the pain of migraine, it is conceivable that a localized surgical lesion at that point, possibly by percutaneous cordotomy, could impair or destroy visceral afferent pain sensation arising from the vessels that mediate headache, without causing a loss of cutaneous pain and temperature sensation.

I can forsee the need for us all to meet again in a few years' time when we have answers to some of these questions.

References

Markowitz, S., Saito, K., and Moskowitz, M.A. (1987). Neurogenically mediated leakage of plasma protein occurs from blood vessels in dura mater but not brain. *Journal of Neuroscience*, **7**, 4129–36.

Markowitz, S., Saito, K., and Moskowitz, M.A. (1988). Neurogenically mediated plasma extravasation in dura mater: effect of ergot-alkaloids. A possible mechanism of action in vascular headache. *Cephalalgia*, **8**, 83–91.

Markowitz, S., Saito, K., Buzzi, M.G., and Moskowitz, M.A. (1989). The development of neurogenic plasma extravasation does not depend upon the degranulation of mast cells in the rat dura mater. *Brain Research*, **477**, 157–65.

Index

75. Ю